THE WORKING BACK

THE WORKING BACK
A Systems View

WILLIAM S. MARRAS, Ph. D.

Professor
The Ohio State University

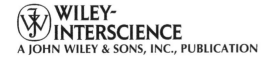

WILEY-INTERSCIENCE

A JOHN WILEY & SONS, INC., PUBLICATION

Library of Congress Cataloging-in-Publication Data:

Marras, William S. (William Steven),
   The working back : a systems View / William S. Marras.
      p. ; cm.
   Includes bibliographic references.
   ISBN 978-0-470-13405-4 (cloth)

1. Backache–Etiology. 2. Low back pain–Risk factors. 3. Occupational diseases. 4.
Human engineering. I. Title.
   [DNLM: 1. Low Back Pain–prevention & control. 2. Occupational
Diseases–prevention & control. 3. Biomechanics. 4. Ergonomics. WE 750 M358w 2008]
   RD771. B217M36 2008
   617. 5′64–dc22   2007035518

CONTENTS

ACKNOWLEDGMENTS

THIS BOOK represents a compilation of learning and discovery about low back pain over the past quarter of a century. Much of this discovery was inspired by numerous individuals and groups both within and outside the scientific community who have helped me transition my thinking from a traditional biomechanical approach to more of a systems view of causality. I am, therefore, indebted to many who helped make this project possible. First, I must thank my family (Jillian and Alex) and my friends who inspired (and tolerated me) during the lengthy process of digesting and interpreting the volumes of information considered for this book. I would like to thank my late father, Steven W. Marras, who instilled in me the value of science and the scientific process. I am grateful to Dr. Stuart McGill, my friend, colleague, and fishing buddy for encouraging me to "tell my story." Second, I owe a large debt of gratitude to my current and former students who actively participated in many of the studies mentioned in this book, including Drs. Steven Lavender, Carolyn Sommerich, Gary Mirka, Kevin Granata, Sue Ferguson, Sudhakar Rajulu, Fadi Fathallah, Gary Allread, Kermit Davis, J-Y Kim, Mike Jorgensen, and Sean Gallagher as well as my current colleagues and students who have continued this pursuit including Greg Knapik, Gang Yang, Riley Splittoesser, Lee Mazurek and Kim Vandlen. My colleagues within the field have also played a large part in my thinking about low back pain causality. I am grateful to - Drs. Don Chaffin, Eb Kroemer, Al King, and Tom Rockwell for helping me to shape my thinking. It is also important that I recognize members of the medical and surgical community who have helped me appreciate how biomechanical concepts could integrate with clinical issues. My thinking has been stimulated by many prominent surgeons and physicians including Drs. Alf Nachmeson, Gunnar Anderson, Tapio Videman, John Frymoyer, Purnendu Gupta, Josue Gabriel, and Ehud Mendel. Third, a project like this would not be possible without technical and administrative support. I am deeply appreciative of the efforts of Ms. Candi McCain for her coordination of the manuscript and figures and the efforts of Mr. Ben Ramsey who produced some of the artwork for this book. Finally, I must thank the Ohio State University and the Department of Integrated Systems Engineering for providing me the environment and time to work on this project.

CHAPTER 1

INTRODUCTION

*T*HIS CHAPTER *begins with a discussion indicating that much is unknown about low back pain causality, especially its relationship to work. This chapter is intended to calibrate readers' expectations so that they understand the difficulties in making definitive statements about low back pain causality due to work. Second, an argument is made for why we must view the body of knowledge as a series of puzzle pieces that must be put together to form a "picture" or system. This section indicates that this will be done in a relatively nontechnical manner and the audience for the book is identified. Third, a discussion indicates that there are several work (physical, psychosocial, and organizational) factors as well as nonwork (genetic) factors that constitute the "puzzle pieces." Workers are exposed to these factors regularly and the key to understanding is to determine how these factors interact and lead to back pain. Fourth, a high level conceptual model is proposed that suggests how physical and nonphysical work factors might interact with personal factors to affect the forces that are experienced by the spine subsequent back pain. Finally, the organization of the book is discussed and the reader is reminded that the book will provide a framework for how one should think about low back pain causality. The objective of the book is to place the reader in a position to reason through various workplace design issues as opposed to providing a "cookbook" formula for low back pain prevention.*

What causes low back pain? Does work cause low back pain or would it occur regardless of work activities? No one knows the answers to these questions beyond a shadow of a doubt. I repeat, *no one knows for sure*! Numerous publications have attempted to explain various causes of back pain (referred to as causal pathways) including genetics, stability, acute trauma, repetitive stress to the tissue (cumulative trauma), aging, cardiovascular problems, psychological problems, organizational and social (psychosocial) problems, among others. However, no one has been able to *prove* or definitively *disprove* any of these theories. Realistically, the causal pathways are probably more complex than any single one of these pathways suggests. In all likelihood, there are probably numerous means by which low back pain can be initiated. Furthermore, one would expect that many of these pathways develop simultaneously and perhaps even interplay with each other.

The focus of this book concerns the many factors that can contribute to low back pain. However, this book is unique because it concentrates on the factors that *lead to* low back pain from a multidisciplinary and interdisciplinary perspective. While thousands of books have been written about the treatment of low back pain and how to manage back pain once it occurs, this book is different in that it is concerned with the ways in which back pain can be initiated and considers the factors that are within our control to minimize the risk of an initial or recurring back problem due to work-related factors.

Causality of health problems, such as low back pain, in real-life situations is extremely difficult to study and prove for a variety of experimental and ethical reasons. Some suggest that causality can be proven in what are referred to as *randomized controlled trials* such as what is done to test the efficacy of a new drug. In a typical randomized controlled trial, a population of people with an ailment is divided into different groups. Some are randomly given the drug of interest and others are randomly given a placebo. If the improvement rate among the "drug" group is statistically better compared to that of the "placebo" group, then the drug is deemed effective.

However, *causality* of a back disorder is very different from *treatment* of a low back disorder. Causality cannot be proven in the same way as the effectiveness of a drug can be proven. The literature over the past 50 years has suggested that many factors may influence low back pain. Therefore, it is difficult to isolate the issues that increase risk. In addition, contemporary studies are indicating that many of the categories of risk factors interact strongly. Thus, it becomes even more difficult to understand how these factors react in combination with each other. Furthermore, there are several scientific, practical, and ethical problems with applying such a model to low back causality and specifically to workplace interventions in the actual workplace. For example, almost everyone works, ages, and is exposed to a variety of forces through work, sports, accidents, and so on. It, therefore, becomes nearly impossible to compare people who are exposed to these multidimensional risk factors to those who are not, as would be necessary to prove causality in a randomized controlled trial. So how does one isolate the potential effect of forces resulting from work compared to spine forces resulting from other exposures? It becomes extremely difficult and, potentially, unethical to do so.

In addition, not many employers are willing to allow their facilities to be used in long-term studies of low back pain. The priority in industry is to make money. Very few industries are amenable to exposing part of their work force to different work risk conditions to prove a scientific point. Would you allow half of your employees to be exposed to suspected risk factors while not allowing the other half? Besides, word travels quickly in work environments, and psychological effects would quickly contaminate the study.

Similar problems also exist in drug treatment studies. Since few researchers are able to accurately and quantitatively measure the *extent* of low back pain, how does one assure that everyone starts the study at the same state of impairment? You cannot. Instead one must recruit very large populations of patients and hope that the samples are large enough so that low back pain severity is equally likely in each group. Finally, few physicians are willing to randomize treatments among their patients. Could you imagine going to your physician to have your back pain treated and then finding out that your treatment was part of a placebo group? Recently, a study randomized surgical treatment versus conservative treatment for back pain. Those patients who agreed to the randomization of treatment were enrolled in the "randomized" study where they did not become part of an "observational" group. Different effectiveness of surgery was reported depending upon group membership (1,2). However, it was clear that those in the observational group had much more severe pain than the randomized group. This study illustrates the difficulty with randomized controlled trials.

Hence, the traditional "rules" of science are difficult to apply in this complex, multidimensional problem we call low back pain in the "real-world" environment. Since low back pain is so complex, no one study will ever prove or disprove the causal pathway. Most individual studies simply explore one or, in rare cases, the interaction between two potential causal pathways. One way to gain faith in a causal mechanism is to repeat studies several times and observe whether the studies all arrive with the same conclusions. This way of thinking (looking for many studies arriving at the same conclusion) is called looking at the *preponderance* of evidence. While a preponderance of evidence assures us that a risk factor is important, this type of rationale is often unable to assess and account for the interaction of various causal factors. A major tenet of statistical reasoning states that the interaction of causal factors can be far more powerful in determining the outcome than any single causal factors. In other words, it is common for factors to combine in unique ways and dictate the effects of causal factors. Therefore, instead of looking at low back pain causality from a singular, myopic viewpoint, we will examine the potential interactions in risk factors by examining the *pattern of evidence* associated with work-associated low back pain. It will try and build a case for how the multidimensional components of low back pain can interact and most likely influence low back pain risk.

My experience in low back pain and work comes from 25 years of research into low back biomechanics, experience examining hundreds of jobs associated with back pain, practical experience changing the jobs, and determining what works and why it works in reducing back pain risk at work, as well as personal experience with low back pain. Thus, this book is a practical explanation of the factors that influence the low back pain experience and a discussion of what tools and ability we have to influence a certain percentage of back pain that may be due to work.

The goal of this book is to provide the reader with a functional understating of how we think back pain is influenced by various work and nonwork factors. While various assessment tools will be discussed, it should be obvious that there are no "cookbook" solutions or "magic bullets." However, if one has a reasonable understanding of the causal pathways involved with low back pain as well as an appreciation for how these pathways can be activated by various individual and workplace exposures, then one should be armed with the knowledge to assess a given work environment and prescribe effective interventions given the situation.

1.1 AUDIENCE FOR THE BOOK

This book is intended for a diverse audience. This book is intended to interpret the science in such a way that it is understandable for people of diverse backgrounds. The key to understanding low back pain causality is to understand how the various concepts fit together and interact as opposed to understanding the sophisticated scientific techniques that form the basis of the individual studies. These scientific techniques are simply tools to mine the knowledge that is inherent to the study. Thus, instead of delving into the minute details of the various studies, an attempt will be made to show how the major contributions of various studies fit together to form a pattern or picture of how low back pain might occur.

Hence, this book is intended for a broad audience consisting of anyone interested in low back pain causality. The book should be of interest to several groups including

1. those who either design work, dictate work processes and schedules, or perform the work that might lead to low back pain;
2. those who attempt to determine how return to work will influence the risk of low back pain recurrence or exacerbation;
3. those suffering from low back pain who are interested in the mechanisms behind low back pain; and
4. researchers who are interested in a more global view of how low back pain might be associated with work.

1.2 APOLITICAL CAUSALITY ASSESSMENT

Besides being difficult to explore from a scientific inquiry perspective, the low back pain causality controversy is also clouded by political and monetary incentives. Low back pain can be very expensive and can cost companies and medical providers millions of dollars. Low back treatment is also big business with surgical supply companies charging huge amounts for equipment, implants, and treatment procedures for low back pain. Since large amounts of money are at stake, workers' compensation insurance and legal issues can become the objective of a workplace risk assessment instead of attempts to resolve and mediate the risk of low back pain associated with a job task. In addition, once monetary incentives are in place, compensation rather than resolution of the back pain can become the objective (3,4). This makes some suspicious that those suffering from low back pain are malingering or striving for secondary (often monetary) gain. The suspicious nature of a work investigation can further escalate the level of distrust among the worker and further magnify the emotional component of the pain and serve to further enhance the pain. Hence, the low back pain business is costly for all involved.

The costly nature of the work-related low back pain environment provides an opportunity for low back pain experts to cash in on their opinions. Experts claiming that the work task was a likely cause of a low back disorder can secure a lifetime settlement for a worker. Likewise, experts who contend that there is no relationship between work and low back pain can potentially save a company millions of dollars in workers' compensation costs. Either way, when large sums of money are involved there are always incentives for bias on the part of the experts. In addition, national politics have also been entangled in the debate. Large corporations and unions have a great deal of money at stake and both groups place political pressure on elected representatives to "spin" the science in a direction that benefits their cause. Thus, rulemaking is often influenced by politics more than scientific integrity (5).

This book will strive to set aside political and monetary incentives, cut through the literature base that is motivated by such concerns, and provide a realistic view of how the various bodies of knowledge regarding low back pain causality might fit together to form a logical explanation of how low back pain occurs under work conditions. As we will soon see, there is evidence to support the contention that there are numerous pathways to low back pain. The work task might be simply the initiating event in a long chain of events leading to low back pain and the work can either mediate or enhance the problem.

1.3 A SYSTEMS VIEW OF LOW BACK PAIN CAUSALITY

While many of the studies that form the underlying logic in this book involve complex methodologies and techniques, the basic concepts underlying the ideas are fairly straightforward. The point of the book is to show how various influences or risk factors might be considered collectively, or in combination, to influence the risk of low back pain at work. The idea here is to assess how the multiple dimensions of risk can interact and combine to set the stage for low back pain to occur. One can consider this type of thinking as a jigsaw puzzle with the different pieces of the puzzle representing the different aspects of risk. When pieces of the puzzle are viewed in their correct orientation and in perspective, the overall picture, or in this case, causality pathway becomes clearer. It is the goal of this book to show how the pieces of the puzzle or the *pattern of evidence* fit together so that we might better understand low back pain causality at work.

1.4   THE REALITY OF WORK

To be realistic, the pattern of evidence associated with exposure to physical work must consider not only the effects of exposure to physical work characteristics also the effects of many other factors that might exacerbate or mediate the influence of physical work characteristics. The effects of exposure to the organizational stress issues associated with work as well as the unique characteristics of the individual worker and their individual response to physical and psychological stresses should be considered. This book is about considering how these factors can interact in a systematic manner.

Individual characteristics of the worker may mediate or accentuate the intensity of the load imposed upon a tissue due to work and may also play a role in how the worker's tissues are able to tolerate the tissue load. To make matters worse, it is possible that this relationship can change over time. Age, conditioning, genetics, lifestyle habits, psychological state, personality, and the current state of tissue degeneration can all influence the rate at which tissue is stressed and how the body tissues handle the stress. The ability of the body to induce forces upon a tissue as well as the ability of the body to withstand tissue load have all been well documented in the literature (6), but their interactive influence of loads in combination with psychological stress and individual variation in responses has not been well documented in the literature and is not well understood.

The influence of time can also profoundly affect the influence of physical loads imposed on the body. The ability of the body to withstand physical loading can change dramatically over time. Cumulative loading and adaptation to loading can alter our interpretation of risk depending upon the magnitude of the accumulated load, the temporal nature of the cumulative exposure, and the ability of the body to compensate for the tissue insult.

Factors such as physical factors, psychosocial factors, and organizational factors can all play a role in defining risk. Traditionally, it has been the physical workplace factors that have been explored and associated with increased tissue loading, particularly when the biomechanical characteristics of the work were properly and specifically addressed (6). However, there continues to be controversy as to the contributions of psychosocial factors and organizational factors. Some have argued that increases in low back pain reporting can be explained through work dissatisfaction, organizational factors, or the availability of compensation (7). However, most studies have not considered the explanatory power of these factors relative to that of the load–tolerance relationship. Some of the classic psychosocial studies, when re-examined, have been found to explain a very small percentage of variability in low back pain reporting (8). Analyses have shown that when biomechanical evaluations are considered collectively along with psychosocial evaluations, the explanatory power associated with the psychosocial studies is greatly reduced (9). More recent findings have also shown that psychosocial factors have an interactive effect with biomechanical loading (10) and that individual factors, such as personality, can explain much of the variation in the magnitude of the loading forces experienced across individuals (11).

Collectively, this pattern of evidence suggests that no single factor fully explains the presence or absence of cumulative trauma and its association with low back pain. Furthermore, it is also clear that researchers often find only what they are looking for. If one does not bother to properly measure the influence of a potential risk factor, they certainly will not find a significant association with that factor, and they are therefore, not justified in suggesting there is no causality associated with a factor they did not properly explore.

Traditionally, the literature has taken the approach of examining single-risk factors *in isolation*, in trying to explain back pain. Large bodies of literature exist that argue for the

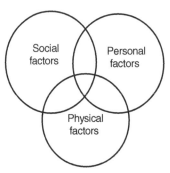

Figure 1.1 Interaction between various dimensions of risk factors contributing to cumulative trauma and low back pain.

influence of each type of risk factor independently. However, if we consider the components of the system, it is likely that physical factors, individual characteristics, organizational factors, and psychosocial factors *all* influence the load–tolerance relationship that is at the core of cumulative trauma. The evidence suggests that cumulative exposure to loads when combined with other risk factors can contribute to low back disorders above and beyond the influence of aging or genetics alone. However, the magnitude of the effect of cumulative trauma above and beyond aging and genetics is not well understood. In addition, it is not known how cumulative trauma responds in conjunction with other risk factors.

The pattern of evidence suggests that we must consider how the *system* behaves in order to appreciate the influence of any one or any combination of risk factors in the etiology of low back pain. Instead of continuing to explore low back pain causality within the confines of specific disciplines (e.g., biomechanics, psychosocial, physiology, genetics, etc.), we must more fully explore the interactions between these disciplines as proposed in Fig. 1.1. The pattern of evidence suggests that the explanatory power inherent to the interaction between these disciplines may very well overpower the influence of any main effects. Thus, in order to understand the amount of variability that is accounted for by any one of the risk factors we must also understand the nature of the interactions between the risk factors. The research community has already begun to quantify the degree of interaction between many of these risk factors, yet much more work is required before we fully understand these interactions. These interactions represent the current research "gaps" as well as opportunities for future research direction.

When considering the pattern of evidence for low back pain, if all the components of plausibility are considered in perspective, a picture emerges that logically supports the relative influence of various risk factors associated with the etiology of low back disorder.

1.5 HOW MIGHT THE DIFFERENT ASPECTS OF WORK BE ASSOCIATED WITH BACK PAIN

How could a conceptual model be developed that can integrate the different bodies of literature associated with low back pain occurrences? This issue was debated by the National Research Council and the Institute of Medicine within the National Academy of Sciences in two studies exploring the work relatedness of musculoskeletal disorders (6,12). In these studies, the literature was thoroughly evaluated and explored and a unifying model was developed based upon the interaction of potential causal factors suggested by Fig. 1.1. This model is further expanded in Fig. 1.2. This model suggests a pain pathway that is shown in the right hand box labeled "PERSON" in Fig. 1.2. The PERSON box indicates the possible

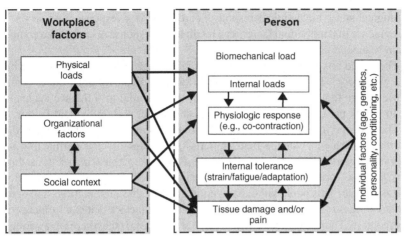

Figure 1.2   Conceptual model relating potential workplace risk factors to the development of low back pain. (Adapted from reference 12).

work-related pathways and processes that could occur within the person including the biomechanical load–tolerance relationship and the factors that may mediate this relationship (e.g., individual factors and adaptation). This pathway suggests that at the heart of this system, work-related low back pain must be initiated by a biomechanical response (forces) to one of many (physical, psychological, psychosocial, etc.) conditions found in the workplace that is capable of exceeding a tissue tolerance. The biomechanical load "box" indicates that physical force and motion factors must be of sufficient magnitude to cause the body to develop sufficient internal (to the body) forces upon the spinal tissues. These can often be magnified by muscle coactivation, hence, biomechanical analyses must be sensitive enough to consider this means of loading in order to accurately consider work-related spinal tissue loading.

Forces or loads imposed on the back are compared to internal (tissue) tolerances within the back. Tolerances can take many forms in this model including tolerances relative to the structural strength of the tissues including endplate strength, disc fiber strength, ligament strength, muscle tolerance, and so on that result in tissue strain. Another form of tolerance that must be considered is biochemical tolerance. Structural tolerances are most likely preceded by biochemical reactions. For example, cytokines are strong initiators of inflammatory responses that can be upregulated by repetitive insult to a tissue. In addition, as we will see, these responses can be mediated or exacerbated by physiologic adaptation, former experiences that alter muscle recruitment, and cognitive factors. Hence, "internal tolerance" in this model can include many forms of tolerance.

The next block in this sequence suggests that pain can result from these tolerances being exceeded. The inflammatory responses, tissue damage, and so on can lead to pain-sensitive tissues (nociceptors) being activated, which initiates the sequence of pain. It should also be noted that arrows flow in both directions in these last two boxes. This indicates that the individual tolerances and pain experiences can be either exacerbated once exposed or may help adaptation. In either case, significant feedback loops can complicate the sequence of events.

The model in Fig. 1.2 shows that the pain pathway just described can also be influenced by the specific characteristics and conditions of the individual. These conditions and characteristics include genetic factors, personality, physical capacity and conditioning, psychological state, biochemical response, cardiovascular response, and so on. There is strong evidence that individual factors can mediate the response of each of the components in this pain sequence.

The dotted box in the left-hand portion of the figure indicates the potential influences of the workplace. These include physical factors, organizational factors, and social influences. Note that each of these factors has the potential to influence each component of the low back pain pathway sequence and can interact with individual factors.

This model is the governing concept behind this book's logic. The chapters that follow review the pattern of evidence that supports this means of considering low back pain causality and work. While this model suggests many complex interactions through the various "arrows," one should not be overly concerned if this system of interactions is not clear at this stage. This book will expand upon many of these interactions and demonstrate how many of these factors can influence the system of factors that can influence low back pain perception. The important thing to realize at this stage is that there are a variety of work and nonwork factors that can play a role via this web of influences.

1.6 ORGANIZATION OF THE BOOK

The goal of this book is to explain the potential avenues of low back pain and show how they could be related to work exposure. Our knowledge of low back pain has advanced rapidly over the past several decades. It is unlikely that the major cause of most modern work related low back pain is simply lifting a load that is too heavy, which causes a structure to break. While it is possible, for the majority of workers, this is probably not the mechanism of pain for most work-related low back pain. The literature now suggests that there are numerous, more complex, potential pathways of pain that may be associated with work tasks.

In order to effectively assess and design workplaces that minimize low back pain risk, one must be armed with an underpinning of causal mechanism logic so that one could understand the initiators of sequences of events that can lead to persistent low back pain. Therefore, instead of simply listing the numerous pathways to low back pain, it is important to develop an appreciation of how these pathways might interact with the physical and social work environments as well as with the individual attributes of the worker. Hence, we are talking about a *system*. It would be easy to simply list a set of rules of dos and don'ts for work. However, invariably, one will quickly run into a situation that has not been described in the "list" and in reality the work situation would probably contain several different trade-offs between risk factors. This situation would lead to a conclusion that one should automate the process. Automation is costly and is often not effective from a production efficiency standpoint. However, if one has an understanding of the spectrum of underlying mechanisms involved in low back pain, it is more likely that one can reason through the work situation and devise a feasible intervention to minimize the pain. Therefore, this book will attempt to lay the ground work for a systems approach to understanding the causes and pathways of low back pain.

Given these goals, this book is organized in a manner that will provide the basis of understanding in the spectrum of topics that are important to understanding work-related low back pain. While each chapter is designed to be relatively independent so that it can be read by itself, maximum understanding will be gained if one considers each chapter in the context of the entire system and, thus, it is recommended that one read the entire book and build the knowledge base as one progresses from chapter to chapter.

Chapter 2 reviews the magnitude of the low back pain problem and explores factors that may contribute to low back pain from an observational (as opposed to causal) standpoint. The chapter reviews statistics (in terms of magnitude, trends, and costs) indicating the extent to which back pain impacts society. The chapter also reviews the epidemiologic (surveillance) findings to suggest the degree to which physical, psychosocial, and individual risk factors have been associated with low back pain. Epidemiology is the science of observing trends in the workplace. It has the advantage of going beyond theoretical relationships and can show that if certain conditions are present, the probability for low back pain increases. Hence, strong relationships can be found. The disadvantage of epidemiology is that it is often difficult to isolate a specific risk factor of interest and it is often difficult to study interactions between potential risk factors. In addition, the measurement tools used in epidemiologic research are often fairly imprecise. Nonetheless, epidemiology can be a useful tool for identifying historic trends in the workplace. However, as with all scientific approaches, one must consider the limitations of the tools and view the information in perspective.

Chapter 3 will present the basics of anatomy of the low back in a functional manner. Anatomy is presented along with a description of why the anatomy is important to the functioning of the back and spine. An appreciation for anatomy is essential for the understanding of which structures could be involved in the various pathways of injury. Along the same lines, Chapter 4 reviews the mechanisms of pain transmission in the human body. The goal is to help the reader understand that pain perception is influenced not only by physical loading but also by prior (cognitive) experiences. This chapter will show how pain occurs and the roles that physical load and memory play in the pain experience. The influence of biomechanical loads imposed upon tissues and biochemical reactions is discussed in terms of their ability to initiate pain perception.

Based upon the previous three chapters, Chapter 5 articulates the various pain pathways that are possible as a function of work exposure. The chapter begins by discussing how our understanding about back pain perception has changed over the years and discusses why traditional views (suggesting that tissue damage must be present) may not be realistic. This chapter outlines the various sequences of events that we believe occur within the human during the back pain experience and, where available, thresholds for tissue damage and pain initiation are described. The chapter describes how muscle tensions within the low back can activate the various pain pathways. This chapter also establishes that understanding how work and nonwork factors influence muscle tensions is the key to understanding pain pathway initiation.

Chapter 6 provides an overview of occupational biomechanics. Biomechanical analyses are often used to assess workplaces in order to assess risk of low back pain. However, biomechanical assessments have evolved rapidly over the past few decades. This chapter reviews the progression of commonly used biomechanical assessments and concepts and will discuss state-of-the art techniques that have the ability to precisely evaluate tissue stress associated with various work-related exposures.

The results of biomechanical assessments performed on potential physical work factors will be reviewed in Chapter 7. This chapter will show how physical work factors affect both spine forces and muscle tension.

Psychosocial and organizational influences on the biomechanics of spine loading and muscle recruitment patterns are discussed in Chapter 8. Several recent studies have shown that these cognitive environment factors affect spine loading and muscle activities in much the same way as physical load exposure.

Chapter 9 reports on the biomechanical behavior of the spine that is associated with individual factors such as gender and personality. Since the systems approach must consider biomechanical effects of the unique characteristics the worker brings to the job, this chapter evaluates the extent to which tissue loads are influenced by these unique individual characteristics.

The next chapter, Chapter 10, reviews the quantitative biomechanical literature that has been able to investigate the interaction between the workplace factors, psychosocial/organizational factors, and individual factors. This chapter emphasizes that the low back pain is the result of a system of interactions that must be considered if back pain is to be controlled in the workplace.

Interventions intended to control low back pain are discussed in Chapters 11 and 12. We have no ability to control individual factors at work, so the focus in these two chapters is on what we can control from a work perspective. Chapter 11 discusses ways that one can control and intervene in the physical risk factors associated with work, whereas Chapter 12 discusses the options for controlling the psychosocial and organizational environment at work.

Chapter 13 will show case studies of how physical and psychosocial/organizational aspects the workplace have been manipulated to minimize the occurrence of low back pain and lead to optimal working health.

A major challenge to the working environment involves assimilating workers back into the workplace once low back pain has occurred. Chapter 14 will review some of the biomechanically relevant literature associated with the previously described pain pathways and secondary (recurring) low back pain. Finally, Chapter 15 consolidates the information from the previous chapters into system logic to stimulate the reader to consider whatever new (yet unexplored) factors might also influence this systems approach to understanding low back pain.

REFERENCES

1. WEINSTEIN JN, LURIE JD, TOSTESON TD, SKINNER JS, HANSCOM B, TOSTESON AN, HERKOWITZ H, FISCHGRUND J, CAMMISA FP, ALBERT T, DEYO RA. Surgical vs nonoperative treatment for lumbar disk herniation: the Spine Patient Outcomes Research Trial (SPORT) observational cohort. J Am Med Assoc 2006;296:2451–2459.

2. WEINSTEIN JN, TOSTESON TD, LURIE JD, TOSTESON AN, HANSCOM B, SKINNER JS, ABDU WA, HILIBRAND AS, BODEN SD, DEYO RA. Surgical vs nonoperative treatment for lumbar disk herniation: the Spine Patient Outcomes Research Trial (SPORT): a randomized trial. J Am Med Assoc 2006;296:2441–2450.

3. HADLER NM. Back pain in the workplace. What you lift or how you lift matters far less than whether you lift or when. Spine 1997;22:935–940.

4. HADLER NM. The disabled, the disallowed, the disaffected and the disavowed. J Occup Environ Med 1996;38: 247–251.

5. MOONEY C. The Republican War on Science. New York (NY): Basic Books; 2005.

6. NRC. Musculoskeletal disorders and the workplace: low back and upper extremity. Washington (DC): National Academy of Sciences, National Research Council, National Academy Press; 2001.

7. HADLER NM. Back pain in the workplace. What you lift or how you lift matters far less than whether you lift or when [editorial]. Spine 1997;22:935–940.

8. VOLINN E, SPRATT KF, MAGNUSSON M, POPE MH. The Boeing prospective study and beyond. Spine 2001;26:1613–1622.

9. DAVIS KG, HEANEY CA. The relationship between psychosocial work characteristics and low back pain: underlying methodological issues. Clinical Biomechanics 2000;15:389–406.

10. DAVIS KG, MARRAS WS, HEANEY CA, WATERS TR, GUPTA P. The impact of mental processing and pacing on spine loading: 2002 Volvo Award in biomechanics. Spine 2002;27:2645–2653.

11. MARRAS WS, DAVIS KG, HEANEY CA, MARONITIS AB, ALLREAD WG. The influence of psychosocial stress, gender, and personality on mechanical loading of the lumbar spine. Spine 2000;25:3045–3054.

12. NRC. Work-related musculoskeletal disorders: report workshop summary, and workshop papers. Washington (DC): National Academy of Sciences, National Research Council, National Academy Press; 1999.

CHAPTER 2

BACK PAIN MAGNITUDE AND POTENTIAL RISK FACTORS

*T*HIS CHAPTER *reviews work-related low back pain statistics from an observational (as opposed to causal) standpoint. It documents the frequency of back pain occurrences in society and reviews the literature indicating associations with the presence of potential work factors. Thus, there are two main thrusts to the chapter. The first thrust reviews statistics (in terms of magnitude, trends, and costs) indicating the extent to which back pain impacts society. The second thrust reviews the epidemiologic (surveillance) findings to suggest the degree to which physical, psychosocial, and individual risk factors have been associated with low back pain.*

2.1 WHAT IS BACK PAIN?

According to the American Society of Orthopaedic Surgeons (1), back problems can take many forms, including degenerative and rheumatic disorders, disk problems, and injuries such as sprains, strains, and fractures. Many of these disorders can contribute to back pain. Hence, back pain definitions cover a broad range of pain-generating sources that can encompass everything from a mild muscle strain to serious disc problems. This broad definition of low back pain also makes it difficult to study and interpret.

2.2 HOW COMMON IS BACK PAIN?

Back pain is extremely common. Some believe that because it is so common, we should be accepting low back pain as just part of life. Others believe that because of the back's unique structure, where forces are concentrated in a small area, the spine is more vulnerable to pain and, thus, one could design activities to minimize the magnitude of the load imposed on the spine and the resultant risk of low back pain. Much of what follows in the forthcoming chapters will address these issues.

The following are some facts and figures indicating how common back pain has become. These details are presented to help place the magnitude of the low back pain problem in perspective.

- Over the course of a lifetime, up to 80% of Americans will suffer from at least one episode of back pain (2).
- Low back pain represents the second most common symptom-related reason for visits to a physician (3).

The Working Back: A Systems View, by Williams S. Marras
Copyright © 2008 John Wiley & Sons, Inc.

- Fifteen to twenty percent of Americans will report back pain yearly (2).
- In 1998, total health care expenditures incurred by individuals with back pain in the United States reached $90.7 billion (2).
- Those with back pain incurred health care expenditures about 60% higher than individuals without back pain (2).
- Back pain results in a loss of over 100 million workdays per year (4).
- Twenty-one percent of workers with back reports were away from work for 3–5 days, 14.3% reporting back problems lost 6–10 days of work, and 29.6% of workers reporting back pain missed 3 or more weeks away from work (5).
- In 2002, there were over 345,000 back injuries requiring time away from work (5).
- Between 20% and 35% of Americans report experiencing severe low back pain in the past 3 months. Figure 2.1 shows that low back pain reports are extremely common regardless of age, gender, race, or income level (6).
- Nearly 21 million physician visits for back pain occurred in 2003. Table 2.1 shows this breakdown according to gender and office visit category or code (1).
- Work-related low back pain represents about 20% of the Workers' Compensation Claims yet nearly 40% of the costs (7). Thus, low back problems are disproportionately expensive.

2.3   BACK PAIN AT WORK

It should be stated up front that since most people work, workplace risk factors and individual risk factors are difficult to separate (8). However, back pain patterns can be identified through surveys of working populations. In the United States back disorders are associated with more days away from work than lost workdays attributable to any other part of the body (9). Recent studies of 17,000 men and women of a working age population in Sweden (10) indicated that 5% of workers sought care for a new (no recurring) low back pain episode over a 3-year period. They also found that many of these cases eventually became chronic.

Evaluation of data from the National Health Injury Survey (NHIS), a large sample of U.S. households, found that back pain accounts for about one quarter of the workers' compensation claims in the United States (11). Two thirds of the low back pain cases were attributed to occupational activities. Prevalence (the percentage of a population affected with a particular condition at a given time) of lost workdays due to back pain were found to be

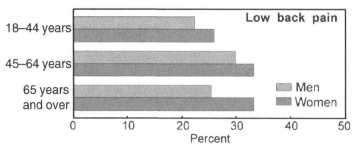

Figure 2.1   Age and gender of people reporting severe low back pain in past three months, 2003. (From reference 6).

TABLE 2.1   Number of Physician Visits for Back and Low Back Pain in 2003 (From Reference 1)

Reason for visit (reason for visit code)	Total no. of patients	No. of female patients	No. of male patients
Back symptoms (1905.0–1905.6)	20,845,000	12,425,000	8,420,000
Back pain (subset symptoms; 1905.1)	19,697,000	11,947,000	7,750,000
Low back symptoms (1910.0–1910.6)	10,665,000	6,448,000	4,217,000
Low back pain (subset symptoms; 1910.1)	10,429,000	6,304,000	4,124,000

Source: National Ambulatory Medical Care Survey (2003).

4.6% (12). Certain occupations were also found to be significantly linked to greater rates of low back pain reporting. Risk appeared to be highest for construction laborers (prevalence 22.6%) and nursing aides (19.8%) (11). Figure 2.2 summarizes the findings of a National Institute for Occupational Safety and Health (NIOSH) analysis of work-related low back disorders (9). This figure indicates that the proportion of people experiencing low back pain at any one time (prevalence) was greatest in the service industry followed by the manufacturing sector. These account for nearly half of all occupationally related low back disorders. Further analysis also indicates that handling of containers as well as worker motions and positions during work were the conditions most often associated with low back reports in U.S. industry. Hence, these cross-sectional data strongly suggest that occupational factors appear to be related to risk of low back disorders.

2.4   EPIDEMIOLOGY OF WORK RISK FACTORS

Epidemiology is the science of exploring associations between risk factors and medical conditions based on observations within the population of interest. A review of previous occupationally related epidemiologic studies has demonstrated that the findings of epidemiologic studies vary greatly depending on the dependent (observed) measure of interest (e.g., discomfort versus incidence versus lost time, etc.). For example, Figure 2.3 indicates how the percentage of positive associations between risk factor categories and low back pain changes depending on whether low back pain is defined as the presence of symptoms, a self proclaimed injury, a reported incident, an incident involving lost time or an incident

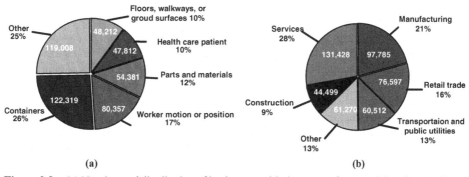

(a)   (b)

Figure 2.2   (**a**) Number and distribution of back cases with days away from work in private industry by industry division during 1997 (8). (**b**) Number and distribution of back cases with days away from work in private industry by source of the disorder during 1997. (From reference 4).

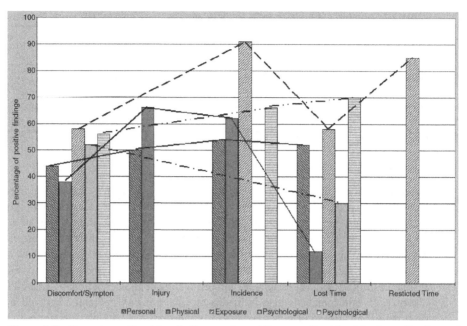

Figure 2.3 Percentage of positive findings and trend lines on all epidemiologic studies for each surveillance measure and risk factor combination. Note the generally increasing percentage of positive findings as the surveillance measure moves from discomfort/symptoms to incidence. (From reference 13).

involving restricted time (13). Thus, depending on which measure one is studying, a very different profile of low back pain can be observed.

A potential problem with some epidemiologic studies is that the observation point of the study (discomfort versus incident versus lost time, etc.) all occur at very different times during the progression of a low back reports and are influenced by the degree to which the low back pain interferes with the ability of the person to perform their job function (disability). Figure 2.4 shows how the typical sequence of low back pain events occur over time. As can be seen the different reporting measures (e.g., discomforts versus lost or restricted time) can occur at very different points in time. Differences in job demands associated with various professions can easily confound this picture. For example, a college professor may have the same level of low back impairment as a laborer; however, the professor may not perform any tasks that would exacerbate the discomfort and, thus, would never report the pain. Since the pain never interferes with the job function, this back pain would go unreported. However, a warehouse worker might be employed in a job that results in repeated exacerbation of the symptoms due to the nature of the work resulting in increased levels of pain. It would be far more likely for the low back incident to be reported as an incident or disability in this case or the worker may simply quit the job due to pain and never report it.

In most epidemiologic study designs, it is difficult to investigate the interaction among potential risk factors. This is particularly true given the variable exposures and work rotation schedules present in the modern workplace. Hence, although epidemiologic studies can provide valuable insight into which singular risk factors might be associated with risk of low back pain at work, it is difficult for these study designs to account for the more in depth interactions between classes of risk factors that might be responsible for the low back pain report. The information derived from these studies very often does not address the

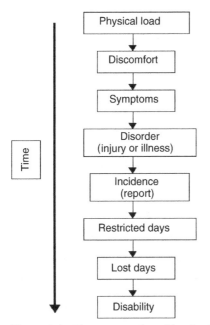

Figure 2.4 Time progression of low back disorders. (From reference 13).

multidimensional nature of the risk and, thus, interventions based on these single risk factor studies may be insufficient to effectively control a complex, multidimensional problem such as low back pain at the worksite.

Control of low back disorder risk in the workplace requires knowledge beyond simple identification and elimination of risk factors. It requires a much deeper understanding of how risk of low back pain occurs in the work setting amongst all of the various physical and nonphysical factors actively interacting. Control requires an understanding of "how much exposure to the various risk factors is too much exposure." In addition, one needs an understanding of how the risky exposure levels would change when risk factors are present in combination. Practically, our knowledge can only develop to this level of sophistication when we are able to quantify the means by which risk is increased. Our understanding of risk also needs to progress to the point where we can begin to understand how and why some people are at greater risk of developing low back pain when exposed to the same level of work risk as others. In other words, we need to begin to develop a better understanding so that the variability between individuals can be better understood. Only then can we answer the question: how much exposure to risk is too much exposure to risk for a given individual?

Occupational risk control requires tools that have high levels of both sensitivity and specificity. Sensitivity is a measure of how well the risk factor indeed identifies the risk for the condition of interest (low back pain). Specificity, however, is a measure of how well the measure can reject a situation where risk is not present. In other words, high levels of sensitivity would not miss many situations where risk of low back pain was present, and high levels of specificity would not sound false alarms when the risk of low back pain was not present. Measures of risk that are used to incorporate interventions for the control of occupational low back pain that are not sensitive will not be able to identify those work situations that would increase the risk to the worker. On the contrary, measures that are not specific might suggest interventions that needlessly indicate that work situations need to be changed. Given today's highly competitive industrial society, it is important that interventions are applied only when needed and are likely to be effective. Most industries can ill afford to incorporate control measures that do not have both high sensitivity and specificity. Such tools would waste valuable resources without justification. Recent studies have shown that our current low back pain risk control tools need to be better developed and validated so that risk can be optimally minimized (14,15).

2.5 EPIDEMIOLOGY OF PHYSICAL RISK FACTORS

Several epidemiologic reviews have identified specific individual risk factors that increase the risk of low back pain in the workplace. The NIOSH performed a critical review of the epidemiologic evidence associated with musculoskeletal disorders (16) (Table 2.2). Five categories of risk factors were evaluated. The critique concluded that strong evidence existed for an association between low back disorders and lifting/forceful movements and low back disorders and whole body vibration. Significant evidence was found for the associations between heavy physical work and awkward postures and back problems. The review concluded that evidence was insufficient to make any conclusions between static work postures and low back disorder risk. In a methodologically rigorous review, one team of researchers (17) were, in general, able to support these conclusions. They found that manual materials handling, bending and twisting, and whole-body vibration were risk factors for back pain.

While these studies have verified the existence of physical risk factors, they have been of limited usefulness in identifying the degree of exposure to a risk factor that becomes problematic (dose). In addition, we would expect that the dose would vary on the basis of different interactions with other factors.

Several studies have been carried out in search of a dose–response relationship among work risk factors and low back pain. Two studies (19,20) suggest that cumulative loading of the spine might be associated with risk of low back disorder at work. One study (21) suggested that the relationship might not be as straightforward as a linear relationship would suggest. When examining the relationship between back pain, history of physical loading, and occupation in cadaveric specimens, the study concluded that the risk relationship between low back disorder risk and loading was "J-shaped" with sedentary jobs being associated with moderate levels of risk, heavy work being associated with the greatest degree of risk, and moderate exposure to loading being associated with the lowest level of risk (Fig. 2.5). Another study (22) has recently suggested that the combination of occupational lifting, trunk flexion, and duration of the activities significantly increased risk. This study supports the idea that risk is interactive and multidimensional in nature. Another review (23) suggests little epidemiologic support for the notion that sitting at work was associated with low back pain. These findings suggest that risk is certainly not linear and is indeed complex in

TABLE 2.2 Epidemiologic Evidence of Causal Association Between Physical Risk Factors and Low Back Pain (From Reference 18)

Risk factor	Strong evidence (+++)	Evidence (++)	Insufficient evidence (+/0)	Evidence of no effect (−)
Lifting/Forceful movement	√			
Awkward posture		√		
Heavy physical work		√		
Whole body vibration	√			
Static work posture			√	

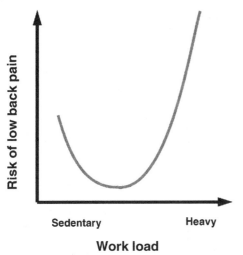

Figure 2.5   Suspected relationship between the intensity of exposure to heavy work and the risk of low back pain.

nature. Hence, we must begin to consider the collective and interactive exposure to risk factors if low back pain is to be controlled at the worksite.

This review of the epidemiologic evidence associated with physical work factors should serve to reinforce the view of low back pain risk as a pattern of evidence or jig saw puzzle as described in the previous chapter. If one looks at the big picture, we can see that most of the epidemiologic studies available today offer only a partial view of the risk picture since the interactions between risk factors is not well documented by these studies.

Recent rigorous epidemiologic reviews of the literature performed by the National Research Council (8) have also concluded that there is a clear relationship between back disorders and physical load imposed by manual material handling, frequent bending and twisting, physically heavy work, and whole-body vibration. The risk attributable to these risk factors is summarized in Table 2.3. This analysis indicates that the vast majority of high-quality epidemiologic studies have associated low back pain with these risk factors and up to two thirds of risk can be attributed to physical activities. Hence, it is clear that at least a portion of the risk of low back pain can be due to the nature of the work to which workers are exposed. As a result of these epidemiologic analyses, it was concluded that preventive measures may reduce the exposure to risk factors and reduce the occurrence of back problems.

The significance of considering the interaction of physical factors with other factors has also come to the attention of epidemiologic studies. The multidimensional nature of risk can be reinforced by considering the effective preventive strategies for secondary prevention of low back disorder (preventing recurrent back problems). Studies have begun to explore the interaction between low back pain, physical exposure factors, and psychosocial factors. Several studies (25–27) have noted that much of low back pain treatment for recurrence is multidimensional. Only recently have epidemiologic studies exploring the role of variables in primary prevention of work-related low back pain suggested that multiple dimensions, such as physical stressors and psychosocial factors, play a role in low back pain risk (28). A recent study has also demonstrated that the interaction of low social support at the workplace and bending at work were strongly associated with extended work absence due to low back pain (29).

TABLE 2.3 Summary of Epidemiologic Studies with Risk Estimates of Null and Positive Associations of Work-Related Risk Factors and the Occurrence of Back Disorders (Adapted From Reference 24)

	Risk estimate					
	Null association[a]		Positive association		Attributable fraction (%)	
Work-related risk factor	n	Range	n	Range	n	Range
Manual material handling	4	0.90–1.45	24	1.12–3.54	17	11–66
Frequent bending and twisting	2	1.08–1.30	15	1.29–8.09	8	19–57
Heavy physical load	0		8	1.54–3.71	5	31–58
Static work posture	3	0.80–0.97	3	1.30–3.29	3	14–32
Repetitive movements	2	0.98–1.20	1	1.97	1	41
Whole-body vibration	1	1.10	16	1.26–9.00	11	18–80

Notes: n = number of associations presented in epidemiologic studies.

[a]Confidence intervals of the risk estimates included the null estimate (1.0). In only 12 of 16 null associations was the magnitude of the risk estimate presented.

2.6 EPIDEMIOLOGY OF INDIVIDUAL (PERSONAL) RISK FACTORS

One can also learn much about the factors associated with increased risk of low back pain by examining the epidemiologic literature associated with individual or personal risk factors. Several trends are apparent from this body of work. First, personal factors play a role in risk of experiencing a low back pain. It is important to separate personal factors from occupational factors so that one can distinguish risk associated with work from that associated with factors that are inexplicably bound to the individual. A review of 57 original industrial-based surveillance studies (30) indicated that personal factors were the most frequently investigated risk factor for low back pain. Of these studies, previous back injury history and income were most often associated with risk (Table 2.4). Low back disorders typically begins at a relatively young age with the highest frequency of symptoms occurring between the ages of 35 and 55, while lost workdays typically increase with increasing age (31). Gender also appears to be an interactive factor in determining who experiences low back disorders. The risk for men peaks at about 40 years of age, whereas the greatest prevalence and incidence for women occurs between the ages of 50 and 60.

2.6.1 Age

In general, the literature indicates that back pain begins early in life with symptoms occurring between the ages of 35–55 (32). Recent studies have shown a link between age and spinal instability (33) indicating that there are associations between muscle control and risk that change over time. Figure 2.6 indicates how the reporting of low back pain changes as a function of age for both males and females.

2.6.2 Gender

The literature regarding the influence of gender on low back pain reveals a mixed pattern. In general, females report more back pain than males (34) (Fig. 2.1). However, when occupation is considered, a review of the literature has concluded that there was strong evidence that males are at a higher risk of low back pain than females (35). One study concluded that females were at a higher risk of back pain in white collar work as well as blue

TABLE 2.4   Percentage of Studies Finding a Positive Association with Personal Risk Factors (From Reference 13) (Note: Headache Involved Only One Study with Two Outcomes)

Personal risk factors	% Studies finding relationship
Age	35
Sex	8
Previous history	87
Intelligence/Education	40
Duration of pain	*
Race	0
Number of years experience/Seniority	14
Marital status	25
Household income/unemployment	66
Exercise/Recreational activity	30
Smoking	44
Length of time off	*
Headache	100
Distance to work	*
Car ownership	*
Total (percent positive)	
Prospective studies (percent positive)	

Note: References in the risk factor column were independent measures, covariates, or associated with another risk factor.

*One observation, therefore percentage was not calculated.

collar work; however, the risk is equivalent among service industry workers (36). Some of this may be a result of documented differences in lifting patterns and work methods between males and females (37,38).

2.6.3   Anthropometry

Anthropometry concerns the study of the physical size, shape, and mobility of people. Several studies have explored the relationship between physical body dimensions and low back pain.

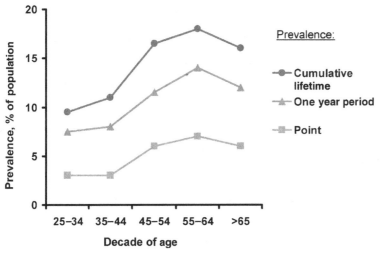

Figure 2.6   Changes in low back pain prevalence as a function of age for males and females in the United States (Deyo, R.A. and Y.J. Tsui-Wu, Descriptive epidemiology of low-back pain and its related medical care in the United States. Spine, 1987, 12(3): p 264–268).

One report suggests that relative risk of low back pain increased for males over 180 cm and females over 170 cm tall compared to those 10 cm shorter (39). This study also suggests that those with greater body mass are also at greater risk. A review of obesity and low back pain (40) indicated that 32% of the studies show a significant but weak association between low back pain and obesity. Another study (41) reports an association between low back pain and body weight but only for the 20% most obese portion of the population. Leg length discrepancies have also been considered as an individual risk factor for low back pain (42).

One study attempting to find physical correlates to back pain found that decreased lateral range of motion, a long back, decreased lordosis (low back curvature), psychological distress, and previous low back pain reports could explain up to 12% of first time low back pain reports (43). Decreases in flexibility have been noted in low back pain patients but the differences have been so small they are of little practical value (44). A study in a large manufacturing facility concluded that low back pain symptoms associated with straight leg raises were the only physical ability that was associated with future low back pain. This relationship was enhanced in women when age and weight were considered and in men when previous back complaints were considered (45).

It has been suggested (32) that individual factors simply set the stage for problems by interacting with other types of risk factors as opposed to being the idiopathic initiator of low back pain. Again, this view reinforces the multidimensional and interactive nature of low back pain risk.

2.6.4   Fitness/Strength

Historically, an association between strength, fitness, and low back pain risk has been assumed by many employers. This assumption has resulted in some employers performing preemployment testing and hiring only workers who were the strongest workers or most fit for employment. While many studies have examined the association between *recovery* from low back pain and strength and/or fitness, far fewer studies have explored the relationship between these factors and the occurrence of an initial low back pain episode.

Two studies of fire fighters examined the relationship between low back pain occurrence and fitness (46,47). Fitness measures included task-specific strength, spine flexibility, isometric strength, and cardiovascular conditioning. Both of these studies reported a monotonic relationship between increased fitness/strength and a reduction in low back pain. A study of industrial workers reported a slight association between increased isometric strength and increased reporting of low back pain (48). However, this study did not examine back strength relative to job demands.

Another study examined 27 years of field surveillance studies that attempted to examine the relationship between back pain reports and back strength (49). This review reported limited evidence that exercises to strengthen back or abdominal muscles and to improve overall fitness can decrease the incidence and duration of low back pain episodes. However, the study concluded that there was some evidence that exercise can prevent low back pain in asymptomatic individuals.

Collectively, this information suggests that at least part of the low back pain causality component concerns the strength and fitness of the worker. Thus, for optimal low back health, it is important to maintain at least a basic level of fitness as defined by strength, coordination, and cardiovascular fitness.

2.6.5   Alcohol

The role of alcohol in association with back pain has not been well established. The literatures show both increased low back pain with increased consumption (50) and no association between low back pain and alcohol consumption (51). However, it is not uncommon for back surgeons to encourage moderate alcohol consumption to help relieve stress.

2.6.6   Smoking

Numerous studies suggest a link between cigarette smoking and low back pain. An association has been identified between smoking and nonspecific low back pain (41,52), smoking and sciatica (53), smoking and spine damage (54), and adolescent smoking and low back pain (55). Smoking and degeneration of the entire lumbar spine can be responsible for an 18% increase in disc degeneration (56). Most studies suggest that smoking interferes with nutrition delivery to the spinal structures. However, some analyses have not been able to determine whether the smoking precedes the low back pain event (52). Such a trend would make the trend more significant. Studies have also reported greater work absenteeism in smokers as well as increased productivity and decreased absenteeism in former smokers (57).

2.6.7   Heredity/Genetics

Much of the recent literature has attempted to assess the degree to which low back pain was associated with heredity. A recent study (58) showed that disc height and disc bulge were related to heredity. Disc degeneration was studied using MRI among twins. The combination of genetics, age, and occupation was able to explain up to 77% of the variability in degeneration in the upper lumbar spine. Leisure physical loading, age, and familial history were able to explain 43% of the variability in the lower lumbar levels (59). Recent investigations of genetics and back pain have reported that between 30% and 39% of back problems could be associated with genetic factors depending upon the definition of back pain (60). Others have also found a relationship between low back pain and heredity explaining 44% and 40% of the variability among males and females, respectively; however, a genetic interaction with age was also emphasized (60,61).

Another recent review of the literature observed heredity factors and disc degeneration and found a large variation in the reported findings. However, this review suggested that heredity can explain up to 74% of variability in disc degeneration observations (62).

While studies exploring the link between MRI findings and heredity are certainly interesting and provoke some fascinating hypotheses, one must consider these findings in light of the fact that very few (less than 20%) reports of low back pain have imaging evidence of pain (63). Until stronger links between pain and MRI findings are established, we must not over interpret the findings of such studies.

2.6.8   Social Class and Psychological Factors

Social class has been observed as a potential risk factor for low back pain. Low or intermediate social class and blue collar occupations have been associated with increased rates of hospitalizations for disc herniations in males. However, psychological distress has been associated with increased reports in females (64). Mental stress has been associated with sciatica in some patients (53). However, when assessing the role of social class, covariates (relationships among factors that cause them to respond together) in risk must be considered. Most obvious is the fact that many work-related risk factors (e.g., lifting) are most often associated with the work most often performed by those of lower socioeconomic classes.

An extensive literature review (65) found that psychological factors played a role in pain perception and that stress, distress, anxiety, mood, cognitive functioning, and pain behavior all

TABLE 2.5 Summary of *Individual Psychosocial* Factors and Back Pain in a Review of 38 Prospective Studies (From Reference 24)

Individual psychosocial factor	Null association	Positive association	Attributable fraction (%)	
	n	n	n	Range
Depression or anxiety[a]	5	17	6	14–53
Psychological distress[b]	0	11	4	23–63
Personality factors	3	4	4	33–49
Fear-avoidance-coping	1	8	1	35
Pain behavior/function[c]	1	6	1	38

[a]Seventeen studies assessed depression only, two studies anxiety only, and three studies both depression and anxiety.

[b]Nine studies assessed psychological distress and two assessed stress.

[c]Four studies assessed pain behavior and three assessed pain-related functioning.

could be significant risk factors for chronic and acute low back pain. This review also indicated that personality factors had mixed results. Psychological factors, by themselves, explained only a small part of the variance. The review stressed that low back pain was a multivariate problem that was only partly explained by most social and psychological factors.

Some believe that *individual psychosocial* factors such as depression or anxiety, psychological distress, personality, fear/avoidance/coping behavior, and pain behavior may be related to the incidence of low back pain. A review of role of individual psychosocial factors in relation to low back pain was published by the National Academy of Sciences (24). Table 2.5 shows the results of this review of 38 prospective studies. As was the case with work-related physical exposure factors, this review calculated the attributable fraction of the back pain that would be reduced if these variables were not present. As can be seen, the range of values associated with the attributable fraction are large with variables ranging from 14% to 63%. The large ranges of attributable fraction emphasize the necessity to consider the low back pain as a multidimensional concern with individual psychosocial factors interacting with other types of risk factors to ultimately define risk.

2.7 EPIDEMIOLOGY OF WORK-RELATED PSYCHOSOCIAL/ ORGANIZATIONAL FACTORS

A large body of literature has also suggested that *work-related psychosocial* factors and organizational factors may be responsible for low back disorders. Work-related psychosocial factors are different from individual psychosocial problems in that they refer to the unique managerial and time demand aspects of work that are unique to a particular organization. One of the early efforts to assess the relationship between psychosocial factors and musculoskeletal disorders reviewed previous studies regarding psychosocial factors (66). This review of the literature suggested that monotonous work, high perceived work load, and time pressure were related to musculoskeletal symptoms. The review also suggested that low control on the job and lack of social support by colleagues are positively associated with musculoskeletal disease. However, this review resulted in a hypothetical model suggesting that individual characteristics and stress symptoms can modify the relationship between psychosocial factors and musculoskeletal disorders. The review also discussed the difficulty in separating psychosocial factors and physical factors at the workplace since these factors often occur simultaneously. Many of these inherent problems in assessing low back pain causality have also been stressed by others (67–69).

TABLE 2.6   Summary of Work-Related Psychosocial Factors and Back Pain: 21 Prospective Studies (From Reference 24)

Work-related psychosocial Factor	Null association	Positive association	Attributable fraction (%)	
	n	*n*	*n*	Range
High job demands	1	5	2	21–48
Low decision latitude/control	0	2		
Low stimulus from work (monotony)	2	4	1	23
Low social support at work	0	7	3	28–48
Low job satisfaction	1	13	6	17–69
High perceived stress	0	3	1	17
High perceived emotional effort	0	3		
Perceived ability to return to work	0	3		
Perceived work dangerous to back	0	2		

Much of the back pain research community took note of studies performed in large manufacturing facilities where subjects who stated that they "hardly ever" enjoyed their job tasks were 2.5 times more likely to report a back injury than subjects who "almost always" enjoyed their job tasks. The study also reported a doubling of reporting for those subjects having high levels of hysteria (70). However, latter reviews of this work suggested that the factors identified accounted for only 7% of the variability in low back pain reporting (71).

As with other categories of risk factors, the National Academy of Sciences has evaluated the attributable risk associated with work-related psychosocial factors through a review of the literature (24). Table 2.6 shows that, similar to the other risk factors discussed, work-related psychosocial/organizational risk factors may account for between 17% and 69% of the variability in reporting based upon a review of 21 prospective studies.

Over the past decade, several studies have assessed the impact of psychosocial factors and some also observed physical factors in the workplace in relation to the risk of low back pain (66,70,72–74). The studies confirmed that monotonous work, high perceived work load, time pressure, low job satisfaction, and lack of social support are related to low back disorder risk. However, an objective analysis of the literature (75) found that the impact of psychosocial factors was diminished, yet still significant, once biomechanical factors were accounted for in the study designs. Although several studies have identified these issues as related to the risk of low back disorders, this review (75) pointed out that few of the studies have properly evaluated physical work risk factors simultaneously. Consideration of biomechanical influence can have a significant impact on the strength of the psychosocial factor findings. Table 2.7 indicates a 20% increase in null results of psychosocial factors when the studies control for biomechanical demands. Thus, it has been impossible to separate the contributions of the physical workplace from that of the psychosocial components of the work.

2.8   POTENTIAL INTERACTION OF PHYSICAL AND PSYCHOSOCIAL FACTORS

As suggested earlier, there is sufficient reason to believe that many of the risk factor categories associated with low back pain interact at different levels of risk factor intensity to define overall risk. One potential way in which individual psychosocial factors and workplace biomechanical factors might interact is depicted in Fig. 2.7. Few can argue that

TABLE 2.7 Relationship (Percentage of Studies Reviewed) of Psychosocial Variables with Positive, Negative, Null, or Mixed Findings as a Function of Controlling for Biomechanical Variables (B) or Unadjusted for Biomechanical Influences (U) (From Reference 75)

Psychosocial variable	Low job satisfaction		Lack of variety and skill		Lack of influence over work		Poor social relations		Pool supervisor relations		Poor coworker relations		High concentration demands		High work demands		High responsibility		High feeling of stress		Multicomponent variables	
	U	B	U	B	U	B	U	B	U	B	U	B	U	B	U	B	U	B	U	B	U	B
Positive association	50	35	32	20	33	13	18	20	30	17	22	0	36	50	47	36	33	0	50	40	54	18
Negative association	0	6	6	0	0	0	0	0	0	0	11	25	0	0	0	0	0	0	0	0	0	0
Null association	35	53	50	60	46	80	53	60	60	67	56	75	46	33	37	64	67	100	20	40	31	64
Positive and null association	14	6	18	20	21	7	29	20	10	17	11	0	18	17	16	0	0	0	30	20	15	18

These authors used a case-referent design.

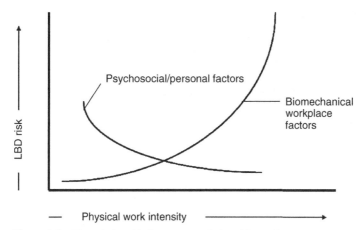

Figure 2.7   The relationship between workplace biomechanical factors and psychosocial/personality factors that may account for observed "J" relationship of low back disorder (LBD) risk and work intensity.

heavy biomechanical loading can lead to high rates of low back pain. This trend is indicated by the increasing trend in risk due to biomechanical workplace factors in the figure that indicates at high physical work intensities risk is dominated by biomechanical loading due to the work design. However, at low levels of physical work intensity, the figure indicates that individual psychosocial- and personality-related factors may play a greater role in defining low back pain risk. The interaction of the influence of these categories of risk factors yields a J-shaped curve of risk that has been observed in epidemiologic studies (Fig. 2.5).

KEY POINTS

- Back pain is very common and the general categorization of back pain referred to in the literature encompasses the whole spectrum of back pain from minor sprains to serious disorders requiring surgery.
- The costs associated with back pain are proportionally more expensive than those associated with other musculoskeletal disorders.
- Over 100 million workdays are lost to back pain every year.
- The U.S. government estimates that two thirds of low back pain cases are attributed to occupational activities.
- Literature reviews indicate that the physical components of work are associated with low back pain risk and include the factors of manual handling of material, frequent bending and twisting, heavy physical work, and whole-body vibration. The relationship between static postures and risk is less clear.
- Numerous literature reviews associate many individual (personal) factors with risk. Among the more frequently cited risk factors are age, smoking, genetics, and individual psychosocial factors (anxiety, distress, and personality). Some believe that these individual factors "set the stage" for physical factors to become more potent risk factors for some workers.
- A literature review has also demonstrated associations between low back pain and organizationally based psychosocial risk factors. These psychosocial factors include

high job demands, low decision latitude/control, low social support at work, and low job satisfaction. A review of the literature has also suggested that these factors may be surrogates for physical work factors and that their influence would be diminished if biomechanical demands were simultaneously evaluated.

- Collectively, the epidemiologic literature suggests that low back pain is multidimensional in terms of risk and there may be significant interactions between these risk dimensions.

REFERENCES

1. American Academy of Orthopaedic Surgeons (AAOS). Back Pain and Back Problems; 2005 [cited].
2. Luo X, *et al.* Estimates and patterns of direct health care expenditures among individuals with back pain in the United States. Spine 2004;29(1):79–86.
3. Deyo RA, Weinstein JN. Low back pain. N Eng J Med 2001;344(5):363–370.
4. Atlas SJ, *et al.* Primary care involvement and outcomes of care in patients with a workers' compensation claim for back pain. Spine 2004;29(9):1041–1048.
5. Bureau of Labor Statistics (BLS). Lost-worktime injuries and illnesses: characteristics and resulting days away from work, 2002. Bureau of Labor Statistics; 2004.
6. National Center for Health Statistics. Health, United States, 2006: with Chartbook on Trends in the Health of Americans with Special Feature on Pain. CDC :Atlanta (GA); 2006.
7. Hamrick C. CTDs and Ergonomics in Ohio. in International Ergonomics Association (IEA) 2000/Human Factors and Ergonomics Society (HFES) 2000 Congress. San Diego, CA: Human Factors and Ergonomics Society; 2000.
8. N.R.C. Musculoskeletal disorders and the workplace: low back and upper extremity. Washington (DC): National Academy Press; 2001.
9. NIOSH, Worker Health Chartbook Department of Health and Human Services (DHHS), Public Health Service, Centers for Disease Control, National Institute for Occupational Safety and Health (NIOSH), Cincinnati (OH); p. 250 2000.
10. Vingard E, *et al.* Seeking care for low back pain in the general population: a two-year follow-up study: results from the MUSIC-Norrtalje Study. Spine 2002; 27 (19):2159–2165.
11. Guo HR, *et al.* Back pain among workers in the United States: national estimates and workers at high risk. Am J Ind Med 1995;28(5):591–602.
12. Guo HR, *et al.* Back pain prevalence in US industry and estimates of lost workdays. Am J Public Health 1999;89 (7):1029–1035.
13. Ferguson SA, Marras WS. A literature review of low back disorder surveillance measures and risk factors. Clin Biomech 1997;12:211–226.
14. Marras WS, *et al.* The effectiveness of commonly used lifting assessment methods to identify industrial jobs associated with elevated risk of low-back disorders. Ergonomics 1999;42(1):229–245.
15. Waters TR, *et al.* Evaluation of the revised NIOSH lifting equation. A cross-sectional epidemiologic study. Spine 1999;386–394, discussion 395.
16. National Institute for Occupational Safety and Health. Musculoskeletal Disorders and Workplace Factors. Department of Health and Human Services (DHHS), National Institute for Occupational Safety and Health (NIOSH). 1997.
17. Hoogendoorn WE, *et al.* Physical load during work and leisure time as risk factors for back pain [see comments]. Scand J Work Environment and Health 1999;25 (5):387–403.
18. National Institute of Occupational Safety and Health. Musculoskeletal Disorders and Workplace Factors: a critical review of epidemiologic evidence for work-related musculoskeletal disorders of the neck, upper extremity, and low back. Bernard BP, editor. Cincinnati, (OH): Department of Health and Human Services (DHHS), Public Health Service, Centers fir Disease Control, National Institute for Occupational Safety and Health (NIOSH); 1997.
19. Norman R, *et al.* A comparison of peak vs cumulative physical work exposure risk factors for the reporting of low back pain in the automotive industry. Clin Biomech (Bristol, Avon) 1998;13(8):561–573.
20. Kumar S, Cumulative load as a risk factor for back pain. Spine 1990;15(12):1311–1316.
21. Videman T, Nurminen M, Troup JD. 1990 Volvo Award in clinical sciences. Lumbar spinal pathology in cadaveric material in relation to history of back pain, occupation, and physical loading. Spine 1990;15(8):728–740.
22. Seidler A, *et al.* The role of cumulative physical work load in lumbar spine disease: risk factors for lumbar osteochondrosis and spondylosis associated with chronic complaints. Occup Environ Med 2001;58(11):735–746.
23. Hartvigsen J, *et al.* [Does sitting at work cause low back pain?]. Ugeskr Laeger 2002;164(6):759–761.
24. NRC. Musculoskeletal disorders and the workplace: low back and upper extremity, Panel on Musculoskeletal Disorders at the Workplace. Washington (DC):

National Academy of Sciences, National Research Council, National Academy Press; p. 492.2001.

25. WADDELL G. The Back Pain Revolution. Edinburgh: Churchill Livingstone; 1999.

26. WADDELL G. Biopsychosocial analysis of low back pain. Baillieres Clin Rheumatol 1992;6(3):523–557.

27. FRANK JW, et al. Disability resulting from occupational low back pain. Part II: what do we know about secondary prevention? A review of the scientific evidence on prevention after disability begins. Spine 1996;21 (24):2918–2929.

28. KRAUSE N, et al. Psychosocial job factors, physical workload, and incidence of work- related spinal injury: a 5-year prospective study of urban transit operators. Spine 1998;23(23):2507–2516.

29. TUBACH F, et al. Risk factors for sick leave due to low back pain: a prospective study. J Occup Environ Med 2002;44(5):451–458.

30. FERGUSON SA, MARRAS WS. A literature review of low back disorder surveillance measures and risk factors. Clin Biomech (Bristol, Avon) 1997;12(4):211–226.

31. ANDERSSON GB. The epidemiology of spinal disorders. In The Adult Spine: Principles and Practice, FRYMOYER, JW, editor. Philadelphia: Lippincott-Raven Publishers; 1997;93–141.

32. LEBOEUF-YDE C, Back pain – individual and genetic factors. J Electromyogr Kinesiol 2004;14(1): 129–133.

33. IGUCHI T, et al. Age distribution of three radiologic factors for lumbar instability: probable aging process of the instability with disc degeneration. Spine 2003;28 (23):2628–2633.

34. ZWERLING C, et al. Occupational injuries: comparing the rates of male and female postal workers. Am J Epidemiol 1993;138(1):46–55.

35. HOOFTMAN WE, et al. Gender differences in the relations between work-related physical and psychosocial risk factors and musculoskeletal complaints. Scand J Work Environ Health 2004;30(4):261–278.

36. GLUCK JV, OLEINICK A. Claim rates of compensable back injuries by age, gender, occupation, and industry. Do they relate to return-to-work experience?Spine 1998;23 (14):1572–1587.

37. LINDBECK L, KJELLBERG K. Gender differences in lifting technique. Ergonomics 2001;44(2):202–214.

38. van der BEEK AJ, et al. Gender differences in exerted forces and physiological load during pushing and pulling of wheeled cages by postal workers. Ergonomics 2000;43(2):269–281.

39. HELIOVAARA M. Body height, obesity, and risk of herniated lumbar intervertebral disc. Spine 1987;12(5):469–472.

40. LEBOEUF-YDE C. Body weight and low back pain. A systematic literature review of 56 journal articles reporting on 65 epidemiologic studies. Spine 2000;25 (2):226–237.

41. DEYO RA, BASS JE. Lifestyle and low-back pain. The influence of smoking and obesity. Spine 1989;14 (5):501–506.

42. KAKUSHIMA M, MIYAMOTO K, SHIMIZU K. The effect of leg length discrepancy on spinal motion during gait: three-dimensional analysis in healthy volunteers. Spine 2003;28(21):2472–2476.

43. ADAMS MA, MANNION AF, DOLAN P. Personal risk factors for first-time low back pain. Spine 1999;24(23):2497–2505.

44. BATTIE MC, et al. The role of spinal flexibility in back pain complaints within industry. A prospective study. Spine 1990;15(8):768–773.

45. BATTIE MC, et al. Anthropometric and clinical measures as predictors of back pain complaints in industry: a prospective study. J Spinal Disord 1990;3(3):195–204.

46. CADY LD, et al. Strength and fitness and subsequent back injuries in firefighters. J Occup Med 1979;21 (4):269–272.

47. CADY LD Jr, THOMAS PC, KARWASKY RJ. Program for increasing health and physical fitness of fire fighters. J Occup Med 1985;27(2):110–114.

48. BATTIE MC, et al. Isometric lifting strength as a predictor of industrial back pain reports. Spine 1989;14(8):851–856.

49. LAHAD A, et al. The effectiveness of four interventions for the prevention of low back pain. J Am Med Assoc 1994;272(16):1286–1291.

50. GORMAN DM, et al. Relationship between alcohol abuse and low back pain. Alcohol 1987;22(1):61–63.

51. LEBOEUF-YDE C. Alcohol and low-back pain: a systematic literature review. J Manipulat Physiol Therap 2000;23(5):343–346.

52. GOLDBERG MS, SCOTT SC, MAYO NE. A review of the association between cigarette smoking and the development of nonspecific back pain and related outcomes. Spine 2000;25(8):995–1014.

53. MIRANDA H, et al. Individual factors, occupational loading, and physical exercise as predictors of sciatic pain. Spine 2002;27(10):1102–1109.

54. SCOTT SC, et al. The association between cigarette smoking and back pain in adults. Spine 1999;24 (11):1090–1098.

55. FELDMAN DE, et al., Smoking. A risk factor for development of low back pain in adolescents. Spine 1999;24 (23):2492–2496.

56. BATTIE MC, et al., 1991 Volvo Award in clinical sciences. Smoking and lumbar intervertebral disc degeneration: an MRI study of identical twins. Spine 1991;16(9):1015–1021.

57. HALPERN MT, et al. Impact of smoking status on workplace absenteeism and productivity. Tobacco Control 2001;10(3):233–238.

58. SAMBROOK PN, MACGREGOR AJ, SPECTOR TD. Genetic influences on cervical and lumbar disc degeneration: a magnetic resonance imaging study in twins. Arthritis Rheum 1999;42(2):366–372.

59. BATTIE MC, et al. 1995 Volvo Award in clinical sciences. Determinants of lumbar disc degeneration. A study relating lifetime exposures and magnetic resonance imaging findings in identical twins. Spine 1995;20 (24):2601–2612.

60. BATTIE M, *et al.*Heretability of low back pain and the role of disc degenerationOrthopaedics Research Society 53rd Annual Meeting; San Diego, CA;2007.

61. HESTBAEK L, *et al.* Heredity of low back pain in a young population: a classical twin study. Twin Res 2004;7 (1):16–26.

62. BATTIE MC, VIDEMAN T, PARENT E. Lumbar disc degeneration: epidemiology and genetic influences. Spine 2004;29(23):2679–2690.

63. JARVIK JG, DEYO RA. Imaging of lumbar intervertebral disk degeneration and aging, excluding disk herniations. Radiol Clin North Am 2000;38(61):255–1266, vi.

64. HELIOVAARA M, KNEKT P, AROMAA A. Incidence and risk factors of herniated lumbar intervertebral disc or sciatica leading to hospitalization. J Chronic Dis 1987;40 (3):251–258.

65. LINTON SJ. A review of psychological risk factors in back and neck pain. Spine 2000;25(9):1148–1156.

66. BONGERS PM, *et al.* Psychosocial factors at work and musculoskeletal disease. Scand J Work Environ Health 1993;19(5):297–312.

67. DERSH J, POLATIN PB, GATCHEL RJ. Chronic pain and psychopathology: research findings and theoretical considerations. Psychosom Med 2002;64 (5):773–786.

68. FEUERSTEIN M, *et al.* From confounders to suspected risk factors: psychosocial factors and work-related upper extremity disorders. J Electromyogr Kinesiol 2004;14 (1):171–178.

69. FRANK JW, *et al.* Occupational back pain – an unhelpful polemic. Scand J Work Environ Health 1995;21(1):3–14.

70. BIGOS SJ, *et al.* A prospective study of work perceptions and psychosocial factors affecting the report of back injury [published erratum appears in Spine 1991 Jun;16 (6):688]. Spine 1991;16(1):1–6.

71. VOLINN E, *et al.* The Boeing prospective study and beyond. Spine 2001;26(14):1613–1622.

72. KARASEK R, *et al.* The Job Content Questionnaire (JCQ): an instrument for internationally comparative assessments of psychosocial job characteristics. J Occup Health Psychol 1998;3(4):322–355.

73. van POPPEL MN, *et al.* Risk factors for back pain incidence in industry: a prospective study. Pain 1998;77(1): 81–86.

74. HOOGENDOORN WE, *et al.* Systematic review of psychosocial factors at work and private life as risk factors for back pain. Spine 2000;25(16):2114–2125.

75. DAVIS KG, HEANEY CA. The relationship between psychosocial work characteristics and low back pain: underlying methodological issues. Clin Biomech (Bristol, Avon) 2000;15(6):389–406.

CHAPTER 3

FUNCTION, STRUCTURE, AND SUPPORT OF THE BACK

THIS CHAPTER presents a basic overview of back anatomy in a functional manner. Anatomy is presented along with a description of why the anatomy is important to the functioning of the back and spine. This chapter assumes no prior physiology or anatomy background. The goal is to present only enough detail so that the reader can understand the causal pathways presented in later chapters.

This chapter is intended to provide the reader with a basic functional (yet nontechnical) working knowledge of anatomy and function of the human back and spine. It is *not* intended to be a comprehensive description of spinal anatomy. There are many books available that have described the anatomy of the spine very well (1–4). Instead, the goal of this chapter is to describe the functional structure of the spine in enough detail so that the reader can appreciate how the anatomy might affect the functioning of the spine and potentially, lead to back pain. In addition, it is important to understand the anatomy of the back so that we can understand how work-related factors might be related to the experience of low back pain.

3.1 BODY COORDINATES

To describe movements and motions of the body in precise terms, it is necessary to describe the directions of motion relative to a coordinate system. Direction of motion is described relative to the three cardinal planes (coordinate system) shown in Fig. 3.1. The sagittal plane of the body divides the body into the right and left halves and describes movements such as forward flexion and extension toward the rear. The lateral plane divides the body into the front and back and is used to describe sideways or lateral motion to either the left or right. Finally, the transverse plane separates the body into the top and lower halves of the body and is used to describe twisting motion, either clockwise (CW) or counter clockwise (CCW). By describing movements in combinations of these planes, it is possible to describe any movement or motion of the spine.

3.2 BONY STRUCTURES OF THE SPINE

The spine is constructed of a series of building blocks or vertebral bones that are stacked upon one another to form the spinal column that runs from the pelvis to the head. Twenty-six of these bones are vertebral bones. A vertebral bone or vertebrae is

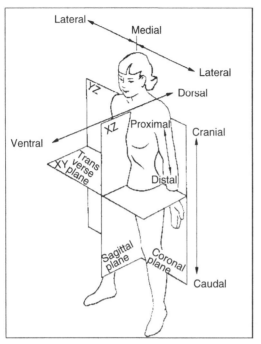

Figure 3.1 The primary cardinal planes of the body. Movement of the body and specifically the spine is referenced relative the sagittal, frontal, and transverse planes as shown. (NASA-STD-3000 260 (Rev A), msis.jsc.nasa.gov/sections/section03.htm)

shown in Fig. 3.2. The large round portion of the bone is the *vertebral body* and is the major load-bearing structure in the spine. The outer portion of this bone is constructed of a thin layer of very strong and stiff cortical bone. Cortical bone, also called compact bone, forms a protective outer shell around every bone in the body. Cortical bone has a high resistance to bending and torsion and provides strength where bending would be undesirable. The inner portion of the bone is spongy matrix of cancellous bone. Cancellous bone is less dense and more elastic than cortical bone. This type of bone

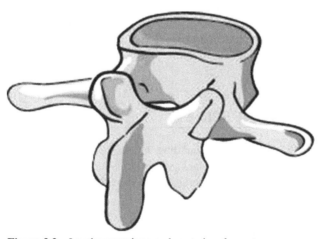

Figure 3.2 Lumbar vertebrae and posterior elements.

forms the interior scaffolding and helps the bone to maintain their shape despite compressive forces. The bone is rigid but appears spongy. It is composed of bundles of short and parallel strands of bone fused together.

Just posterior (towards the rear) of the vertebral body are bony structures that make up the *posterior elements* and help form a protective channel or opening for the spinal cord. These bony protrusions consist of the transverse processes and the spinous process. The spinous processes are the bones that can be seen on a person's back and appears to be a series of "bumps" under the skin. The transverse processes and spinous processes form a guidance system for the back that keep the bones aligned and also serve as mechanical "stops" to prevent the spine from twisting excessively. In addition, they share in load support under some conditions.

The posterior elements also provide attachment points for both ligaments that connect bone to bone and tendons that connect muscles to bone. These muscles and ligaments provide rigidity to the system of bones as well as provide feedback as to body as to its position in space by way of the muscles and muscle–tendon junction.

3.3 THE DISC (AND THE SPINAL JOINT)

The vertebral bodies are connected by disc that serve three purposes. First, they serve as shock absorbers between the vertebrae. Second, they transmit load between vertebrae. Third, they permit and govern motion between the vertebrae. The disc consists of two parts. The outer portions of the disc consist of alternating layers of fibers that are oriented at a 65° angle relative to the vertical. Seventy to 90 layers of fibers make up concentric "rings" that define the disk also called the *annulus fibrosus* (Fig. 3.3). Within the annulus fibrosis is a gelatinous core named the *nucleus pulposus* (Fig. 3.3). Collectively these structures form a shock absorption system. However, the integrity of the system changes throughout the day. The disk absorbs water while one is sleeping, which makes the system stiffer when one wakes up in the morning. Conversely, when one is upright, water is squeezed out of the disk and the structure becomes more lax.

3.4 FUNCTIONAL SPINAL UNIT

Two vertebral bones along with their connecting disc are referred to as a *functional spinal unit* (Fig. 3.4). When these functional spinal units are considered along the length of the spine, the spinal column is formed (Fig. 3.5). As shown in Fig. 3.5, there are four subcategories of vertebrae (cervical, thoracic, lumbar, and sacral) that are associated with

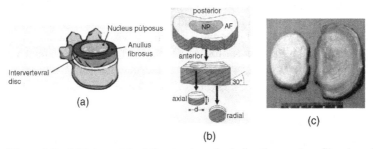

Figure 3.3 (a) Intervertebral disc structures including the annulous fibrosis and the nucleus pulposus. (**b** and **c**) Alternating layers of disk fibers. (Courtesy of James Iatridis, http://www.cems.uvm.edu/~iatridis/research)

Functional Spinal Unit

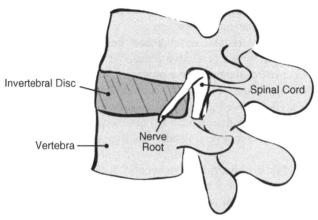

Figure 3.4   The functional spinal unit consisting of two vertebrae and one disc.

four physiologic curves. Seven cervical vertebrae comprise the neck, 12 vertebrae define the thoracic spine, and 5 vertebrae form the lumbar spine. In addition, the sacrum is defined by five immobile or "fused" vertebrae and the coccyx (often referred to as the tailbone) is a fusion of four coccygeal vertebrae at the very base of the spine. Each vertebra is numbered according to its vertical position along the spine (beginning with the vertebrae closest to the head) along with the subcategory name of the vertebrae. Disk levels are also named relative to the vertebral levels surrounding the disk. For example, the lowest lumbar vertebra (fifth lumbar vertebra or L5) is adjacent to the first sacral vertebra (S1) and the disc between these vertebra is referred to as L5/S1.

Several curves are also apparent in the upright spine (Fig. 3.5). The cervical and lumbar curves are referred to as cervical lordosis and lumbar lordosis, whereas the thoracic and sacral curves are called thoracic kyphosis and sacral kyposis since these curves bow in the opposite direction of the lordotic curves. Collectively, these curves form a stable system that maintain the center of gravity in a balanced state.

3.5   SPINE SUPPORT

The stack of bones comprising the spinal column is stable and strong while in compression (see Fig. 3.6) but can be easily toppled with a small force directed from the side (shear shown in Fig. 3.6). Therefore, the integrity of the spinal column must be offered by supporting structures within the trunk. Support for the spinal column occurs by way of the muscles and ligaments connecting the vertebral structures and the pelvis. The structures stabilize the spine by providing anterior/posterior (forward/backward) as well as lateral (sideways) support in much the same way as guy wires support a tall antenna or stays support the mast of a ship (Fig. 3.7).

3.6   LIGAMENTS

Ligamentous support is provided by the anterior longitudinal ligament and posterior longitudinal ligament that run the length of the spine in front and in back of the spine,

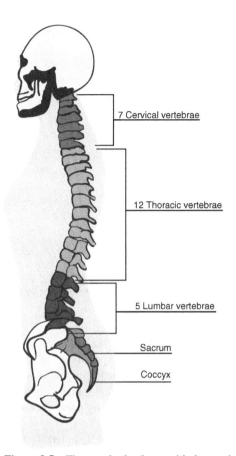

Figure 3.5   The vertebral column with the cervical, thoracic, lumbar, sacrum, and coccyx vertebrae identified. Note the curves of the spine also named according to region.

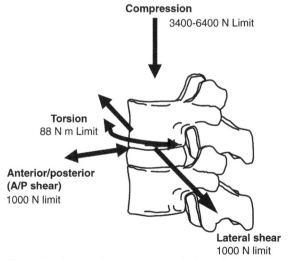

Figure 3.6   Loads imposed on the lumbar spine.

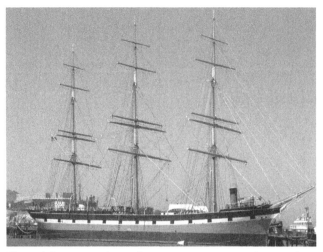

Figure 3.7   Support for a tall structure such as a mast is most efficiently provided by guy wires called stays and shrouds on a sailing ship. In a similar fashion, spine support is provided by the muscles and ligaments that run the length of the spine.

respectively. These longitudinal ligaments are located close to the vertebrae and prevent the vertebrae from separating as well as contain the disc within its space (see Fig. 3.8). However, the posterior longitudinal ligament narrows considerably at the lower lumbar levels. Several ligaments run between the vertebrae (intertransverse ligaments, interspinous ligaments, supraspinous ligament, and facet capsulary ligaments). These ligaments resist forces that would pull the spine out of alignment.

Another important supporting structure of the spine is the ligament flavum shown in Fig. 3.8. This ligament provides support to the posterior elements of the spine and helps form the spinal canal through which the spinal cord runs.

Ligaments provide passive support or force to the spine in that they only provide support when they are under tension and usually provide force when the torso is in a nonneutral or deviated posture. Recent studies have also shown that the ligaments are

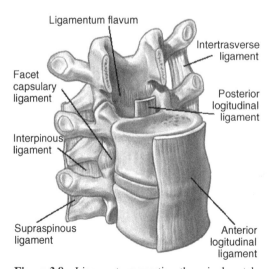

Figure 3.8   Ligaments supporting the spinal vertebrae. (Courtesy of: Stewart Eidelson, MD).

capable of providing feedback to the musculoskeletal system and can actually initiate muscle activities if they are stretched sufficiently (5–7).

3.7 MUSCLES

The other support mechanism for the spine involves the muscles within the torso. There are over 30 muscles that support and load the spinal column. Some of these muscles are large, power-producing muscles that span large sections of the spinal column, while others are small and attached between the vertebral segments. Some believe that these small muscles are not powerful enough to apply significant force to the spine but simply serve as a sophisticated feedback mechanism (4). The muscles that have sufficient mechanical advantage to support or load the spine consist of multifidus, erector spinae, internal oblique, external oblique, and the rectus abominus muscle pairs and are shown in Fig. 3.9. Note that these muscles are located *both* posteriorly (behind the spine) and anteriorly (in front of the spine), thereby surrounding the spine to offer support and stability. Given the distance from the spine, each of these power-producing muscles has a different mechanical advantage relative to the spine that permit it to both support and load the spine. One should also realize that even though the muscle area is shown in cross section, the muscles are oriented at various angles that allow them to impose compression, shear, and torsion forces on the spine.

Unlike ligaments, muscles provide active support to the spine. Muscles activate and generate force in response to the loads imposed on a structure from outside (external to) the body, such as when one is lifting or pushing a load. The muscles must counteract these external forces and must do so while at a mechanical disadvantage (due to the shorter lever arm relative to the spine). Therefore, muscles are capable of imposing very large loads on the spine and are an important component in defining the loads that are experienced by the spine during activities. Since there are many muscles within the torso, the sequence in which muscles are recruited and exert force becomes an important factor in defining spine loading during an exertion. The manner in which the muscles are recruited is referred to a *motor control*. Motor control patterns vary greatly between individuals and are influenced by life experiences and injury to the musculoskeletal system, training, the work environment, and worker attitudes (8–10). The pattern of muscle recruitment indicates whether the muscles are recruited in sequence or simultaneously. During heavy exertions or when highly controlled exertions are performed, the torso recruits many of the muscles simultaneously in an attempt to protect the spine or exert high levels of control on the movement. When muscles are recruited simultaneously during an activity, they can oppose or "fight each other" (referred to biomechancially as cocontraction or coactivation), which results in greater loading of the spinal structures. Thus, understanding the motor control pattern associated with activities is an important component of understanding how the spine is loaded during an activity.

3.8 FASCIA

Fascia can be defined as a sheet of fibrous connective tissue that envelops, separates, or binds together muscles, organs, and other soft structures. Within the thoracolumbar spine, it is believed that the fascia plays a role in transmitting force and supporting the spine. Abdominal fascia is shown over the rectus abdominis muscle in Fig. 3.10. The thoracolumbar fascia consists of three layers that envelop the muscles. The anterior layer is thin and attached to the quadratus lumborum. The middle layer lies behind the quadratus lumborum and is attached to the lumbar transverse processes and attaching to the intertransverse ligaments. Finally, the

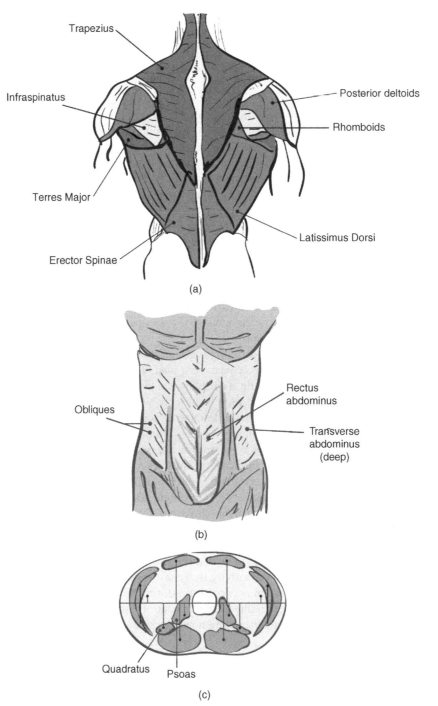

Figure 3.9 (**a**) Back muscles, (**b**) abdominal muscles, and (**c**) a cross-sectional view of muscles that support (and load) the spine. Note the different lever arm distances and the differences in mechanical advantage of the various muscles in (**c**).

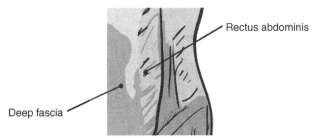

Figure 3.10   Fascia within the trunk helps connect tissue.

posterior thoracolumbar fascia surrounds the back muscles. It begins at the spinous processes and wraps around the back muscles and joins with the throacolumbar fascia along the lateral portion of the iliocostalis lumborum. It is the posterior layer of the fascia that is believed to play the greatest role from a biomechanical standpoint (11,12).

3.9 NERVES

An elaborate network of nerves passes along the length of the spine. The main communication connection between the brain and the rest of the body consists of the spinal cord that resides within the spinal canal. The spinal canal is located just behind (posterior to) the vertebral body and in front of the posterior elements forming a channel along the length of the spine. Nerves branch out at each level of the spine forming nerve roots that distribute and receive information to and from the various tissues of the body (Figure 3.11a). Above the L1 level, nerve roots branch off from the spinal cord and pass through an area called the radicular canal beyond which the nerve branches out further to form of peripheral nerves and serve various parts of the body. The lumbar nerve roots are labeled relative to the vertebral body at which they exit the spinal canal. Thus, the nerve root exiting just below the second lumbar vertebrae is called the L2 nerve root. Within the lumbar spine, the nerve roots exit the spinal cord at L1 and continue individually as nerve roots within the spinal canal down the lumbar spine to form the cauda equina.

The spinal cord is connected to the spinal nerves by the dorsal root and ventral root. The dorsal root transmits afferent (traveling to the brain) sensory information to the brain, whereas the ventral root transmits efferent (away from the brain) motor control information to the muscles. Just before the dorsal root and ventral root exit the intervertebral foramen, they join to form the spinal nerve root, which is very short. However, just before the roots unite, a bump is seen on the dorsal root called the dorsal root ganglion (see Fig. 3.11b). The dorsal root ganglion consists of cell bodies of the sensory fibers within the dorsal root. As the spinal nerve exits the spinal column, it immediately divides again into the ventral ramus and dorsal ramus. After this point, peripheral nerves are formed that serve specific parts of the body. Figure 3.12 shows the spinal nerve roots and the parts of the body that are affected by damage to the nerve root at each level.

Within the lumbar spine, as the dorsal rami exit the spinal column, they form nearly right angles from the lumbar spinal nerves. As they move toward the transverse processes, the dorsal rami between L1 and L4 divide into two to three branches that are presented at each level. This arrangement may provide opportunities for pressure to be imposed on the nerve.

Nerve intervention to the disk was originally thought to be nonexistent. However, we now know that the outer third of the annulus contains a network of complex nerve endings

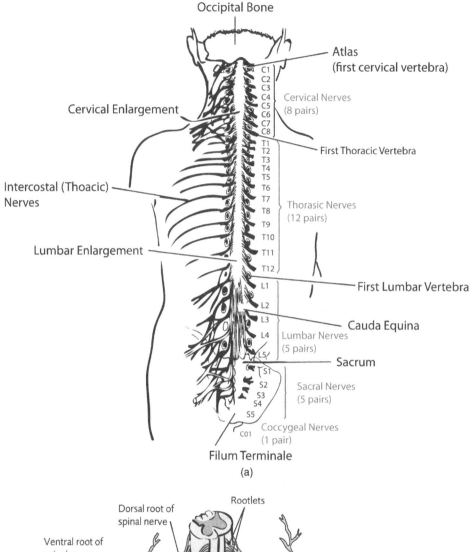

(a)

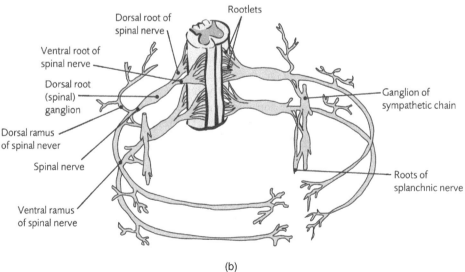

(b)

Figure 3.11 The organization of the spinal nerves (**a**) along the length of the spine and (**b**) as they surround the torso.

Effects of spinal injury

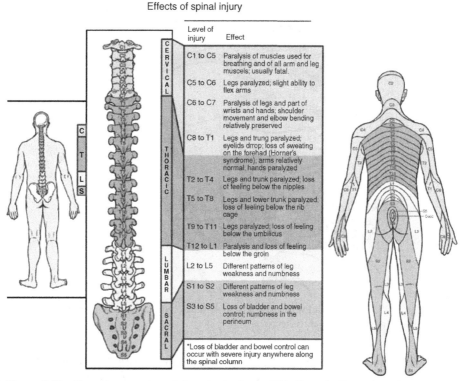

Level of injury	Effect
C1 to C5	Paralysis of muscles used for breathing and of all arm and leg muscels; usually fatal.
C5 to C6	Legs paralyzed; slight ability to flex arms
C6 to C7	Paralysis of legs and part of wrists and hands; shoulder movement and elbow bending relatively preserved
C8 to T1	Legs and trung paralyzed; eyelids drrop; loss of sweating on the forehad (Horner's syndrome); arms relatively normal; hands paralyzed
T2 to T4	Legs and trunk paralyzed; loss of feeling below the nipples
T5 to T8	Legs and lower trunk paralyzed; loss of feeling below the rib cage
T9 to T11	Legs paralyzed; loss of feeling below the umbilicus
T12 to L1	Paralysis and loss of feeling below the groin
L2 to L5	Different patterns of leg weakness and numbness
S1 to S2	Different patterns of leg weakness and numbness
S3 to S5	Loss of bladder and bowel control; numbness in the perineum

*Loss of bladder and bowel control can occur with severe injury anywhere along the spinal column

Figure 3.12   Nerve intervention of the spinal column. This figure indicates how function can be effected if the various spinal nerves are compromised (from The Merck Manual of Medical information - Second Edition, p. 562, edited by Mark H. Beers. Copyright 2003 by Merck & Co., Inc., Whitehouse Station, NJ. Available at http://www.merck.com/mmhe/sec06/ch093/ch0932.html)

that are capable of transmitting pain signals. Pain receptors are not uniformly distributed, with the greatest number of endings residing in the lateral regions of the disk.

3.10 BLOOD VESSELS

Blood delivery is important to maintain the health of biologic tissue. In addition, blood regulation is involved in the perception of pain. It is important to appreciate the anatomy of blood supply within the spine. Lumbar spine blood supply is provided by the lumbar arteries and drainage is accomplished via the lumbar veins (Fig. 3.13).

A pair of lumbar arteries originate from the back of the aorta in front of the lumbar vertebrae. The lumbar arteries then run backward around the vertebral body. Once the artery reaches the point of the intervertebral foramen, it further divides into several branches. Lateral branches of the artery continue on to the psoas and quadratus lumborum muscles. Other branches run along side the ramus and dorsal ramus of the spinal nerve and innervate the paravertebral muscles. The posterior branches of the lumbar artery form a network of blood vessels around the zagapohysial joints. Three medial branches initiate from the lumbar artery. One of these branches crosses the disk and circumvents the pedicle to form a network along with vessels from higher segments.

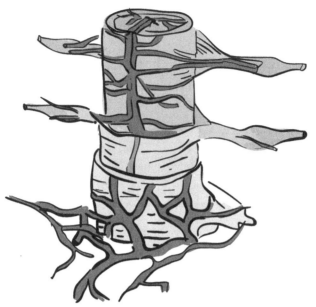

Figure 3.13   Artery and venous blood supply delivered to the spinal cord, nerve roots, and surrounding muscles and tissues.

A number of veins surround the lumbar spine and serve a drainage mission. These veins include the lumbar veins and the venous plexuses. The lumbar veins drain into the inferior vena cava. The venous plexus is a variable series of vessels that interconnect to the lumbar veins. Blood supply to the spinal nerve roots is received form the vessels emanating from the spinal cord and from radicular branches of the lumbar arteries.

3.11   END PLATES AND NUTRITION

An important consideration for low back pain generation is the nutritional supply to the intervertebral disk. Although the annulus fibers are biologically active and require nutrition for their survival, the intervertebral disks have no arterial supply. Only small branching arteries innervate the very outermost fibers of the annulus. Thus, to remain viable, the intervertebral disk must receive nutrition via diffusion from the outer annulus and from the capillary branches beneath the vertebral end plates. Hence, for nutrition to reach the nucleus pulposus, nutrition in the form of oxygen, sugar, and other molecules must diffuse across the end plate or through annulus fibrosus. Motion of the vertebral bodies relative to the disk appears to play a positive role in diffusion and the delivery of nutrients to the intervertebral disc (13).

3.12   FACETS

The joints compromising the posterior elements of the spine are referred to as the articular facet joint. These joints are engaged when spinal curvature in present in the lumbar spine and become disengaged when the spine is flexed. When engaged, these joints are capable of bearing about one third of the load of the spine. However, when disengaged, all the load supported by the spine is transferred to the disk. Because of their ability to support load as well as guide motion, these joints play an important role in defining contact forces within the bones, ligament, muscles, and ultimately, the loading experienced by the nerves.

3.13 THE SYSTEM

This brief description of spinal and back anatomy should emphasize that although there are many individual components that define the anatomy of the back, there are many opportunities for these components to interact. The functioning of any one of the various components can have an impact on the functioning of the other components. Thus, when considering the anatomy of the back, we must consider this an active *system* and the interaction of the various system components must be considered when assessing function.

KEY POINTS

- The anatomical features of the spine and trunk form a complex and intricate system of support and movement within the back.
- A series of bony structures (vertebrae) define the spine and provide structural support, limit motion, and protect the nervous system residing within the structure. Due to the complex, multifunctional nature of the system, there are many opportunities to compromise nerves, blood supply, and active and passive support tissues.
- The many muscles within the trunk represent the only truly active generators of force within the trunk. The recruitment pattern of the various muscles dictates the load history experienced by the various structures of the spine. Passive support is provided primarily by the ligaments, fascia, facet joints, and elongated muscles.
- The disk separates the vertebral bodies, provides shock absorption, and permits spine motion. Disk damage results in the potential to compromise nerve volume. The end plates play a key role in disk nourishment and disk health. However, because of a greatly reduced intervention of nerves within the disk, perception of spine load is greatly compromised.

REFERENCES

1. BOGDUK N, TWOMEY. Clinical Anatomy of the Lumbar Spine. New York: Churchill Livingtsone; 1987.
2. GRACOVETSKY S. The Spinal Engine. New York, (NY): Sringer-Verlag Wien; 1988.
3. McGILL S. Low Back Disorders: Evidence-Based Prevention and Rehabilitation. Champaign, (IL): Human Kinetics; 2002.
4. McGILL S. Ultimate Back Fitness and Performance. Waterloo (Canada): Wabuno Publishers; 2004.
5. SOLOMONOW M. Ligaments: a source of work-related musculoskeletal disorders. J Electromyogr Kinesiol 2004;14:49–60.
6. SOLOMONOW M, EVERSULL E, HE ZHOU B, BARATTA RV, ZHU MP. Neuromuscular neutral zones associated with viscoelastic hysteresis during cyclic lumbar flexion. Spine 2001;26:E314–324.
7. SOLOMONOW M, ZHOU BH, BARATTA RV, LU Y, HARRIS M. Biomechanics of increased exposure to lumbar injury caused by cyclic loading: Part 1. Loss of reflexive muscular stabilization. Spine 1999;24:2426–2434.
8. DAVIS KG, MARRAS WS, HEANEY CA, WATERS TR, GUPTA P. The impact of mental processing and pacing on spine loading: 2002 Volvo Award in biomechanics. Spine 2002;27:2645–2653.
9. MARRAS WS, DAVIS KG, HEANEY CA, MARONITIS AB, ALLREAD WG. The influence of psychosocial stress, gender, and personality on mechanical loading of the lumbar spine. Spine 2000;25:3045–3054.

10. MARRAS WS, PARAKKAT J, CHANY AM, YANG G, BURR D, LAVENDER SA. Spine loading as a function of lift frequency, exposure duration, and work experience. Clin Biomech (Bristol, Avon) 2006;21:345–352.

11. BOGDUK N, MACINTOSH JE. The applied anatomy of the thoracolumbar fascia. Spine 1984;9:164–170.

12. GRACOVETSKY S, FARFAN HF, LAMY C. The mechanism of the lumbar spine. Spine 1981;6:249–262.

13. BOGDUK N, TWONEY L. Clinical Anatomy of the Lumbar Spine.Singapore: Livingston; Churchill 1987.

CHAPTER 4

THE PROCESS OF PAIN

*P*AIN PERCEPTION *is discussed in this chapter. The goal is to help the reader understand that pain perception is influenced not only by physical loading but also by prior (cognitive) experiences. Difference between peripheral and central pain is discussed and the ability of the various spinal structures and tissues to experience pain is considered. Finally, the influence of biomechanical loads imposed on tissues and their biochemical reactions is discussed in terms of their ability to initiate pain perception.*

4.1 WHAT IS PAIN?

To understand how back pain might be related to the work we do, we must first understand: what is pain? Pain is a rather complex reaction to tissue state that is also influenced by cognition (the way you think), emotion, and behavior. Pain has been described as "an unpleasant sensory and emotion experience associated with actual or potential tissue damage, or described in terms of such damage" (1). In other words, pain is a *perception*, just like sound or sight. It is *not* a sensation. Pain perception involves sensitivity to chemical changes in the tissue and an interpretation of these tissue changes in such a way that they are judged to be harmful. Since pain is a perception, the perception is real whether or not damage has occurred to the tissue (2). It is possible to experience pain as a result of damage to a tissue, but it is also possible to experience pain once the tissue damage has healed.

Cognition refers to the mental processing that occurs in the brain in light of a persons experiences, beliefs, and desires. Cognition can influence or shape the perception of pain. Therefore, cognition can lead to emotional and behavioral reactions to tissue stimulation (2). We have all heard of heroic sports feats where a sports figure successfully completes an athletic event only to find out that she had finished the event with a broken bone. This demonstrates how our mind has the ability to filter sensations and refocus our attention on our goals. Similarly, in the absence of such goals or objectives, it is also possible to refocus on our attention on our well-being and magnify the perception of pain. Hence, it is important to realize that even though much of the pain experience can be initiated by a physical insult to the biological system, it is also possible for pain to be perceived due to a disturbance of any part of the biopsychosocial system we call the human experience. As we shall see, when assessing risk of low back pain related to work, we must consider the work requirements, the person's perception of the situation, and their interpretation and beliefs relative to the causality of the pain.

4.2 ORIGINS OF PAIN

Pain can originate from injured tissue or it can be experienced in the central nervous system (CNS). Pain originating from a damaged tissue site is called *peripheral pain* or *nociceptive pain*. To experience peripheral pain, a tissue must be connected to the nervous system. This type of pain is often referred to a joint or muscle pain and indicates tissue disruption in these structures. This typically originates in the motion-associated components of the musculo-skeletal system such as the muscles, tendons, and ligaments or in the peripheral nerves.

Nociceptors (pain sensors) reside in different parts of the body at different densities. The sensory endings of the nociceptors are very thin fibers and are embedded in the tissue. Fat tissue has very few nociceptors and is thus insensitive to mechanical load. However, the interface between ligament and bone or tendon and bone is richly innervated with nociceptors, making these insertion points prime pain-generating locations. Nociceptor pain is believed to be primarily responsible for work-related pain to the low back.

Central pain originates in the nerves and is typically due to a dysfunction of the CNS. This can be due to maladaptive cognitive processes resulting in *psychogenic* pain, but most likely it is due to structural changes in the spinal tissues as a result of spinal cord injury, multiple sclerosis, stroke, or epilepsy (3). Thus, central pain is typically associated with a lesion or dysfunction of the CNS. Neuropathic pain refers to pain occurring at structural or functional nervous system *adaptations* that are secondary to injury and take place either centrally or peripherally (4). Neurogenic pain refers to an injury to the peripheral nerve without any neuropathy or degeneration of the nervous system. Neuropathic pain is often described in terms of abnormal sensations such as cold, shocking, burning, or numbness.

One of the problems associated with chronic work-related musculoskeletal pain such as back pain is that once the pain sequence has been initiated, and if it continues, the pain can become *persistent pain*. Persistent pain may continue even in the absence of the initiating stimulus (after the tissue has healed) because of a CNS dysfunction. However, CNS dysfunction is secondary to long-term peripheral pain. In other words, if pain is consistently perceived from nociceptors, it can result in changes in the CNS that can change the pain from peripheral pain to central pain. Hence, persistent back pain can be complex and can expand from the original sites of pain to more central pain "persistent" sites.

4.3 PAIN TRANSMISSION

Nociceptive pain occurs when normal nerves transmit information to the CNS about trauma to the tissue. Nociceptors are pain-sensing receptors located in the skin, muscles, viscera, blood vessels, bones, and joints, which, when stimulated, transmit a signal to the brain (see Fig. 4.1). Nociceptors can be as long as 1 m between the receptor site with their synaptic ending located in the dorsal horn of the spinal cord. The cell body (somata) of most nociceptors is located at the dorsal root ganglion (DRG) on either side of the vertebrae.

A nociceptor's function is to trigger biochemical responses. When nociceptors signals are blocked, wound healing is delayed. Thus, nociceptors appear to play a role in healing as well as neuroimmune responses. Activation of nociceptors can also initiate a release of vasoactive peptides that instigate redness and increase permeability of the blood vessels. Since nociceptors can serve deep tissues that provide convergent input to the spinal cord, this organization is also believed to be responsible for referred pain or pain felt at a site other than where the cause is situated.

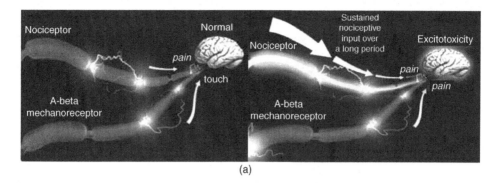

(a)

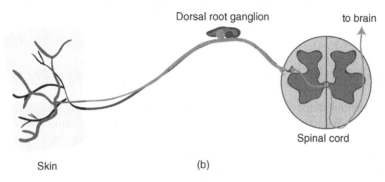

(b)

Figure 4.1   (**a**) Nociceptors' peripheral pain route and (Illustrations by Donald Bliss, NIH Med Arts, with permission) (**b**) path to the central nervous system.

The nocicpetor's sensory ending typically respond to strong stimuli. When a strong stimulus activates a sensory cell, the stimulus typically acts directly on a transduction channel by opening the channel resulting in depolarization and electrical excitation of the neuron. Different types of transduction channels are activated by heat, mechanical stimulation, or chemical stimuli. Low back pain would be expected to involve primarily mechanical stimulation that would be expected to activate specific mechanically sensitive transmission channels (degenerin or DEG).

Pain-sensing nociceptors are also capable of activating when the stimuli are not strong if the nociceptors become sensitized. Sensitization occurs through inflammation of the tissues at the site of the nociceptors. When inflammation occurs, the sensory endings are much more reactive to stimulation to the point where normally nonpainful stimuli become painful (allodynia) and perception of painful stimuli becomes intensified (hyperalgesia). It is believed that this sensitization is a result of the chemical modification of the transduction channels at the sensory endings. Inflammatory mediators such as bradykinin and prostaglandins can enhance sensitization though this mechanism, thereby increasing pain perception (5).

Synapses from the nociceptors occur within the dorsal horn of the spinal cord (Fig. 4.2). Here, the pain signal enters the central nervous system. Voltage-gated calcium channels are opened when neurotransmitters are released and synaptic transmission of the pain signal occurs. However, the pain transmission is modifiable at this point. The synapse is controlled by a system shown in Fig. 4.3. Specific interneurons within the dorsal horn are able to use endorphins as transmitters that act to block the transmission of the pain signal. The interruption of the pain signal is mediated by morphin receptors that act by inhibiting presynaptic activity of the voltage-gated calcium channels (5).

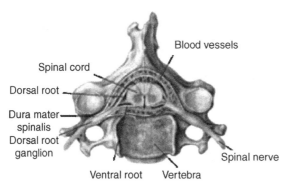

Figure 4.2 Dorsal horn of spinal cord where signals enter the central nervous system. Note the close tight fit of the dorsal root ganglion as it enters the spinal canal. (From reference 5).

4.4 THE PAIN PROCESS

Our understanding of the mechanisms involved in back pain has advanced significantly over the past decade. We now understand that back pain is a set of complex cellular, molecular, and functional adaptations that are initiated by stimulation of nociceptors at the peripheral nervous system site. Nociceptors trigger a signal that ascends to the dorsal ganglion neuronal cell body and adjacent dorsal horn palisading interneurons, then to the brainstem medullary structures, and finally projects signals to widespread regions of the cortical and subcortical central nervous system. Pain is fundamentally a *sensitization* of tissue. However, this sensitization can occur at the pain receptor or the sensitization can extend through the various components of the nervous system and even affect the brain responses. Thus, while pain appears to be initiated by compromise of tissue through the application of force, this is only

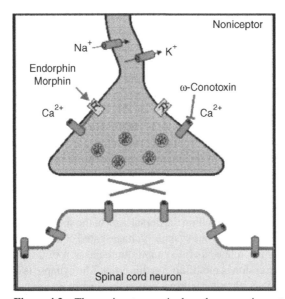

Figure 4.3 The nociceptor – spinal cord synapse is controlled by a system shown here. Specific interneurons within the dorsal horn are able to use endorphins as transmitters that act to block the transmission of the pain signal. (From reference 5).

the beginning of a system of responses that we interpret as pain. While older theories of pain sensitization considered sensitization as anatomic variations and injuries, newer theories consider pain sensitization to be functional in nature and thereby shaped by the person's exposures and experiences. Pain can be thought of as a continuum that can progress from peripheral pain to chronic pain. The characteristics of each type of pain described in this section along with the probable pain mechanisms are summarized in Table 4.1.

Peripheral pain is typically the simplest pain and indicates that the nociceptive receptors in the peripheral nervous system are being exposed to a stimulus. Nociceptors can be stimulated either directly or can be trigged by adjacent or even remote tissue injury. Nociceptor stimulation projects toward and is altered by a dynamic and complex CNS system that interprets the experience of pain. To understand the influence of work in back pain, it is important to recognize that the nociceptor is the initiating factor of pain and it can initiate central pain responses. However, it is also important to understand that the nociceptor is just one component of a multidimensional interactive nervous system.

Neuropathic pain describes pain that is typically initiated by stimulation of peripheral tissue or a nerve injury, yet stimulation of the tissue is no longer necessary to maintain the pain sensation. Hence, pain persists with this condition, even though the magnitude of the tissue or nerve stimulus would not be expected to result in a painful response. Under these conditions, the stimulus is often repetitive in nature. Thus, the tolerance to stimulation is significantly reduced under these conditions.

Pain is referred to as *central pain* when abnormally behaving neurons are located within and throughout the CNS. Thus, central pain refers to central nervous system

TABLE 4.1 The Relationship Between Sources of Pain and the Various Types of Pain

	Pain		
	Acute		Chronic
Pain Mechanism	Peripheral	Neuropathic	Central
Direct tissue stimulation of nociceptors at site of tissue insult	X		
Adjacent or remote tissue stimulation (increased stimulation via involvement of more nociceptors)	X		
Cytokine upregulation (increased sensitization via biochemical response— nociceptors react more easily)	X	X	X
Tissue stimulation no longer necessary			
Inflammatory cascade (increased sensitization via biochemical sensitization and increased pressure on nociceptors)		X	X
Tissue stimulation no longer necessary			
Pain response patterns imprinted in brain			X
Tissue stimulation no longer necessary			

sensitization. The key to understanding pain is to understand how sensitization can occur. Sensitization can occur peripherally or centrally.

4.5   THE INFLAMMATORY PROCESS (CYTOKINES)

One of the more important discoveries regarding back pain in recent years has been the defining the roles of cytokines. A cytokine is a regulatory protein, such as interleukin (or lymphokine), that is released by cells of the immune system and acts as intercellular mediator in the generation of an immune response. Studies have found that when cytokines are upregulated, a cascade of inflammatory responses are initiated that can enhance the sensitivity of nociceptors (6–10), and thus, result in a greatly increased sensitivity to pain. Specifically, within the spine, interleukin-1 a/b (IL-I a/b), interleukin-6 (IL-6), and tumor necrosis factor alpha (TNF-a) have been found to greatly increase pain sensitivity (8).

The logic of how cytokines play a key role in the development of musculoskeletal disorders have been well described (6). According to this theory, loads imposed on tissues due to activities provoke physiological responses that can influence the tissue tolerance. Loads imposed on the tissue below the tissue tolerance preserve the integrity of the tissue. However, loads imposed above the tissue tolerance initiate a series of physiologic responses that can lead to inflammation. This sequence of events is referred to as the *overexertion* theory of musculoskeletal disorders. Tissue microtruama can result in an inflammatory reaction of the tissue. In the case of repetitive tasks (such as highly repetitive work tasks), the tissue loads are superimposed on the inflamed tissue where the increased pressure leads to increased nociceptors stimulation. A cycle of injury, further inflammation, and motor dysfunction follow. It is this inflammatory response of the tissue that leads to a vicious cycle or cascade of chronic tissue sensitivity and a reduction of tissue tolerance to the repetitive task.

The role of tissue inflammation is to protect tissue from further damage and initiate tissue regeneration. Inflammation attempts to engulf and destroy a hostile threat to the tissue. Phagocytes are released that serves as an important bodily defense mechanism against infection by microorganisms and against occlusion of mucous surfaces or tissues by foreign particles and tissue debris. During repetitive tasks that may or may not include high force exertions, tissues are overstretched and/or compressed, and these tissue loads can lead to oxygen deprivation in the tissue (11). This tissue abuse can cause mechanical disruption of the cellular membranes and intracellular structures, leading to a localized release of proteins including cytokines. The extent of tissue damage and the length of time since damage occurred dictate the nature of the inflammatory response (6).

Initial acute inflammation typically occurs suddenly and follows the sequence described in Fig. 4.4 (6). According to this sequence, small artery twigs in the capillary bed (arteriolar) are initially constricted, followed by vasodilation, which increases permeability of the endothelium, diffusion of fluid and plasma proteins, and migration of leukocytes from the vessels into the injured tissues. The vasodilation results in tissue heat, redness, and an increase in tissue mass. The increase in tissue pressure on the nerves (due to edema) can result in pain and loss of function. One of the more long-term results of increased vascular permeability is the influx of inflammatory mediators such as TNF-a and IL-1 released from injured cells when vessels have been overstretched or compressed. Since IL-1 and TNF-a are proinflammatory agents, several reactions can occur. First, *neutrophils* respond during the acute inflammatory response within the first 24 h and can be present for

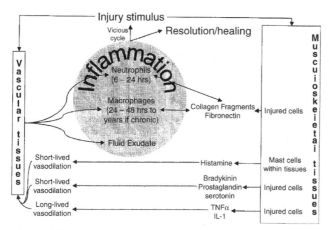

Figure 4.4 Cytokine upregulation and the role of the vascular tissue in the inflammatory process. (From reference 6).

up to 5 days. Neutrophils are white blood cells that are highly destructive to microorganisms. When a tissue is damaged, neutrophils go to the site of the injury and defend the injured tissue from invading bacteria. In this context, neutrophils can be thought of as the body's "security force." Second, the neutrophils also signal *macrophages* to clean up the injury site. Macrophages consume dead and damaged tissue so that the remaining healthy tissue can regenerate. Monocytes and macrophages, the predominant immune cells, respond to tendon and muscle injuries within the next 24–48 h. Changes in chemical concentrations resulting from these reactions can increase concentrations of cytokines such as IL-1a and IL-6 that can cause further inflammation. Finally, the tissue can undergo adaptation. The inflammation and tissue damage are eventually resolved and normal function is restored. However, if the tissue is not able to adapt, persistent inflammation may occur, which can result in additional tissue damage and set the stage for chronic pain (12).

Acute inflammation can result in either (1) complete repair and return of function, (2) healing along with scar formation, or (3) development of chronic fibrosis. With mild insult to the tissue, complete repair is often possible. However, scar formation can occur with more significant tissue insult in tissues that have little capacity for regeneration. Such is the situation in muscle tissue after long periods of edema. Formation of connective tissue can further lead to new stress points within the tissue and the further exacerbation of nociceptors, which will be prolonged and result in chronic fibrosis.

Chronic inflammation can begin shortly after an acute response and can last for years as a result of a continued exposure to the stimulus, repeated acute inflammation events, or interference with normal healing. Systemic effects due to acute and chronic inflammation can expand the influence of cytokines to other parts of the body through the circulatory system and can even cause fever if cytokines reach parts of the brain. Ultimately, inflammation is intended to repair injured tissue or replace the tissue with scar tissue. However, repeated insult to the tissue, inadequate blood supply, nutritional insufficiency, infection, or metabolic disorders can mediate the quality of the healing response (6).

There appears to be a clear link between biomechanical tissue loading and cytokine response. Statistically significant correlations have been found between the level of cytokines and the degree of tissue deformation at injury (13). This indicates a direct link between the injury magnitude and nociception. Furthermore, much of the recent literature has demonstrated how work-related activities can serve as the initiating stimulus behind

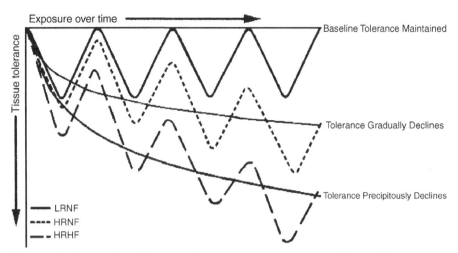

Figure 4.5   The relationship between long-term exposure to repeated tissue inflammation and tissue tolerance (LRNF = low repetition, negligible force (baseline); HRNF = high repetition, negligible force; HRHF = high repetition, high force). (From reference 6).

the sequence of events involved in the inflammatory process and the increased sensitivity to pain. Increased vascularity with accompanying edema, hypervascularization with functional decline, and decreased tissue tolerance have been noted in tissues exposed to mechanical loading (14–16). Chronic inflammation of the tendons and muscles has been reported as a result of highly repetitive tasks (17–19). These studies have shown that highly repetitive tasks, even without high force output, can result in increases in inflammation in the involved muscles as well as those muscles that are not directly involved in the task. These studies further demonstrate the systemic nature of the cytokine upregulation influence.

The inflammatory process has been shown to clearly follow a dose–response relationship (18). The literature demonstrates that tissue tolerance is influenced more by an overexertion (increased load) than by increases in repetition (cumulative trauma). However, both factors interact strongly. The inflammatory response of tissue has been monitored and shows how tissue tolerance decreases gradually as a function of exposure to high repetition tasks, and tolerance declines precipitously when the high repetition tasks are combined with high force tasks (Fig. 4.5).

4.6   PERIPHERAL NERVOUS SYSTEM SENSITIZATION

Three primary neurophysiologic mechanisms have been identified following peripheral nerve injury by which sensitization can occur (20). First, spontaneous discharge of neighboring axons can occur. Neighboring axons can be chemically and electrophysiologically sensitized and begin to fire simply because of their proximity relative to the damaged cells (21). As a result of this firing, the spinal cord dorsal horn becomes sensitized. This sensitization, in turn, leads to a loss of firing inhibition and can result in chronic pain (22).

Second, receptor sensitivity can increase and sensitize the peripheral tissue. This occurs through a change in the biochemical behavior that governs the synapses at the receptors. N-Methyl-D-aspartic acid (NMDA) and alpha amino-3-hydroly-5-methyl-4-

isoxazole-propionic acid (AMPA) receptors can produce exaggerated discharge of low-threshold receptors (20,23). Repetitive stimulation can activate automatic rhythmic discharge in the dorsal root ganglion and can modify synaptic activity.

Third, neuronal sensitivity can increase through coupling of somatic primary afferent and sympathetic neurons. This occurs interneuronally and through local blood flow resulting in an increase in epinephrine output (20,24). This abnormal sympathetic neuronal activity results in heightened sensitivity and is called complex regional pain syndrome. This syndrome can include abnormalities in blood flow.

While these mechanisms are believed to enhance sensitization at the peripheral site, it is not clear whether these responses are a result of exposure or predispose a person to these reactions. It is also important to recognize that peripheral tissue stimulation is not mandatory for CNS sensitization. Central mechanisms can be affected by a central processing disorder such as myofascial pain.

4.7 NEUROPATHIC PAIN: THE CYTOKINE CASCADE AND NERVE SENSITIZATION

Damage to peripheral tissue triggers a cytokine induced local physiologic response. For example, a tear in the annulus can lead to cytokine upregulation at that site. The cytokine upregulation can be a response to continual overactivation of the nerve and can cause the peripheral nerve to behave abnormally. Proinflammatory cytokines act on the peripheral neurons and the spinal cord dorsal horn to induce and facilitate inflammatory neuropathic pain and causes excessive sensitization. When the peripheral nerve becomes overly sensitized, it overstimulates the spinal dorsal horn lamina and can induce central sensitization (20). Cytokines, such as TNF-a, can initiate an inflammatory cascade as it inserts across the neuronal cell membrane and destabilize cellular ionic status and increases spontaneous neuronal discharge (25). Animal models have demonstrated how TNF-a applied to peripheral nerves can cause neuropathic pain (26) and how blockage of TNF-a can relieve neuropathic pain (27). Cellular response to proinflammatory cytokines can be further amplified by abnormal efferent input, causing a cycle of pain escalation. The neuropathic inflammation further aggravates the peripheral nociceptor by causing neuron-stimulated release of even more inflammatory cytokines. Hence, a vicious cycle of pain can be initiated and can be self perpetuating when cytokine-induced sensitization occurs at the peripheral nerve.

4.8 PAIN MECHANISMS OF THE CENTRAL NERVOUS SYSTEM

Repeated dorsal ganglion afferent discharge occurring at the dorsal horn can lead to abnormal behavior of the central nervous system (20). As cytokines act to sensitize peripheral neurons, the neurons can generate a cascade of abnormal nociceptive signals to the dorsal horn of the spinal cord. These signals can then trigger abnormal medullary and cerebral responses in the brain. This process represents the initiation of central sensitization. Repetitive discharge of sensory fibers can cause escalation of action potential discharge that can maintain hypersensitivity of the central nervous system (24).

Brainstem structures have also been implicated in facilitating the mechanisms of chronic pain through chemical manipulation of pain-inhibiting pathways (28). These

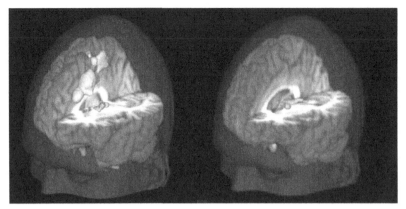

Figure 4.6 Difference in brain activity in subjects who are overly sensitive to peripheral pain (left image) compared to a normal response (right image) (R.C. Coghill et al., Neural correlates of interindividual differences in the subjective experience of pain. PNAS 2003, 100 (14), 8538–8542. (Copyright 2003, National Academy of Sciences, USA.)

pathways can be managed through the use of antidepressants, thereby demonstrating central sensitization involvement.

Central pain has also been documented via altered brain function activity in response to peripheral nociceptive activation in patients with chronic low back pain. Changes in the brain function in the cerebral regions of the brain in response to mechanical pressure pain as well as imagined pain have been documented through the use of functional MRI (fMRI) (29). Figure 4.6 shows the difference in brain activity between a patient who is overly sensitive to peripheral pain compared to a patient who is not. This central pain response clearly is manifested through changes in brain activity. When comparing normal patients to those suffering from back pain and fibromyalgia, the patients suffering from back pain and fibromyalgia report greater pain in response to similar mechanical pressure as well as show very different brain mapping in response to the same peripheral nociceptive stimulus (30).

Recent theories about brain functioning no longer consider the brain to be subdivided into discrete centers that operate independently from sensory and emotional simulation. Current thinking suggests that widespread areas of the brain are actively involved in nearly all components of the conscious sensory and emotional experience. The brain continuously modulates a stream of neuron regulatory input and therefore plays a major role in pain perception. Thus, pain is a central nervous system process. The interpretation of pain is determined only after the complex pathways project through the brain (20). Hence, once the brain becomes sensitized to pain, the experience of pain can persist long after the physical injury has healed. However, it is important to realize that the complex processes described are *initiated by a physical insult to the tissue*. Neurophysiology suggests that "the post injury central nervous system becomes sensitized by the injury or other predisposing factors" (20).

4.9 ROLE OF THE ENVIRONMENT IN CENTRAL SENSITIZATION

As has been demonstrated, pain is a complex and dynamic phenomenon that includes peripheral stimulation of a nociceptor, sensitization at the peripheral site, and neuropathic and/or central pain pathways. Nerve cells can be either transformed by a prior injury or predisposed to respond to sensations as abnormally painful.

Once the pain becomes central in nature, interaction with brain activities can shape and modulate the pain experience. Thus, it should be no surprise that anxiety and fear can lead to exaggerated pain responses and fear-avoidance behavior. Emotion can activate the central nervous system differently in response to somatosensory input compared to a less affect-sensitive brain (31,32). Thus, to the extent that psychosocial and organizational factors in the workplace can induce an emotion response, it is conceivable that the neural pathways associated with central pain sensitization can provide a plausible pathways for work-related back pain.

4.10   IMPLICATIONS FOR LOW BACK PAIN

The previous sections have reviewed the different types of pain that can be perceived by the body. The following section shows how these concepts can be applied specifically to the tissues believed to be associated with low back pain transmission.

4.11   NERVES AT RISK OF SENSITIZATION

To understand which tissues within the spine may be responsible for the initiation and transmission of a pain stimulus, it is important to briefly describe the neuroanatomy of the functioning spine. The spinal canal contains the spinal cord, and branches out at the various levels of the spine into nerve roots. The dorsal root of the spinal nerve transmits information from the sensory fibers running through the spinal nerve to the spinal cord. The ventral root mostly relays information in the other direction from the spinal cord to the spinal nerve. The dorsal and ventral nerve roots exit the spinal cord and join to form the spinal nerve as it exists the spinal column at the intervertebral foramen. The spinal nerves branch out to serve various parts of the body, where there are many opportunities for the nerves to become compromised and potentially serve as sources for pain. As the nerve root exits the intervertebral foramen, it branches off into the ventral and dorsal rami. These anatomical constraints result in very short spinal nerves that provide opportunities for stretching and compression of the nerves (33).

As the spinal cord branches out at each spinal level, one encounters an enlarged portion of the nerve called the DRG. This structure contains cell bodies of the sensory fibers in the dorsal root and has been described as "the brain of the functional spinal unit" (see Fig. 3.11) (34). The DRG serves as a communication link between the internal and external environments and the spinal cord, since it receives information from the tissues and transmits this information to the brain as well as back from the brain. However, since this structure resides within the spinal column, it can easily be compressed by a bulging disc. Even slight pressure on the DRG has been shown to increase nerve activity well after the nerve stimulation has ended (35). The DRG is important since it can manufacture several neruogenic peptides that can increase sensitivity to pain (34).

4.12   TISSUES AT RISK OF SENSITIZATION

Given that pain-generating tissues must be connected to the nervous system, it should be possible to identify the specific tissues and structures that are capable of initiating pain in the low back. Several studies have attempted to document the pain pathways in the low back by stimulating certain tissues and "mapping" the nature and location of the reported pain as a result of the stimulation. One landmark study (36) studied the reactions of 193 patients who were given progressive local anesthesia. The patients had undergone surgery for spinal disc herniation, stenosis, or both. During the surgery, these researchers stimulated various tissues to observe the sources of pain. The lumbar fascia was not sensitive to the stimulation when touched or even cut. However, pressure on the supraspinous ligament produced some pain. No pain resulted from pressure applied on the muscles. However, when the base of the muscles was touched at the intersection of the muscle and bone (myotendonous junction), particularly at the site of blood vessels or nerves, localized pain was prevalent in the back.

These findings have lead to the belief that pain arises from blood vessels and nerves as opposed to muscle tissue itself. A nerve root itself is typically insensitive to pressure. However, if the nerve root has been exposed previously to continuous pressure, stretching, and swelling, then stimulation of the nerve root will result in pain and sciatic symptoms (37).

The disc has often been considered as a source of low back pain. However, only the outer regions of the annulus are innervated by pain-sensitive nociceptors. As expected, studies (36) verified that pain occurred only when the outer regions of the annulus were stimulated. Buttock pain was produced with pressure on either the outer annulus or the nerve root. Local anesthesia was often effective in blocking this pain. This study also demonstrated that the central part of the annulus and the posterior longitudinal ligament were capable of producing central back pain, whereas forces applied to the lateral aspects of the ligament resulted in pain on the side where the stimulus was applied.

Further investigations found that the vertebral end plates were pressure sensitive and insult to the end plate resulted in deep low back pain. The facet joints have also been identified as a source of sharp and localized pain. However, the nature of the pain observed in these investigations was not consistent with the often reported deep and dull pain believed to be representative of facet pain. The specific structures found not to result in pain when the ligamentum flavum, epidural fat, nucleus pulposus, bony lamina, the posterior dura, and the spinous processes were stimulated mechanically.

Scarring has also been suggested as a source of pain. However, reports indicate that scar tissue itself is not sensitive to pain compared to the nerve root. This suggests that the pain sensitivity to a scar may be secondary to repair of the nerve that is sensitive to compression and/or tension (37). Hence, this process suggests a major role of the blood delivery system in defining pain.

4.13 DISC AND NERVE ROOTS

Pressure on the disc has been observed to mimic low back pain similar to that of lumbago (38). Some have hypothesized that the disc is most likely the origin of most low back pain; however, evaluation of pain distribution indicted that pressure within the disc does not lead to pain unless disc degeneration or annular disruption is present (39). Hence, the mechanism of pain generation within the disc and nerve roots is more complicated than just the presence of pressure itself.

4.14 FACET JOINTS

Over the last couple of decades, the facet joints have also been implicated as a likely source of low back pain. Neurologic studies have demonstrated that the facet joints contain an extensive distribution of small nerve fibers and endings, high threshold mechanoreceptors, and nerves that become sensitive when exposed to inflammatory agents or algesic chemicals (40). These nerves also innervate the surrounding muscles. The introduction of pressure on the facet joint capsules can result in the production of pain typical of low back symptoms including radiation of pain down the leg (41). However, studies that have blocked communication with the facet through facet block injections have had mixed results (41,42). Therefore, as with the disc and nerve roots, the pain-producing mechanisms within this part of the spine cannot be described entirely on the basis of anatomic compromise.

4.15 MUSCULAR-BASED PAIN

Sprains and strains of the low back represent the most common diagnosis for low back pain (nonspecific low back pain) and are the most common work-related diagnoses for low back pain (43). While it is now known exactly how muscle pain is involved in the low back pain experience, it is generally thought that muscle pain is due to (1) fatigue, (2) fibromyalgia, or (3) muscle damage.

Since there are hundreds of muscle in the body, the timing of muscle recruitment and the magnitude of the force supplied by each muscle are important factors in ensuring a smooth, energy-efficient utilization of the musculoskeletal system. However, the muscle recruitment pattern can be greatly influence by fatigue (44). Nonoptimal muscle recruitment patterns can result in a risk of muscle injury.

Fatigue can be operationally defined as loss of muscle force production. Muscle fatigue is believed to be a result of either central fatigue within the CNS or peripheral fatigue that occurs outside the CNS. Fatigue is associated with a change in the motor unit firing rates (rate of firing), recruitment of fibers, as well as chemical changes in the muscle that affect the muscle's ability to utilize oxygen.

It has also been suggested that another potential injury pathway related that muscle recruitment anomalies involves tension myositis syndrome (TMS). This concept (45,46) suggests that increased states of muscle tension in the back can be initiated by way of the autonomic nervous system. This increased muscle tension can significantly reduce blood flow to the muscles, nerves, tendons, and ligaments, thereby depriving them of the necessary nutrition needed to sustain healthy tissues. Oxygen deprivation can lead to several painful pathways. First, muscle spasm can lead to acute pain. Second, Fig. 4.7 indicates that the

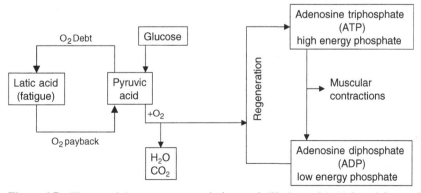

Figure 4.7   The muscle's energy system during work (Krebs cycle). (Adapted from reference 47).

disruption of oxygen content can lead to a decrease in ATP, which is needed to produce a significant muscular contraction. Thus, the chemical balance of the muscle is disrupted with an increase in lactic acid leading to muscle discomfort. Third, oxygen deprivation is also believed to be related to fibromyalgia. Fibromyalgia has been observed in those with low back pain and can result in trigger points that have been identified as sites of increased upregulation of cytokine which could lead to increased inflammation and increased stimulation of surrounding nociceptors. Finally, muscle tension can deprive the nerves, running through the muscle, of oxygen which can lead to significant pain. Nerves are far more sensitive to oxygen deprivation than are muscles for normal functioning.

4.16 LUMBAR NERVE ROOTS

Nerve roots are typically not sensitive to pressure when stimulated (48). However, compressed and inflamed nerve roots can become sensitive to mechanical manipulation (49). It is generally accepted that when a nerve root is stretched, compressed, or swollen, pain is reported by nearly all subjects. In addition, only when these compromised structures were stimulated was sciatica reported by patients (36). Hence, for a nerve root to become a source of pain, the nerve root must have experienced an insult and force must be imposed on the structure.

4.17 RELATIONSHIP BETWEEN TISSUE LOADING AND PAIN

Several studies have demonstrated how loads applied to various tissues within the spine can affect neural responses in proportion to the magnitude of the biomechanical load. This has been demonstrated for the sciatic nerve and the DRG (50), edema patterns (51), and nerve root loading (52). The magnitude of the load (injury) has also been correlated with the degree of sensitivity (13). Specifically, "the greater the nerve root compression at injury, the worse the clinical symptoms of behavioral sensitivity and pain" (13). Recent work has also been able to define mechanical thresholds for pain based on the degree of nerve root compression (11).

4.18 CONCLUSIONS

It should be clear from this discussion that pain is far from a simple perception of tissue damage. It is also evident that we are in the early phases of understanding the potential complex interactions associated with pain interpretation. While it is clear that injured tissues are capable of being the source of pain, other factors such as psychological factors, the repair process, task exposure, prior experiences, and physiologic responses to the upregulation of proinflammatory agents can all influence the perception and duration of pain.

KEY POINTS

- Pain is complex and is mediated by cognition, emotion, experience, and behavioral factors.

- Pain can originate from either the muscle and joints (nociceptive pain) or from the nervous system (central pain).

- Nonciceptors transmit information about tissue damage and are believed to be the primary mechanism involved in the initiation of work-related pain. If the pain sequence persists, pain can result from changes in the central nervous system even after the original damaged tissue is no longer the source of pain.

- Pressure, stretching, and swelling of tissue normally precede pain generation, suggesting that interference with blood flow to a tissue is often associated with pain.

- Compression of the spinal nerves can result in pain. Spinal nerve compromise can result in pain symptoms in different parts of the body (leg, buttock, back, etc.).

- Facet joints can produce deep and dull pain.

- Scar tissue can interfere with blood flow and can result in muscle pain.

- Muscle disruption can be a source of pain resulting from fatigue, fibromyalgia, and/or muscle damage.

- Cytokine upregulation can lead to inflammation of tissue, interfere with oxygen delivery, and increase nociceptor sensitivity, resulting in pain.

- Anxiety, chronic pain, depression, crises, and memories of pain can make one more receptive to pain transmission.

REFERENCES

1. MERSKEY H. Pain terms. Pain 1986; S211–S215.
2. RAMSEY D. Anatomy of Pain Ontario Inter-Urban Pain Conference; Waterloo, Ontario, Canada;1996 (updated 2001).
3. BOIVIE J. Central pain syndromes. In CAMPELL J, editor. Pain 1996 – An Updated review. Seattle: IASP Press; 1996. p. 23–29.
4. JENSEN T. Mechanisms of neuropathic Pain. In CAMPELL J, editor. Pain 1996 – An Updated review. Seattle: IASP Press; 1996. p. 77–86.
5. University of Heidelberg, 2006. Department of Molecular Physiology, Pain Research website – http://www.molekulare-physiologie.de/int_pain_intro.html.
6. BARR AE, BARBE MF. Inflammation reduces physiological tissue tolerance in the development of work-related musculoskeletal disorders. J Electromyogr Kinesiol 2004;14:77–85.
7. BARR AE, BARBE MF, CLARK BD. Systemic inflammatory mediators contribute to widespread effects in work-related musculoskeletal disorders. Exercise Sport Sci Rev 2004;32:135–142.
8. DINARELLO CA. Proinflammatory cytokines. Chest 2000;118:503–508.
9. RANG HP, BEVAN S, DRAY A. Chemical activation of nociceptive peripheral neurones. Br Med Bull 1991; 47:534–548.
10. IGARASHI A, KIKUCHI S, KONNO S, OLMARKER K. Inflammatory cytokines released from the facet joint tissue in degenerative lumbar spinal disorders. Spine 2004; 29:2091–2095.
11. WINKELSTEIN BA, DELEO JA. Mechanical thresholds for initiation and persistence of pain following nerve root injury: mechanical and chemical contributions at injury. J Biomech Eng 2004;126:258–263.
12. BARBE MF, BARR AE. Inflammation and the pathophysiology of work-related musculoskeletal disorders. Brain Behav Immun 2006;20:423–429.
13. WINKELSTEIN BA, RUTKOWSKI MD, WEINSTEIN JN, DELEO JA. Quantification of neural tissue injury in a rat radiculopathy model: comparison of local deformation, behavioral outcomes, and spinal cytokine mRNA for two surgeons J Neurosci Methods 2001;111:49–57.
14. ARCHAMBAULT JM, HART DA, HERZOG W. Response of rabbit Achilles tendon to chronic repetitive loading. Connect Tissue Res 2001;42:13–23.
15. MESSNER K, WEI Y, ANDERSSON B, GILLQUIST J, RASANEN T. Rat model of Achilles tendon disorder. A pilot study. Cells Tissues Organs 1999;165:30–39.
16. SOSLOWSKY LJ, THOMOPOULOS S, TUN S, FLANAGAN CL, KEEFER CC, MASTAW J, CARPENTER JE. Neer Award 1999. Overuse activity injures the supraspinatus tendon in an animal model: a histologic and biomechanical study. J Shoulder Elbow Surg 2000;9:79–84.
17. BARBE MF, BARR AE, GORZELANY I, AMIN M, GAUGHAN JP, SAFADI FF. Chronic repetitive reaching and grasping results in decreased motor performance and widespread

tissue responses in a rat model of MSD. J Orthop Res 2003;21:167–176.

18. BARR AE, SAFADI FF, GORZELANY I, AMIN M, POPOFF SN, BARBE MF. Repetitive, negligible force reaching in rats induces pathological overloading of upper extremity bones. J Bone Miner Res 2003;18:2023–2032.

19. CLARK BD, BARR AE, SAFADI FF, BEITMAN L, AL-SHATTI T, AMIN M, GAUGHAN JP, BARBE MF. Median nerve trauma in a rat model of work-related musculoskeletal disorder. J Neurotrauma 2003;20:681–695.

20. TAUBEN D. Central nervous system modulation of spinal pain: pain sensitization and implications for surgical selection. SpineLine; 2005. 7–12.

21. RAJA S, MEYER R, CAMPBELL J. Hyperalgesia and sensititzation of primary afferent fibers. In FIELDS H, editor. Pain Syndromes in Neurology. Boston (MA): Butterfield-Heinemann, Boston; 1990. p. 19–45.

22. WOOLF CJ, MANNION RJ. Neuropathic pain: aetiology, symptoms, mechanisms, and management. Lancet 1999;353:1959–1964.

23. KAWASAKI Y, KOHNO T, ZHUANG ZY, BRENNER GJ, WANG H, Van Der MEER C, BEFORT K, WOOLF CJ, JI RR. Ionotropic and metabotropic receptors, protein kinase A, protein kinase C, and Src contribute to C-fiberinduced ERK activation and cAMP response element-binding protein phosphorylation in dorsal horn neurons, leading to central sensitization. J Neurosc 2004;24:8310–8321.

24. WOOLF CJ, THOMPSON SW. The induction and maintenance of central sensitization is dependent on *N*-methyl-D-aspartic acid receptor activation: implications for the treatment of post-injury pain hypersensitivity states. Pain 1991;44:293–299.

25. SOMMER C, KRESS M. Recent findings on how proinflammatory cytokines cause pain: peripheral mechanisms in inflammatory and neuropathic hyperalgesia. Neurosci Lett 2004;361:184–187.

26. SOMMER C, LINDENLAUB T, TEUTEBERG P, SCHAFERS M, HARTUNG T, TOYKA KV. Anti–TNF-neutralizing antibodies reduce pain-related behavior in two different mouse models of painful mononeuropathy. Brain Res 2001;913:86–89.

27. SORKIN LS, DOOM CM. Epineurial application of TNF elicits an acute mechanical hyperalgesia in the awake rat. J Peripheral Nervous Syst 2000;5:96–100.

28. IKEDA H, HEINKE B, RUSCHEWEYH R, SANDKUHLER J. Synaptic plasticity in spinal lamina I projection neurons that mediate hyperalgesia. Science 2003;299:1237–1240.

29. DERBYSHIRE SW, WHALLEY MG, STENGER VA, OAKLEY DA. Cerebral activation during hypnotically induced and imagined pain. Neuroimage 2004;23:392–401.

30. GIESECKE T, GRACELY RH, GRANT MA, NACHEMSON A, PETZKE F, WILLIAMS DA, CLAUW DJ. Evidence of augmented central pain processing in idiopathic chronic low back pain. Arthritis Rheum 2004;50:613–623.

31. GIESECKE T, GRACELY RH, WILLIAMS DA, GEISSER ME, PETZKE FW, CLAUW DJ. The relationship between depression, clinical pain, and experimental pain in a chronic pain cohort. Arthritis Rheum 2005;52:1577–1584.

32. VLAEYEN JW, LINTON SJ. Fear-avoidance and its consequences in chronic musculoskeletal pain: a state of the art. Pain 2000;85:317–332.

33. BOGDUK N, TWOMEY L.Clinical Anatomy of the Lumbar Spine, Melbourne: Churchill Livingstone;1987.

34. WEINSTEIN J. Pain. In FRYMOYER J, editor. The Adult Spine. 2nd ed. Philadelphia: Lipppincott-Raven Publishers; 1997. p. 381–400.

35. HOWE JF, LOESER JD, CALVIN WH. Mechanosensitivity of dorsal root ganglia and chronically injured axons: a physiological basis for the radicular pain of nerve root compression. Pain 1977;3:25–41.

36. KUSLICH SD, ULSTROM CL, MICHAEL CJ. The tissue origin of low back pain and sciatica: a report of pain response to tissue stimulation during operations on the lumbar spine using local anesthesia. Orthop Clin North Am 1991;22:181–187.

37. WEINSTEIN J. Basic pain mechanism and its control. In NORDIN M, ANDERSSON G,POPE M,editors. Musculoskeletal Disordrs in the Workplace: Principles and Practice. St. Louis: Mosby-Year Book, Inc. 1997. p. 45–50.

38. HIRSCH C, INGELMARK BE, MILLER M. The anatomical basis for low back pain. Studies on the presence of sensory nerve endings in ligamentous, capsular and intervertebral disc structures in the human lumbar spine. Acta Orthop Scand 1963;33:1–17.

39. MOONEY V. Presidential address. International Society for the Study of the Lumbar Spine. Dallas, 1986. Where is the pain coming from? Spine 1987;12:754–759.

40. CAVANAUGH JM, OZAKTAY AC, YAMASHITA T, AVRAMOV A, GETCHELL TV, KING AI. Mechanisms of low back pain: a neurophysiologic and neuroanatomic study. Clin Orthop Relat Res 1997;166–180.

41. MOONEY V, ROBERTSON J. The facet syndrome. Clin Orthop Relat Res 1976;149–156.

42. LILIUS G, LAASONEN EM, MYLLYNEN P, HARILAINEN A, GRONLUND G. Lumbar facet joint syndrome. A randomised clinical trial. J Bone Joint Surg (Br) 1989;71:681–684.

43. ANDERSSON G. The epidemiology of spinal disorders. In FRYMOYER JW, editor The Adult Spine. Philadelphia: Lippincott-Raven Publishers; 1997. p. 93–141.

44. PARNIANPOUR M, NORDIN M, KAHANOVITZ N, FRANKEL V. Volvo award in biomechanics. The triaxial coupling of torque generation of trunk muscles during isometric exertions and the effect of fatiguing isoinertial movements on the motor output and movement patterns. Spine 1988;13:982–992.

45. SARNO JE. Mind Over Back Pain. New York (NY): Berkley Books; 1982.

46. SARNO JE. Healing Back Pain. New York (NY): Warner Books; 1991.

47. GRANDJEAN E. Fitting the Task to the Man 4th ed. Philadelphia: Taylor and Francis; 1988.

48. SMYTH MJ, WRIGHT V. Sciatica and the intervertebral disc: an experimental study. J Bone Joint Surg (Am) 1958;40-A:1401–1418.

49. GREENBARG PE, BROWN MD, PALLARES VS, TOMPKINS JS, MANN NH. Epidural anesthesia for lumbar spine surgery. J Spinal Disord 1988;1:139–143.

50. RYDEVIK BL, MYERS RR, POWELL HC. Pressure increase in the dorsal root ganglion following mechanical compression. Closed compartment syndrome in nerve roots. Spine 1989;14:574–576.

51. OLMARKER K, RYDEVIK B, HOLM S. Edema formation in spinal nerve roots induced by experimental, graded compression. An experimental study on the pig cauda equina with special reference to differences in effects between rapid and slow onset of compression. Spine 1989;14:569–573.

52. CORNEFJORD M, SATO K, OLMARKER K, RYDEVIK B, NORDBORG C. A model for chronic nerve root compression studies. Presentation of a porcine model for controlled, slow-onset compression with analyses of anatomic aspects, compression onset rate, and morphologic and neurophysiologic effects. Spine 1997;22:946–957.

CHAPTER 5

POTENTIAL PATHWAYS TO BACK PAIN

OUR UNDERSTANDING *of back pain perception has changed over the years. This chapter discusses why traditional views of low back pain (suggesting that tissue damage must be present) may not be realistic. A unifying model of low back pain pathways is presented. Two major pathways are proposed that include (1) a support structure disruption pathway and (2) a muscle function disruption pathway. Numerous minor pathways are also contained within these two major pathways. The bulk of this chapter describes how muscle tensions within the low back can activate the various minor pathways. This chapter lays the ground work for later chapters that describe how both work and nonwork factors influence muscle tensions and subsequent pain pathway initiation.*

The goal of this chapter is to integrate our knowledge of back anatomy (Chapter 3) with information about pain generation mechanisms (Chapter 4), so that we can understand the ways in which pain can be developed in the back. To understand the role that modern work can play in the development of back pain, we must consider the current thinking regarding potential pathways by which pain can be initiated and generated in this complex and intricate structure.

Physiologically, there is no single source of pain. Pain can be initiated by structural damage to the musculoskeletal system, alterations to the nervous system, as well as biochemical changes to the soft tissues of the back. However, these changes are also part of a system. Physical and psychological environmental factors, genetic factors, as well as previous experiences have the ability to intensify or modify the reaction of the musculoskeletal system. Thus, to understand how work influences pain, we must understand how the various system components are influenced individually and collectively in the pain experience. This chapter describes, in more detail, the sequence of events that activate the spine's various pain-sensing pathways. An understanding of these pathways provides an underpinning for an appreciation of how various aspects of work could contribute to low back pain.

5.1 VIEWS OF BACK PAIN CAUSALITY

Several models describing the way in which back pain may be initiated have been discussed and debated by those involved in low back pain research. It is highly likely that there are numerous independent factors that can, by themselves or in combination with other risk factors, trigger a low back pain event. Therefore, there is a benefit to examining these various pathways or theories of back pain development so that we could understand the role that work might play in influencing or initiating these various pathways.

The traditional model of low back pain causality, referred to as the "injury model," suggests that back pain and work disability are a result of exposure to physical factors such as lifting heavy loads, bending, twisting, vibration, as well as slips and falls. This model suggests that overloading of the spine's musculoskeletal system can occur during a single (acute trauma) event (such as a lift) and can lead to structural damage of the bones, ligaments, muscles, discs, and so on. Supporters of this theory point to the large literature base that reports an elevated low back pain incidence rate when workers are exposed to these factors compared to workers who are not exposed to these factors. For much of the public health community, these epidemiologic studies present compelling evidence of risk association. The model certainly is consistent with our knowledge of nociceptive pain transmission. This pathway is also conceptually understandable by the millions of workers who have experience with heavy lifting and have observed that when exposed to certain work conditions, they seem to have more trouble with their backs at the end of the day. Just about anyone who has performed such work has experienced or knows someone who has experienced back pain after performing physically difficult work. For example, recent reports from Iraq have shown that back pain is a common problem for soldiers who wear heavy body armor and must wear heavy backpacks over extended periods (1,2).

However, work has changed over the years, and it is less likely that modern work involves acute damage to the tissue. Yet this change in the nature of work in recent years has not resulted in a corresponding change in low back pain reports. This can be explained through the process of *cumulative trauma* (minor repeated trauma) as a source of low back pain. The cumulative trauma pathway suggests that structural damage to the spinal structures occurs gradually over time and can occur at low magnitudes of loading. Cumulative trauma reasoning argues that some of these disorders are rooted in the exposure to risk factors that contribute to progressive "wear and tear" of the spine structures and tissues.

Significant insight regarding the prevalence of cumulative trauma can be gained by examining the systematic pattern of evidence available from a large body of literature exploring the elements of work-related musculoskeletal disorders. The pattern begins by noting trends in the epidemiologic literature suggesting that cumulative trauma is a common element found in many reports of low back pain associated with the workplace (3–6). This observational literature suggests that cumulative exposure might explain at least part of the low back pain picture. However, while the available epidemiologic evidence can suggest which factors may be significant, it is unable to explain how these factors may interact with other potential risk factors. Nonetheless, these studies do suggest that excessive cumulative exposure to musculoskeletal loads can be considered a potential risk factor, since occupations in which there is cumulative exposure to repetitive biomechanical loading have been shown to increase risk.

A biological plausibility argument also supports the epidemiologic finding. At the heart of the logic of cumulative trauma plausibility is the relationship between loads imposed on a structure and the tolerance of that structure. This concept suggests that when the loads experienced by a structure exceed the tolerance magnitude of a structure, damage occurs; whereas, if the imposed load magnitude is below the structural tolerance magnitude, the loading is safe. In classical mechanical terms, "damage" would indicate structural change, which has been demonstrated to occur in the spine for human and animal models as a result of cumulative trauma (7). However, the tissue load can exceed the tissue tolerance in two ways. The load can increase or the tolerance can decrease. It is likely that under cumulative trauma conditions, the tolerance decreases via tissue reactions. We know that with repeated exposure, the tissue response can change and initiate a pain response at a much lower level of load (lowered tolerance). This can occur due to a release of proinflammatory agents, reduction of blood supply to a tissue, rupture of a muscle, cellular changes, or host of other mechanisms that might lead to pain (8). Hence, exceeding a pain-producing tolerance can trigger a sequence of events that can lead to pain, even though the imposed load is not excessive. Thus, it is possible that moderate loads can exceed the tissue pain tolerance when the ability of the tissue to withstand loads is exceeded because of these physiologic changes.

This construct of back pain has been challenged by some over the last few years who argue that low back pain is primarily hereditary and that back pain is a function of natural aging. It has been suggested that low back disorders are idiopathic and constitute a normal life experience. Some have argued that if back pain is caused by exposure to physical factors, one should find structural disruption evidence of damage in workers via imaging such as X-ray, CT scan, or MRI spine imaging. These imaging techniques often show no obvious damage to the spinal structures when people experience low back pain.

Some have speculated that the high rates of low back pain reporting are a result of the way in which our workers' compensation system is designed. The suggestion has been made that back pain is a psychosocial and societal entitlement problem that claims that work-related back pain is socially acceptable because compensation is available. Those who take this view suggest a *biopsychosocial* model of pain and disability that views pain as a complex and dynamic interaction among physiologic, psychologic, and social factors, which perpetuates and can even worsen the clinical presentation (9). While the biopsychosocial rationale has been proven effective as a pain management and treatment tool for low back pain, some assume that this rationale should be extended to low back pain causality. However, the biopsychosocial model does not necessarily translate into a causal model that negates work as an initiating factor for low back pain. This model does not explain the causal pathway to pain. Instead it can be viewed as a "black box" approach to explaining low back pain.

One of the motivating factors for dismissing the injury model of causality in low back pain involves the common lack of tissue damage as evidenced by imaging of the spine. However, people often report that their back pain is exacerbated when people are exposed to physically stressful conditions that impose larger than normal forces on the back structures such as extended standing, bending, twisting, sitting, and so on. Yet, diagnostic images of the back that presumably can identify structural problems in the spine are typically performed with the patient in a supine (reclined) posture. In the supine posture, the vertebrae are aligned well and minimal force is imposed on each of the individual spinal segments. There is a large amount of soft tissue in the back that is capable of experiencing pain. However, in this recumbent, "lying down" position, the potential to apply loads to this tissue and stimulate the pain-sensitive tissues causing pain is minimized since the spine is not opposing gravity in the same way it does in a typical standing or working posture. Figure 5.1 demonstrates this difference. Thus, it is no wonder that few spine structural anomalies are noted when imaging is performed on an injured worker. Unless natural loading is permitted in the positions that exacerbate pain, it would be premature to conclude that structural problems are not present in the back. In addition, natural loading images are one of the key developments in modern biomechanical modeling of the spine.

Detractors of the role of biomechanical loading as a source of low back pain have also claimed that biomechanical assessments have been previously examined and little association with pain has been discovered. However, few have attempted to explore this relationship using the modern day, sophisticated biologically driven biomechanical models. This appears to be a key to understanding low back pain causality as we shall soon discover.

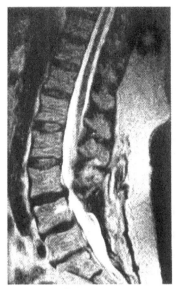 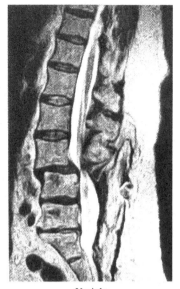

Recumbent   Upright

Figure 5.1   Differences in imaging of the spine in a recumbent (lying down) position compared to an upright standing position. This demonstrates the importance of assessing loads on spinal structures in physiologically meaningful postures. (Courtesy of Fonar, Inc.)

5.2   A UNIFYING MODEL OF LOW BACK PAIN PATHWAYS

Figure 5.2 represents an overview of potential pain pathways that can be involved in low back pain development. As noted in the figure, these pathways begin with the influence of a broadly defined "environment" to which the human responds. Environment may include physical work, social conditions, organizational practices, and leisure activities. The portions of the figure beyond the "environment" are influenced by individual differences that include individual tolerances, unique muscle recruitment patterns, biochemical responses, psychological factors, and so on. There is evidence in the literature that each of these factors has the potential to influence the process described in Fig. 5.2. The response to the environment is initiated in the brain of the worker where control over the musculoskeletal system is managed through changes in the back's tissue tension that is controlled via muscle activities. It is important to realize that the brain responds to both physical and cognitive (psychosocial and organizational) factors in much the same way and involve changes in muscle activities. Key components of these muscle activities involve both the magnitude of the muscle response (force) and the pattern of muscle recruitment.

As indicated in the figure, feedback from the tissues is also capable of influencing future muscle activities via a sophisticated feedback system. These muscle responses to the environment can lead to the two major pathways that can result in pain. One pathway involves disruption of the spine's supporting structures; the other involves a disruption of the back's muscle functioning and "balance" between muscle intensities.

Both of these major pathways terminate in a sequence of events that regulate pain. This sequence is described in the lower portion of Fig. 5.2. As discussed in Chapter 4, a biochemical upregulation of several cytokines is often observed as a result of tissue stress. This upregulation leads to a more vigorous inflammatory response of the tissue. The inflammation in turn can stimulate nociceptors and result in the perception of pain. If this

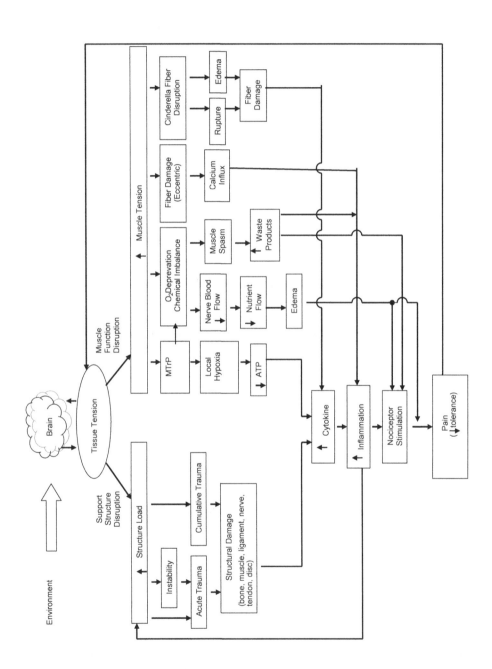

Figure 5.2 Pathways to low back pain generation (*pain feedback loop—given a prior pain experience adjusted responses to the environment can occur).

pain persists, it is possible for changes to occur at the CNS level and the pain can become neuropathic.

5.3   THE SUPPORT STRUCTURE DISRUPTION PATHWAYS

The support structure disruption path indicates that the loads imposed on the spine's supporting structures are large enough to cause breakdown of the tissue. Tissues influenced by the structure loading can include bones, disks, ligaments, tendons, and nerves. The "support structure disruption" sequence of events shown on the left side of Fig. 5.2 describes this pathway. This pathway indicates that tissue damage can be either acute or cumulative. System instability can also lead to an acute trauma event.

Acute trauma occurs when the load imposed on a tissue exceeds the tolerance of the tissue. Typically, acute trauma refers to a tissue disorder that occurs as a result of a single application of force, however, the distinction between acute trauma and cumulative trauma becomes blurred when one considers the fact that even under cumulative trauma conditions, the end point for tissue damage occurs acutely.

This type of trauma results in disruption of the tissue integrity. Under these conditions, bones are cracked or broken, disc end plates suffer microfractures, muscles suffer from fiber tears, and blood flow can be disrupted. In addition, many biochemical studies over the last decade have demonstrated how these types of tissue insults can result in an upregulation of cytokines. This upregulation results in tissue inflammation at much lower levels of load than would occur under normal conditions. The inflammation, in turn, makes nociceptive tissues more sensitive to pain. Hence, the pain end point.

The acute trauma pain pathway figure also indicates that there is a relationship between spine *instability* and acute trauma. Stability refers to the ability of the musculo-skeletal control system to respond to a perturbation and reestablish a state of equilibrium of the spine after a perturbation. Static stability refers to the ability of the spine to refer to its original position after a perturbation. Dynamic stability refers to the ability of the system to reestablish a course of intended movement after a perturbation. Stability is important because it is often the impetus for tissue damage when the system is out of alignment or when the musculoskeletal system overcompensates for a perturbation. When the musculature cannot offer adequate support to a joint (due to improper muscle recruitment, fatigue, structure laxity, or weakness), the structure may move abnormally and create forces on a tissue that are excessive. Hence, this pathway is very similar to the acute trauma pathway but is initiated by a miscalculation of the muscle recruitment pattern.

Cumulative trauma can also be explained via the support structure disruption pathway. As will be explained in more detail in the next chapter, cumulative trauma is distinct from acute trauma in that while the loads imposed on the tissue may be low, the repeated application of load gradually wears down the tissue to the point where the load exceeds the tolerance of the tissue and damage occurs. One can think of cumulative trauma as a factor that has the effect on the body of accelerated aging in that the tissues wear down much more quickly than would be expected (Fig. 5.3). As shown in Fig. 5.2, once the tissue structure is damaged, the remainder of the pathway is similar to that of acute trauma.

One important factor that must be considered in these pathways that might help explain the observed variation is the ability of the body to recover. Much of the biomechanical research on tissue tolerance has been performed on cadaveric specimens. However, one significant difference between cadavers and living tissues is the ability of the living tissue to respond and adapt to loads. Wolff's law states that exposure to loads makes a tissue or structure stronger. However, adaptation has limits. Stress–strain relationships suggest that

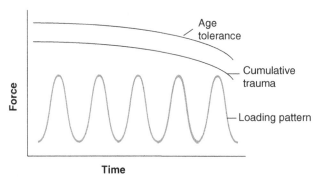

Figure 5.3   Tissue tolerance behavior as a function of cumulative trauma and age.

adaptation increases tissue strength up to and beyond the point at which failure occurs. Body builders are well aware of these concepts. They build muscles by stressing the tissue and then allowing the muscle to rest for at least 24 h. Adaptation ensues and muscle bulk and bone mass increase. However, with some types of repetitive occupational tasks, significant rest may occur only to a limited degree between work shifts and on weekends only if overtime or recreational activities do not interfere with the rest. As is the case with work that consistently exceeds the adaptation limit, the tissue tolerance could drop quickly, making it more susceptible to injury. Therefore, cumulative trauma concepts are simply an extension of accepted concepts of how biological tissue functions.

5.3.1 Support Structure Tolerance

Both the acute and cumulative trauma pathways suggest that the ability of the tissues to withstand (or tolerate) load is exceeded under certain conditions. When tissues are loaded beyond their normal physical strength or beyond their biochemical tolerance, the pain sequence shown at the bottom of Fig. 5.2 can be initiated. This section briefly discusses what is known about the structure tolerances of the spine.

The precise tolerance characteristics of human tissues such as muscles, ligaments, tendons, and bones loaded under various working conditions are difficult to estimate. Tolerances of these structures vary greatly under similar loading conditions. In general, tolerance depends on many other factors such as strain rate (rate of loading), age of the structure, frequency of loading, physiologic influences, heredity, conditioning, as well as other unknown factors. Furthermore, it is not possible to measure these tolerances under in-vivo (live) conditions. Therefore, most of the estimates of tissue tolerance have been derived from various animal and/or theoretical sources. However, these data represent the best estimates of tolerances we have to date for physical tolerance of structures.

The magnitude of spine loading must be compared to the tolerance limits of the spine structures to appreciate causality and risk. Due to ethical considerations, direct tolerance data have been derived from cadaveric tissue. The obvious downfall of this approach is that in-vitro tissue is tested that does not have the ability to adapt or recover (and potentially increase tolerance) as does the human in the workplace. In addition, the material properties of cadaveric tissue vary greatly depending on the specimen preparation. At least one study suggests that tissue failure might occur at levels even below those observed in cadaveric specimens (10). Keeping such potential limitations in mind, it is possible to establish estimates of tissue tolerance that serve as benchmarks for risk. Our previous discussion regarding pain pathways has established that there are many structures within the back that have the potential for initiating chronic low back pain.

Muscle and tendon strain—The muscle is the structure, within the musculoskeletal system, that has the lowest tolerance. The ultimate strength of a muscle has been estimated to be 32 MPa (11). In general, it is believed that the muscle will rupture prior to the (healthy) tendon (12) since tendon stress has been estimated at between 60 and 100 MPa (11,12). There is a safety margin between the muscle failure point and the failure point of the tendon of about twofold (12) to threefold (11).

Ligament and bone tolerance—Ligament and bone tolerances have also been esti-mated. Ultimate ligament stress has been estimated to be approximately 20 MPa. The ultimate stress of bone depends on the direction of loading. Bone tolerance can range from 51 MPa in transverse tension to over 190 MPa in longitudinal compression.

A strong temporal component to ligament recovery has also been identified. One study found that ligaments require long periods of time to regain structural integrity during which compensatory muscle activities are observed (13–20). Recovery time has been observed to be several times the loading duration and can easily exceed the typical work–rest cycles observed in industry.

Contact force tolerance—Low back pain may also be a result of direct stimulation to the facet joints, pressure on the annulus of the disc, or pressure on the longitudinal ligaments. Evaluation of spine loads can assist in the assessment of how work might be related to experiences of back pain. At these sites, inflammatory responses and algesic response typically are involved in the development of pressure and pain. It is much more difficult to specify load tolerance thresholds since the body's individual response to the imposed load collectively define the pressure imposed on the spinal structure. Thus, the tolerance limits for these structures is not well understood at this time.

Disc/end plate and vertebrae tolerance—End plate tolerance has been of particular interest over the last several decades to those involved in low back pain investigations. Even though we can identify specific areas of the spine that experience pain, to properly appreciate the cumulative trauma process, we must view the spinal structures as a system whose components interact with each other. Figure 5.4 shows the sequence of events that are believed to occur during degeneration of the spine. As indicated in the figure, excessive loading, generated from both within and outside the body (internal and external forces), cause microfracturing of the vertebral end plates. These end plates serve as a transport system for nutrient delivery to the disc fibers. If this loading becomes excessive and exceeds the end plate tolerance, a microfracture occurs. This microfracture is typically painless since few pain receptors reside within the disc. This sequence represents one of the major pathways believed to occur for low back disorder. The end plate is a very thin (about 1 mm thick) structure that facilitates nutrient flow from the vertebrae to the disc fibers (annulus fibrosis). The disc has no direct blood supply so it relies heavily on nutrient flow and diffusion from surrounding vascularized tissue for disc viability. Repeated microfracture of this vertebral end plate is thought to lead to the development of scar tissue, which can impair the nutrient flow to the disc fibers. This, in turn, leads to atrophy of the fiber and fiber degeneration. Since the disc contains few nociceptors, the development of microfractures is typically unnoticed by the individual. Since scar tissue is thicker and denser than normal tissue, this scar tissue interferes with nutrient delivery to the disc fibers. Nutrient supply has been found to be critical to the viability of the intervertebral disc (21). This loss of nutrient results in atrophy to the disc fibers and weakens the disc structure. This process represents the beginning of cumulative trauma to the spine and can result in disc protrusions, disc herniation, and instability of the spinal system.

One study (22) demonstrated how disc compression can initiate a number of harmful disc responses that respond according to a dose–response relationship, thus providing further

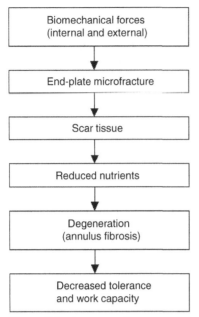

Figure 5.4 Sequence of events associated with repeated trauma leading to disc degeneration.

evidence of a cumulative trauma to the spine. In a normal disc, structural integrity is maintained by the pressure within the disc, and this pressure is a function of the disc's ability to attract and retain water within the disc space. Proteoglycans are biochemicals that help the disc resist compressive loads. These proteoglycans help pull water into the disc and thus maintain disc pressure so that compressive loads can be supported. This pressure also tenses the annulus and ligamentous structures surrounding the disc. These tensions work in conjunction with the facet joints to develop normal spine motion. Thus, this system must be in balance for the spine to move properly and any disruption of the system will have a host of detrimental effects resulting in an imbalance of the system and an inability of the system to support loads or move naturally.

Finally, the role of proinflammatory cytokines must be considered in disc degeneration. Not only can cytokine upregulation lead to tissue degeneration (as described previously), but disc degeneration can also signal an increased upregulation of proinflammatory cytokines. Thus, this can lead to a viscous cycle of degeneration resulting in pain.

Given this process, if one can determine the load level at which the end plate experiences a microfracture, then one can use this information to minimize the effects of cumulative trauma and disc degeneration.

Several studies of in vitro disc end plate tolerance have been reported in the literature. Figure 5.5 shows the range of compressive strength lumbar segment tolerances that have been used to establish tolerance limits for current lifting guides. As can be seen, the data on which these limits are based are varied and often based on relatively small sample sizes.

Figure 5.6 indicates the levels of end plate compressive loading tolerance that have traditionally been used to establish safe lifting situations at the worksite (24). This figure shows the compressive force mean (column value) as well as the compression force distribution (thin line and normal distribution curve) that would result in vertebral end plate microfracture. The figure indicates that, for those under 40 years of age, end plate microfracture damage begins at about 3432 N of compressive load on the spine. If the compressive load is increased to 6375 N, approximately 50% of those exposed will

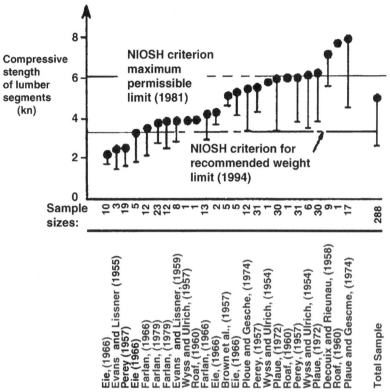

Figure 5.5   Compilation of cadaver compressive tolerance data. (From reference 23).

experience vertebral end plate microfracture. Finally, when the compressive load on the spine reaches a value of 9317 N, almost all of those exposed to the loading will experience a vertebral end plate microfracture. It is also obvious from this figure that the tolerance distribution shifts to lower levels with increasing age (25). In addition, it should be recognized that this tolerance is based on compression of the vertebral end plate alone.

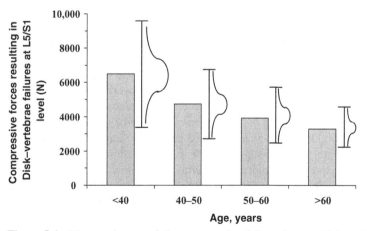

Figure 5.6   Mean and range of disc compression failures by age. (Adapted from reference 26).

TABLE 5.1 Lumbar Spine Compressive Strength (From Reference 27)

		Strength in kN	
Population	N	Mean	SD
Females	132	3.97	1.50
Males	174	5.81	2.58
Total	507	4.96	2.20

Shear and torsional forces in combination with compressive loading could combine to further lower the tolerance at the end plate.

This vertebral end plate tolerance distribution has been widely used to set limits for spine loading and define risk. It should also be noted that others have identified different limits of vertebral end plate tolerance. A review of the available spine tolerance data (27) suggests other compression value limits. Their spine tolerance summary is shown in Table 5.1. They have also been able to describe vertebral compressive strength based on an analysis of 262 values collected from 120 samples. According to these data, the compressive strength of the lumbar spine can be described according to a regression equation:

$$\text{compressive strength(kN)} = (7.26 + 1.88\ G) - (0.494 + 0.468\ G)A$$

$$+ (0.042 + 0.106\ G)C - 0.145L - 0.749S$$

where

A is the age in decade;

G is the gender coded of 0 for female or 1 for male;

C is the cross-sectional area of the vertebrae in cm^2;

L is the the lumbar level unit where 0 is the L5/S1 disc, 1 represents the L5 vertebra, and so on through 10 which represents the T10/L1 disc; and

S is the structure of interest where 0 is a disc and 1 is a vertebra.

This equation suggests that the decrease in strength within a lumbar level is about 0.15 kN of that of the adjacent vertebra and that the strength of the vertebra is about 0.8 kN lower than the strength of the disc (27). This equation can account for 62% of the variability among the samples.

It has also been suggested that spine tolerance limits vary as a function of frequency of loading or loading cycle (28). The risk of disc herniation increases significantly when the disc is subjected to repeated loading (29). Figure 5.7 indicates how spine tolerance varies as a function of spine load level and frequency of loading. This suggests that the tolerance is modulated by additional factors that are significant for workplace assessment purposes. Studies (28) have documented how the spine tolerance is reduced as the frequency of loading increases. Compressive strength of the vertebrae is reduced by 30% with 10 loading cycles and by 50% with 5000 loading cycles. Based these data, a fatigue limit of 30% of ultimate compressive strength has been suggested for living vertebrae (30). This suggests that if workers were not exposed to compressive loading of more than this limit, no fatigue failures would be expected. This work has attempted to address the cumulative trauma or degenerative aspects of work.

The relative position or posture of the spine when the load is applied appears also to be of great significance in defining spine tolerance as well as the ability of the spine to receive

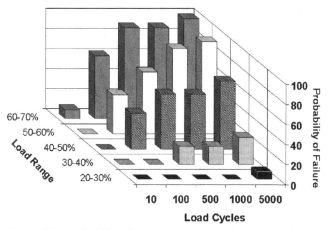

Figure 5.7   Probability of a motion segment to be fractured in dependence on the load range and the number of load cycles. (Adapted from reference 28).

nutrients. A fully flexed spine is much weaker than a spine that is in an upright standing posture (31). Studies (32) have shown that a flexed spine may be as much as 40% weaker than during an upright posture. This point has been emphasized in a recent study that examined the failure strength of the lumbar spine during repeated loading in various lifting postures (33). This study has shown a dramatic difference in spine tolerance as a function of the flexion angle of the spine (Fig. 5.8). Collectively, these studies suggest that for spine tolerance to accurately reflect risk, particular attention must be paid to the angle of the spinal segments while the load is imposed on the vertebral body. As suggested in Fig. 5.8, a load applied to the lumbar spine while the spine is in an upright posture can be tolerated well whereas a load applied while the spine is flexed can be devastating.

There is evidence that disc loading influences the health balance of the disc. A series of studies has documented how mechanical loading of the disc influences mechanical damage to the disc fibers, the electrical charge balance within the disc influencing water content, and the role of disc cell gene expression (34–38). These studies strongly suggest that physical loading of the spine leads to damage in several ways.

Disc degeneration can lead to pain through chemical secretions of the disc leading to an upregulation of cytokines and the subsequent sensitization of nociceptors.

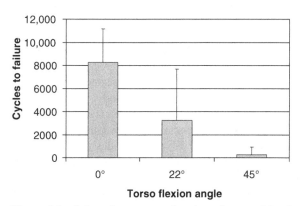

Figure 5.8   Spine tolerance as a function of repeated loading and spine flexion angle. (From reference 33).

TABLE 5.2   Summary of Static Strength for Intact Spinal Segments (Adapted From Reference 30)

Loading mode	Injury mode	Average strength	Notes
Compression	Vertebral end plate fracture	5.2 ($\pm$1.8) kN[a,b]	Dependent on vertebral cross-sectional area and bone density
Shear	Neural arch, facet joint fracture	1.0 kN[c]	Uncertain
Flexion	Posterior ligaments	73 ($\pm$18) Nm	measured with 0.5–1.0 kN compressive preload
Extension	Neural arch	26 ($\pm$9) Nm[d]	Anterior annulus may be damaged
Torsion	Neural arch/facets	25–88 Nm[e]	
Compression plus flexion	Posterior annulus, vertebral body	2.4 ($\pm$1.3) kN[f]	Disc can prolapse under hyperflexion

[a]Brinckmann et al. (1989a,b).
[b]Hutton and Adams (1982).
[c]Miller et al. (1986) and Adams et al. (1994).
[d]Adams et al. (1988).
[e]Farfan et al. (1970) and Adams and Hutton (1981).
[f]Gunning et al. (2001).

Disc hydration has also been identified as an important tolerance factor related to the time of day at which the disc is loaded. The water content of the disc can influence the load sharing among the various structures of the spine. The spinal system is stiffer and more at risk early in the morning compared to later during the workday and some have recommended that lifting not be performed early in the morning (39–41). Thus, tolerance would be expected to vary throughout the workday.

We have long recognized that three-dimensional loading of the spine is important for assessing risk, yet tolerances have only recently been estimated for shear loading of the spine. These are expected to occur between 750 and 1000 N (42). A summary of the static tolerances of the spinal structures is shown in Table 5.2. These tolerances are also expected to be reduced with repetitive loading. It is important to note that these non compression tolerance limits are typically only a fraction of the tolerance due to compressive loading.

Tolerances to combinations of loading have been explored theoretically via finite-element models (43), but little empirical work is available to support these estimates of tolerance. These studies have helped us appreciate that tolerances are reduced when loads occur in combination.

The vertebral spine can fail in several ways. Since vertebral end plate damage is believed to represent a plausible pathway for the occupation-related cumulative trauma to the spine, much of the focus of spine tolerance has centered on the magnitude of forces necessary to result in end plate damage. A recent study has examined the pattern of end plate fractures resulting from controlled loading of vertebrae (44). These are summarized in Fig. 5.9. The study indicated that stellate end plate fractures were associated with increased A–P shear forces and less degenerated discs. Fractures running laterally across the end plate were associated with motion segments with larger interbody volume, and end plate depression was more common in smaller specimens and those experiencing less A–P shear force. Zygapophysial joint damage was more common when the spine was loaded in a neutral posture. These results suggest that prediction of failure modes (e.g., specific end plate fracture patterns) may be possible given knowledge of the spinal loads along with certain characteristics of the lumbar spine.

The longitudinal ligament most frequently is subject to excessive tension resulting in avulsion or bony failure as the ligament can tear away bone from its attachment (42). Faster motions appear to increase the risk of these avulsions. However, the speed of motion

End plate fractures

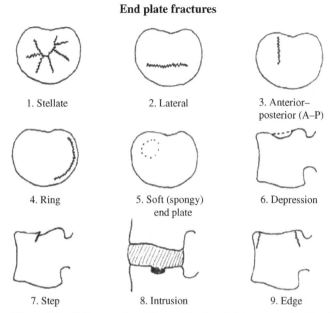

Figure 5.9   Failure modes of the vertebral end plate as a result of loading expected from occupational lifting tasks. (From reference 33).

necessary for such tears is much greater than those typically observed in the workplace unless a sudden slip or fall is responsible for the motion.

The facet joint's neural arch can withstand shear loads of about 2000 N (45) and can also fail in response to torsion loading (31). The loading of these structures depends greatly on the posture of the spine throughout the range of motion. A review of tolerances (46) suggests that significant load sharing occurs between the apophyseal joints and the disc. The proportion of the shared load can change dramatically as the spine changes positions.

5.4   DISC TOLERANCE SUMMARY

This review of the load tolerance literature and its relation to the sensation of pain indicates that pain can be associated with physical loading at multiple sites along the spine. It is also apparent that loading and tolerance are both three dimensional in nature and must be viewed as a system. It is obvious that tolerances to shear and torsion are much lower than those to compression, yet historically our assessment techniques have only concerned themselves with spine compression measures. To make matters more complicated, it appears that the tolerances to injury are modulated by not only load level but also repetition, time of day, and the posture of the spine when the load is applied. It is obvious from this discussion that assessing low back pain causality and controlling risk is far more complex than simply evaluating one dimension of spine loading at a single point in time. To advance our understanding of causality and control of low back disorders, we must begin to develop workplace assessment tools that are capable of realistically evaluating the three-dimensional loading occurring on the spine dynamically throughout the workday in response to a task. Thus, *we must abandon our overly simplistic analysis tools and assess low back disorder risk at the systems level.*

To date, only a limited number of studies have been able to evaluate risk as a function of the complex loading that occurs at the workplace. Quantitative workplace measures (3,47,48) have evaluated the kinematic and kinetic factors associated with jobs that put the worker at a high risk of LBP. These studies have evaluated the three-dimensional factors that are associated with risk. The results of these studies agree well with the issues that most of the load–tolerance models address as well as with the modulating factors mentioned above.

5.5   PAIN TOLERANCE

Over the past decade, we have learned that there are numerous pathways to pain perception associated with musculoskeletal disorders (49–51). Pain tolerance mechanics have been discussed at length in Chapter 4. It is important to understand these pathways since these pathways may be able to be used as tissue tolerance limits as opposed to tissue damage limits. Hence, one might be able to consider the quantitative limits above which a pain pathway is initiated as a tolerance limit for ergonomic purposes. While none of these pathways has been defined quantitatively, they signify an appealing approach since they represent biologically plausible mechanisms that complement the view of injury association derived from the epidemiologic literature.

Several categories of pain pathways are believed to exist that might be used as tolerance limits in the design of the workplace. These categories include structural disruption, tissue stimulation and proinflammatory response, and physiologic tissue tolerance limits.

Each of these pathways is expected to respond differently to mechanical loading of the tissue and thus serve as tolerance limits. Although many of these limits have yet to be quantitatively defined, current biomechanical research is attempting to define these tolerances and it is expected that one will be able to one day use these limits to identify the characteristics of a dose–response relationship.

5.6   THE MUSCLE FUNCTION DISRUPTION PATHWAY

Figure 5.2 indicates that there are several mechanisms by which muscle function disruption can initiate low back pain. From a diagnostic standpoint, by far the largest category of low back pain involves nonspecific or muscle-based low back pain. Many people with low back pain have no identifiable structural impairment, yet they appear to have a functional impairment (52). This is often an indication that the pain is rooted in the muscle as opposed to a supporting structure. Within the muscle-based low back pain category are several interrelated potential low back pain pathways.

Myofascial trigger points (MTrPs) represent a generally underappreciated muscle-related means by which work factors might result in low back pain. This pathway can affect the muscle system behaviors that might lead to local muscle-based pain as well as referred pain. MTrPs have been investigated as a source of musculoskeletal pain for the past century but have not enjoyed the place in mainstream medicine that has occurred with other disorders. The logic behind MTrP pathways related pain has been eloquently described in the literature (53) and will be reiterated here.

The diagnostic history of MTrPs suggests that pain is regional (and often located in the low back) and has an onset consistent with (1) sudden muscle overload, (2) sustained

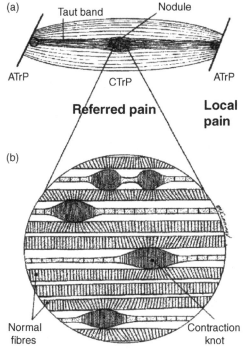

Figure 5.10   (**a**) Relationship between a nodular central trigger point and attachment trigger point. Dark band represents the palpable taut band running through the central trigger point and (**b**) microscopic view of the central trigger paoint with several contraction knots of individual muscle fibers with normal uninvolved muscle fibers among them. (From reference 53).

muscular contraction while the muscle is in shortened positions, and (3) repetitive activity where the symptoms increase with increasing stressfulness of the activity. These factors are consistent with much of the epidemiologically based risk factors associated with work related low back pain (Chapter 2).

A symptom producing a central myofascial trigger point can be described as a hyperirritable nodule of spot tenderness in a taut band of skeletal muscle. Figure 5.10a shows that the trigger point typically consists of a nodule (called the central trigger point or CTrP) that is in line with a taut band within the muscle. At the myotendonous junction interface with the taut band are the attachment trigger points (ATrPs). It is interesting to note that this interface is often the site of pain for many muscular dysfunctions. Clinicians report that pain onset is typically associated with either an acute or chronic muscle overload (53). Chronic overload in this case is defined as either a sustained contraction of the muscle or frequent repetitive movement. It has also been noted that latent MTrPs can be associated with the muscle activated in a shortened state. Figure 5.10b shows a magnified view of the CTrP and indicate that the nodule consists of contraction knots in several of the individual muscle fibers.

Myofascial pain resulting in trigger points has also been documented in the literature and may represent a potential LBP pathway (53). In myofascial pain, an energy crisis is believed to occur in the muscle that results in a sustained contractive activity or "trigger point." The sustained contractive activity increases the metabolic demands and challenges the rich network of capillaries that supply the nutritional and oxygen needs of the tissue region. Circulation in a muscle fails during a sustained contraction that is more than 30–50%

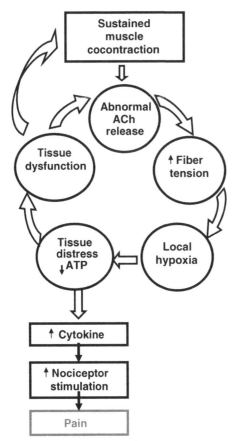

Figure 5.11 Sequence of events associated with myofascial pain. (From reference 53).

of maximum effort. The combination of increased metabolic demand and impaired metabolic supply is thought to produce a severe energy crisis leading to pain (54).

The sequence of events associated with MTrPs is described through the cycle described in Fig. 5.11. This figure represents the "integrated hypothesis" that considers the sequence of events in the development of trigger points (53,54). The sustained or repetitive use of the muscle is believed to act on a central myofascial trigger point. This trigger point is initiated by the release of excessive acetylcholine (ACh). Acetylcholine is a neurotransmitter that is released at the ends of nerve fibers in the somatic and parasympathetic nervous systems and is an essential component in the transmission of nerve impulses. This increased release of acetylcholine represents the first step in the process described in Fig. 5.11. Increased motor end plate noise is believed to be associated with this release (55).

The increased release of acetylcholine initiates the second step in the process that involves increased fiber tension. This can lead to metabolic stress and fiber tension (56).

Next, local hypoxia (a lack of oxygen in the tissue) occurs. Direct measures of hypoxia in the lumbar paraspinal muscles have been noted (53) and serve as evidence of this event. The center of the MTrP nodule has been identified as the region of hypoxia at the center of the nodule. This effect appears to be exacerbated when the muscles are activated at a shortened state.

Third, tissue distress occurs. Tissue ischemia and hypoxia lead to a reduction in the production of adosine triphosphate, a chemical that is necessary for the proper contraction of power-producing muscles (discussed in Chapter 4). The type of hypoxia seen here has been shown to enhance sensitization of nociceptors during contractile activity (57). When this contractile activity is combined with hypoxia of the muscle tissue, distress reactions are intensified.

Fourth, there are interactions with the upregulation of cytokines in the muscle that would increase inflammation and increase nociceptors stimulation (58). Significant differences in the presence of cytokines in subjects suffering from MTrPs compared to asymptomatic subjects have been observed as a result of this process.

Finally, these processes can lead to autonomic nervous system influences on the release of acetylcholine. This triggers a viscous cycle where the process described in Fig. 5.11 is reinforced.

In addition, some have suggested that reprofusion of fluid into the trigger point may occur during rest, resulting in additional stimulation of nociceptors.

Collectively, these steps outline a potential pathway for musculoskeletal pain due to muscle activity in the back that makes sense from a "pattern of evidence" standpoint.

Sustained muscle tension refers to a muscle state where the muscle is in a constant state of low-level tension that is sufficient to disrupt the nutritional cycle of the muscle. Sustained muscle tension typically occurs when there is a high degree of constant coactivation in the trunk musculature. Coactivation occurs when numerous (agonist and antagonist) muscles surrounding the trunk are activated during a task execution even though only the driving (agonist) muscles are needed to perform the task. This coactivation increases the tension in the muscles since the muscles surrounding the trunk oppose or "fight" each other. This high degree of coactivation has been widely observed in those complaining of chronic back pain and results in a disruption of normal motions of the spine (Chapter 14). Cocontraction is related to stability (59–61) and there are trade-offs between the beneficial effects of stability in preventing acute injury events and the detrimental effects of sustained muscle contractions. An appreciation for cocontraction of the trunk musculature represents one of many reasons why an understanding of the recruitment patterns within the trunk is crucial to understanding back pain development.

In any case, this constant low level of contraction can disrupt the natural functioning of the muscle through several potential mechanisms.

Muscle (fiber) damage—When muscles lengthen during the exertion of force, the exertion is called an *eccentric* contraction. These contractions, while requiring less metabolic energy expenditure on the part of the muscles (as when walking down hill), impose relatively large forces on the muscle fibers. A number of studies have demonstrated that when force is applied during these lengthening contractions muscle fiber is likely to be damaged, especially when the muscles are in a lengthened (stretched) state, and the likelihood of damage increases with the duration of the exertion (62–69). In particular, swollen fibers are observed immediately after the activity with the inflammatory process beginning within a few hours after the exertion (70). Damage appears to be a direct result of the material fatigue properties of the muscle (sarcolemma) (71). The sarcomere portion of the tissue can undergo extreme lengthening and the damage caused by this lengthening permits the influx of calcium (66). This process can upset the balance of calcium in the muscle (62,63,72) and result in muscle degradation. Recovery from eccentric contraction-induced injuries has been shown to involve a prolonged recovery process (73).

Tendon overload—Recent studies have also pointed to the tendon as a potential source of pain (74). Nitric oxide has been has been recognized as a regulator of biological processes including tendon degeneration and healing. Current investigations have shown that nitric oxide is upregulated during the chronic overuse of a tendon (74). This process may also initiate inflammatory reactions and subsequent pain.

Lack of rest—Under unstressed conditions, muscle units within the muscle fiber turn on and off under an orderly recruitment strategy so that the muscle fibers can experience adequate rest between firings and maintain their integrity. Typically, muscle recruitment dictates that small motor units are recruited first followed by larger motor units that are necessary for more substantial contractions. However, under prolonged low intensity muscle work "Cinderella" fibers have been identified (75). These fibers are low threshold small fibers that are recruited first during an exertion. Under low force exertions, the larger motor units do not engage, therefore, the Cinderella fibers must be constantly activated and do not turn off or rest. These Cinderella fibers are at greatest risk of injury during low intensity work and may experience fiber damage. Fiber damage (via rupture or edema) is repaired slowly and may even be irreversible. The motor units may also be damaged under these circumstances in that the fibers may lose their ability to contract in response to a motor neuron signal (alpha motor neuron). Either mechanism may result in an increase in cytokine upregulation and greater nociceptor sensitivity. This mechanism suggests that frequent short breaks during work are desirable to allow these fibers to turn off and rest.

Blood flow—Constant tension within the muscle can diminish the flow of blood circulating through the capillaries to the muscles and nerves within the muscle. When muscle tension produces intramuscular pressure that exceeds the capillary closing pressure of about 30 mmHg, muscle ischemia can result (76). The sustained muscular contraction and the sustained reduction in blood flow to the muscle and nerves can result in a reduction of oxygen delivery to the muscles and nerves. Damage according to this mechanism most likely occurs to small muscles (77) and slow twitch fibers (78) during sustained contractions. The increased metabolic demand under these conditions in conjunction with the decreased blood supply due to muscle pressure has been hypothesized to contribute to derangement in intracellular pH/lactic acid, and calcium and potassium balance within the muscle (79–84). Long-term damage as a result of this process can include microvascular and cellular dysfunction (85–87). Chapter 6 also discusses additional pathways of how nutritional flow can be disrupted or regulated through rest. The reduction in oxygen delivery to the muscle can result in muscle spasms (88) and collection of waste products in the muscle (lactic acid) (89), both of which can result in pain. In addition, the nerve is particularly susceptible to the detrimental effects of oxygen deprivation compared to the muscle. A reduction of oxygen to the nerve is believed to be the central problem in carpal tunnel syndrome (90–92). A similar mechanism is believed to affect the nerves in the back. Chapters 7–9 show how physical work factors, psychosocial/organization work factors, and individual characteristics can influence the degree of coactivation occurring in the back, which can set the stage for this blood flow disruption.

Inflammatory response—Another way in which muscle injury occurs is through direct inflammatory response. It is well established that muscle injury can result in such a response (93). Acute inflammation has been noted after eccentric exercise as well as repetitive activity with reperfusion injury after prolonged muscle ischemia (85,87). Recent studies have documented the degree of inflammatory response of the muscles in response to exertions (94). Figure 5.12 shows the dramatic difference in tissue organization and inflammation before and after exertion and demonstrates the degree to which muscles can be affected by prolonged tension that can result from cocontraction of the muscles (94,95).

One hypothesis of muscle-initiated low back pain has been proposed (99–102) and suggests that low level tension in the muscles can lead to tension myositis syndrome (TMS). This hypothesis also suggests that mental states, such as anxiety and anger, can result in the autonomic nervous system limiting the amount of blood available to nourish the muscles, nerves, tendons, or ligaments and resulting in pain and other dysfunctions of the tissues

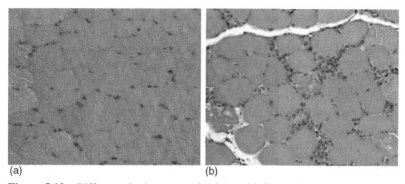

(a)   (b)

Figure 5.12 Difference in tissue organization and inflammation as a function of the number of stretch shortening cycles (SSCs) experienced by the muscle (96–98). (**a**) healthy muscle vs. (**b**) 3 days following intense eccentric exercise (courtesy of T. Best).

(99–102). This pathway appears to be related to the development of fibromyalgia. Studies have demonstrated that oxygenation of the muscle tissue is insufficient in patients diagnosed with fibromyalgia and can result in tissue damage (103–105). While the direct relationship with pain has yet to be explored with this pathway, the pathway certainly makes sense in terms of the "pattern of evidence" criteria.

While myofascial pain sounds similar to fibromyalgia, there are distinct differences. Fibromyalgia is characterized by intensification of nociception that causes deep tissue tenderness that includes deep muscles, whereas myofascial pain is a hypersensitive palpable nodule in a taut band of skeletal muscle due to central zones of oxygen deprivation.

Much of the current thinking of soft tissue disorders involves an increased inflammatory response as a result of cytokine upregulation (increases). Cytokines are proinflammatory agents that occur in the body as a result of both physical and mental loads. Studies have demonstrated that cytokines upregulate as a result of exposure to both acute and cumulative muscle trauma (8,106). Figure 5.2 suggests that constant muscle tension might also initiate an upregulation of cytokine activity that can result in increased inflammation and a subsequent increase in nociceptor stimulation.

Nerve damage—A final potential pathway to pain associated with muscle tension involves the restriction of blood flow to the nerves. Nutritional transport to the nerves is provided by a microvascular system of small blood vessels supplying nutrients from the surrounding tissues. Since there are no lymphatic vessels to drain the space, when edema forms, pressure can increase rapidly and interfere with microcirculation (107). Short-term compression exposure of as low as 20 mmHg has been reported to decrease microvascular flow, and pressures of 30 mmHg can impair axonal transport of nutrients (108). Even at these low pressure levels, formation of edema has been noted 24 h after termination of exposure. Long-term exposure of nerve compression (for up to 2 h) has resulted in edema within 4 h of exposure and damage to the nerve (axonal degeneration and demyelination) are observed 1 week after compression of the tissue (109,110).

While all of these muscle-related pathways can be viewed as independent pathways for pain, there is also some emerging evidence that they are indeed related (53).

5.7 THE ROLE OF INDIVIDUAL DIFFERENCES IN THE PAIN PATHWAYS

A discussion of causal pathways would be incomplete unless the topic of genetic predisposition is addressed. While Chapter 9 discusses individual differences in spine loading patterns and muscle recruitment patterns, this section examines the extent to which the structures and muscle-based responses to these loadings are influenced by an individual's genetic profile (as described in Figs. 1.1 and 1.2). A number of studies have recently reported the extent to which the various pathways to pain may be influenced by inherent (genetic) factors that may be unalterable. Since differences in disease susceptibility and physical characteristics are dictated by specific gene forms (polymorphisms), it is logical to expect that low back pain might be, at least partially, influenced by one's genetic make up.

A *genotype* refers to the genetic "constitution" of an individual, whereas *phenotype* refers to the observable properties of an organism that are produced by the interaction of the genotype and the environment. Much of the diversity among a population is believed to be governed by genetic loci that have quantitative effects on phenotype. These traits are referred to as quantitative trait loci or QTLs. The number of QTLs related to physical performance and health have been explored vigorously over the last several years. These investigations resulted in a rapid increase in the discovery of QTL associations with muscle function over the last few years. In 2000, 29 loci were mapped, in 2001, 71 loci had been included, and in 2002, 90 such QTLs were identified (111). However, in humans, few of the QTLs have been classified as "major" loci, and muscle quantitative trait loci appears to be more complex in humans than in animals (112).

Most of the studies that have explored genetic influences have assessed how genetic classification states or gene forms called polymorphisms might be associated with receptors that govern muscle mass, training, or upregulation of biochemical processes such as cytokine release. As an example of how this process works, Fig. 5.13 indicates how a variety of single muscle-related polymorphism can influence motor neuron survival, muscle fiber development, and muscle regeneration (112).

Genetic mapping is important because it may explain some of the variation in muscle response to load as well as adaptation. Much of the research has endeavored to understand how genetically determined receptors might interact with environmental factors and respond to biochemicals such as cytokines. A major objective of genetics research is to understand how much of an effect is provided by genetic predisposition. For example, it is of interest to

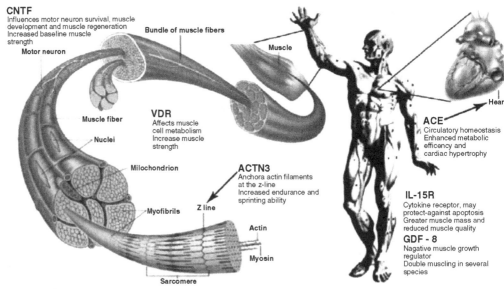

Figure 5.13 Summary of known associations between genetic polymorphisms and muscle phenotypes. (From reference 112).

determine what percent of low back pain (variation) is due to genetics versus occupational factors.

Interleukin-15 is a cytokine that is thought to be associated with the construction process of the muscle metabolism. Studies have shown that IL-15 can increase muscle mass during training. The variation explained by IL-15 has been found to be between 7.1% and 10.6% of the increase in muscle mass (113).

The influence of interactions within the genetic code appear to be fairly complex and situation specific. One recent study found that one ciliary neurotrophic factor receptor gene was associated with increases in fat-free muscle mass and strength and was independent of strength (114), whereas another study found that a similar QTL interaction with a cytokine (interleukin-6 or IL-6) increased mean muscle mass in men but not in women (115). Still another genotype was found to be responsible for increases in muscle strength in women, but only explained 2% of the variation (116). Other genotypes have been identified that influence muscle function in later life (117). And yet another genotype has been identified that affects response of human skeletal muscle to training and muscle overload (118).

Others have found no association between strength and genotype (119). However, much of the literature assessing these associations has been plagued by an inability to replicate findings, small sample sizes, inconsistent analysis methods, and inadequate statistical power. Hence, the role of genetics in the pain pathway is far from clear.

Two interesting studies do indeed shed some light on the role of the interaction between genetic factors and an inflammatory cytokine (120,121). These studies demonstrated an association between interleukin-1 and a genotype in middle-aged men and found that carriers of the gene increased their odds of back pain by two and one half times. However, the studies also compared the role of different occupations and found higher odds ratios associated with differences in occupations compared to differences in genotypes (121).

These investigations confirm the interactive nature of risk factors and low back pain.

5.8 SYSTEM FEEDBACK

To appreciate the self-limiting nature of the low back pain pathways as well as the potential for chronic low back pain, we must also consider the feedback loop (from pain to tissue tension) described in Fig. 5.2. Given a pain experience, we have the ability to remember a muscle recruitment response to a stimulus. Thus, as suggested in Fig. 5.2, when the environmental conditions are received by the human and interpreted as potentially pain provoking (based on the pain experience), the system will anticipate pain and begin increasing muscle tension (in an effort to increase stability and limit nociceptors stimulation). Hence, the pain pathways can be exacerbated by previous experiences as well as environmental stimuli.

5.9 SUMMARY

A particularly appealing aspect of the low back pain pathways presented by the model shown in Fig. 5.2 is that the various pathways have the potential to explain the injury, cumulative trauma, and biopsychosocial views of low back pain. The common element is that all pathways are controlled and activated through brain function that can be influenced by both physical conditions and cognitive (psychosocial/organizational) conditions. Hence, the pattern of evidence can be incorporated into this way of thinking.

It should be clear from this discussion that the key to understanding how the spine tissues are loaded during various work activities is to understand what influence those work activities might have on the recruitment of the muscles and the muscles collective influence on the nature and direction of the forces acting on the various pain-generating structures of the spine. One should also be aware that the *physical work factors interact with a worker's individual factors and psychosocial influences* to ultimately define the risk associated with the performance of work tasks. The following chapters will review the current state of knowledge indicating how physical work factors, individual factors, psychosocial factors, and these interactions can influence the force that is ultimately delivered to the pain-sensitive tissue of the back.

KEY POINTS

- When back structure anatomy is considered along with pain generation processes, several potential back pain pathways are possible.

- The physical and psychological environment provides stimuli to our brains to which we must respond through the recruitment of muscles in order to satisfy a particular objective. The muscle recruitment pattern is unique to an individual. The musculo-skeletal system response defines the forces or loads that act on the back's tissues.

- Tissue loading has the potential to activate two pathways disrupting either the structural support system and/or the muscle function. Muscle function disruption can influence both muscle and nerve function.

- These pathways can result in an upregulation of cytokines leading to an inflammatory response and a sensitization of nociceptors resulting in pain, or they can directly compromise nerve function also resulting in pain.

- A large number of specific structural disruption pathways and muscle function pathways have been identified. The structural disruption load tolerances have been described in the literature, whereas many of the muscle function disruption pathway tolerances have yet to be quantified.

- Genetic factors appear to play a role in defining some of the individual differences in the muscle dysfunction pathways.

REFERENCES

1. COHEN SP, et al. Presentation, diagnoses, mechanisms of injury, and treatment of soldiers injured in Operation Iraqi Freedom: an epidemiological study conducted at two military pain management centers. *Anesth Analg* 2005;104(4):1098–1103, table of contents.
2. WEISE E. Soldiers in Iraq carry extra load: back pain, USA Today; 2005.
3. NORMAN R, et al. A comparison of peak vs cumulative physical work exposure risk factors for the reporting of low back pain in the automotive industry. *Clin Biomech (Bristol, Avon)* 1998;13(8):561–573.
4. HEIKKILA JK, et al. Genetic and environmental factors in sciatica. Evidence from a nationwide panel of 9365 adult twin pairs. *Annal Med* 1989;21(5): 393–398.
5. SEIDLER A, et al. The role of cumulative physical work load in lumbar spine disease: risk factors for lumbar osteochondrosis and spondylosis associated with chronic complaints. *J Occup Environ Med* 2001;58(11):735–746.
6. N.R.C. Musculoskeletal Disorders and the Workplace: Low Back and Upper Extremity. Washington (DC): National Academy Press; 2001.
7. CALLAGHAN JP, MCGILL SM. Intervertebral disc herniation: studies on a porcine model exposed to highly repetitive flexion/extension motion with compressive force. *Clin Biomech (Bristol, Avon)* 2001;16(1):28–37.
8. BARR AE, BARBE MF. Pathophysiological tissue changes associated with repetitive movement: a review of the evidence. *Phys Ther* 2002;82(2):173–187.

9. GATCHEL RJ, BRUGA D. Multi- and interdisciplinary intervention for injured workers with chronic low back pain. *SpineLine;* 2005:8–13.

10. YOGANANDAN N. Biomechanical identification of injury to an intervertebral joint. *Clin Biomech (Bristol, Avon)* 1986;1(3):149.

11. HOY MG, ZAJAC FE, GORDON ME. A musculoskeletal model of the human lower extremity: the effect of muscle, tendon, and moment arm on the moment–angle relationship of musculotendon actuators at the hip, knee, and ankle. *J Biomech* 1990;23(2):157–169.

12. NORDIN M, FRANKEL V. Basic Biomechanics of the Musculoskeletal System.2nd ed.Philadelphia (PA): Lea and Febiger; 1989.

13. SOLOMONOW M. Ligaments: a source of work-related musculoskeletal disorders. *J Electromyogr Kinesiol* 2004;14(1):49–60.

14. SOLOMONOW M, et al. Biomechanics of increased exposure to lumbar injury caused by cyclic loading: Part 1. Loss of reflexive muscular stabilization. *Spine* 1999; 24(23):2426–2434.

15. SOLOMONOW M, et al. The ligamento-muscular stabilizing system of the spine. *Spine* 1998;23(23):2552–2562.

16. STUBBS M, et al. Ligamento-muscular protective reflex in the lumbar spine of the feline. *J Electromyogr Kinesiol* 1998;8(4):197–204.

17. GEDALIA U, et al. Biomechanics of increased exposure to lumbar injury caused by cyclic loading: Part 2. Recovery of reflexive muscular stability with rest. *Spine* 1999;24(23):2461–2467.

18. WANG JL, et al. Viscoelastic finite-element analysis of a lumbar motion segment in combined compression and sagittal flexion. Effect of loading rate. *Spine* 2000;25 (3):310–318.

19. SOLOMONOW M, et al. Neuromuscular disorders associated with static lumbar flexion: a feline model. *J Electromyogr Kinesiol* 2002;12(2):81–90.

20. SOLOMONOW M, et al. Biexponential recovery model of lumbar viscoelastic laxity and reflexive muscular activity after prolonged cyclic loading. *Clin Biomech (Bristol, Avon)* 2000;15(3):167–175.

21. HORNER HA, URBAN JP. 2001 Volvo Award winner in basic science studies: effect of nutrient supply on the viability of cells from the nucleus pulposus of the intervertebral disc. *Spine* 2001;26(23):2543–2549.

22. LOTZ JC, et al. Compression-induced degeneration of the intervertebral disc: an in vivo mouse model and finite-element study. *Spine* 1998;23(23):2493–2506.

23. CHAFFIN D, ANDERSSON BJ, MARTIN B. Occupational Biomechanics.4th ed.Hoboken (NJ): John Wiley & Sons, Inc.; 2006. p. 360.

24. NIOSH Work practices guide for manual lifting Cincinnati (OH): Department of Health and Human Services (DHHS), National Institute for Occupational Safety and Health (NIOSH); 1981.

25. ADAMS MA, et al. Mechanical Initiation of Intervertebral Disc Degeneration. *Spine* 2000;25(13): 1625–1636.

26. NIOSH Work Practices Guide for Manual Lifting. Cincinnati (OH): U.S. Department of Health and Human Services, Public Health Service, Centers for Disease Control, National Institute for Occupational Safety and Health, Division of Miomedical and Behavioral Science; 1981.

27. JAGER M, LUTTMANN A, LAURIG W. Lumbar load during one-hand bricklaying. *Int J Ind Ergon* 1991;8:261–277.

28. BRINKMANN P., BIGGERMANN M. HILWEG D. Fatigue fracture of human lumbar vertebrae. *Clin Biomech (Bristol, Avon)* 1988;3 (Suppl 1):S1–S23.

29. GORDON SJ, et al. Mechanism of disc rupture. A preliminary report. *Spine* 1991;16(4):450–456.

30. NRC. Musculoskeletal disorders and the workplace: low back and upper extremity. Panel of Musculoskeletal Disorders at the Workplace. (DC): Washington National Academy of Sciences, National Research Council, National Academy Press; 2001. p. 492.

31. ADAMS MA, HUTTON WC. Prolapsed intervertebral disc. A hyperflexion injury 1981 Volvo Award in basic science. *Spine* 1982;7(3):184–191.

32. GUNNING JL, CALLAGHAN JP, McGILL SM. Spinal posture and prior loading history modulate compressive strength and type of failure in the spine: a biomechanical study using a porcine cervical spine model. *Clin Biomech (Bristol, Avon)* 2001;16(6):471–480.

33. GALLAGHER S, et al. Torso flexion loads and the fatigue failure of human lumbosacral motion segments. *Spine* 2005;30(20):2265–2273.

34. IATRIDIS JC, et al. Shear mechanical properties of human lumbar annulus fibrosus. *J Orthop Res* 1999;17(5):732–737.

35. IATRIDIS JC, LAIBLE JP, KRAG MH. Influence of fixed charge density magnitude and distribution on the intervertebral disc: applications of a poroelastic and chemical electric (PEACE) model. *J Biomecha Eng* 2003;125 (1):12–24.

36. IATRIDIS JC, MACLEAN JJ, RYAN DA. Mechanical damage to the intervertebral disc annulus fibrosus subjected to tensile loading. *J Biomech* 2005;38(3):557–565.

37. IATRIDIS JC, et al. Compression-induced changes in intervertebral disc properties in a rat tail model. *Spine* 1999;24(10):996–1002.

38. MACLEAN JJ, et al. Effects of immobilization and dynamic compression on intervertebral disc cell gene expression in vivo. *Spine* 2003;28(10):973–981.

39. FATHALLAH FA, MARRAS WS, WRIGHT PL. Diurnal variation in trunk kinematics during a typical work shift. *J Spinal Disord* 1995;8(1):20–25.

40. SNOOK SH, WEBSTER BS, McGORRY RW. The reduction of chronic, nonspecific low back pain through the control of early morning lumbar flexion: 3-year follow-up. *J Occup Rehabil* 2002;12(1):13–19.

41. SNOOK SH. et al. The reduction of chronic nonspecific low back pain through the control of early morning lumbar flexion. A randomized controlled trial. *Spine* 1998;23(23):2601–2607.

42. McGILL SM. The biomechanics of low back injury: implications on current practice in industry and the clinic. *J Biomech* 1997;30(5):465–475.

43. SHIRAZI-ADL A. Strain in fibers of a lumbar disc. Analysis of the role of lifting in producing disc prolapse. *Spine* 1989;14(1):96–103.

44. GALLAGHER S, et al. An exploratory study of loading and morphometric factors associated with specific failure modes in fatigue testing of lumbar motion segments. *Clin Biomech (Bristol, Avon)* 2006;21(3).228–234.

45. CYRON BM, HUTTON WC. The fatigue strength of the lumbar neural arch in spondylolysis. *J Bone and Joint Sur Br* 1978;60(2):234–238.

46. ADAMS M, DOLAN P. Recent advances in lumbar spinal mechanics and their clinical significance. *Clin Biomech (Bristol, Avon)* 1995;10(1):3–19.

47. MARRAS WS, et al. Biomechanical risk factors for occupationally related low back disorders. *Ergonomics* 1995;38(2):377–410.

48. MARRAS WS, et al. The role of dynamic three-dimensional trunk motion in occupationally-related low back disorders. The effects of workplace factors, trunk position, and trunk motion characteristics on risk of injury. *Spine* 1993;18(5):617–628.

49. KHALSA PS. Biomechanics of musculoskeletal pain: dynamics of the neuromatrix. *J Electromyogr Kinesiol* 2004;14(1):109–120.

50. CAVANAUGH JM, et al. Mechanisms of low back pain: a neurophysiologic and neuroanatomic study. *Clin Orthop* 1997; (335):166–180.

51. CAVANAUGH JM. Neural mechanisms of lumbar pain. *Spine* 1995;20(16):1804–1809.

52. JENSEN MC.et al. Magnetic resonance imaging of the lumbar spine in people without back pain. *N Engl J Med* 1994;331(2):69–73.

53. SIMONS DG. Review of enigmatic MTrPs as a common cause of enigmatic musculoskeletal pain and dysfunction. *J Electromyogr Kinesiol* 2004;14(1):95–107.

54. SIMONS DG, TRAVELL JG, SIMONS LS. Travell & Simons' Myofascial Pain and Dysfunction: The Trigger Point Manual. Volume 1, Upper Half of Body. Philadelphia (PA): Lippincott, Williams & Wilkins; 1999. p. 1038.

55. SIMONS DG, HONG CZ, SIMONS LS. Endplate potentials are common to midfiber myofacial trigger points. *Am J Phys Med Rehabil* 2002;81(3):212–222.

56. SIMONS DG, STOLOV WC. Microscopic features and transient contraction of palpable bands in canine muscle. *Am J Phy Med* 1976;55(2):65–88.

57. MENSE S, et al. Lesions of rat skeletal muscle after local block of acetylcholinesterase and neuromuscular stimulation. *J App Physiol* 2003;94(6):2494–2501.

58. SHAH JP, et al. An in vivo microanalytical technique for measuring the local biochemical milieu of human skeletal muscle. *J Appl Physiol* 2005;99(5):1977–1984.

59. CHOLEWICKI J, SIMONS AP, RADEBOLD A. Effects of external trunk loads on lumbar spine stability. *J Biomech* 2000;33(11):1377–1385.

60. CHOLEWICKI J, VANVLIET IJ. Relative contribution of trunk muscles to the stability of the lumbar spine during isometric exertions. *Clin Biomech (Bristol, Avon)* 2002;17(2):99–105.

61. PANJABI MM. The stabilizing system of the spine: Part II. Neutral zone and instability hypothesis. *J Spinal Disord* 1992;5(4):390–396; discussion 397.

62. LOWE DA, et al. Eccentric contraction-induced injury of mouse soleus muscle: effect of varying [Ca2+]. *J Appl Physiol* 1994;76(4):1445–1453.

63. LOWE DA, et al. Muscle function and protein metabolism after initiation of eccentric contraction-induced injury. *J Appl Physiol* 1995;79(4):1260–1270.

64. McCULLY KK. Exercise-induced injury to skeletal muscle. *Federation Proceedings* 1986;45(13):2933–2936.

65. McCULLY KK, FAULKNER JA. Characteristics of lengthening contractions associated with injury to skeletal muscle fibers. *J Appl Physiol* 1986;61(1):293–299.

66. MORGAN DL. New insights into the behavior of muscle during active lengthening. *Biophy J* 1990;57(2):209–221.

67. STAUBER WT. Eccentric action of muscles: physiology, injury and adaptation In: PANDOLF KB, editor. Exercise and Sport Sciences Reviews, Baltimore: Williams and Wilkins; 1989. p. 157–185.

68. STAUBER WT. Factors involved in strain-induced injury in skeletal muscles and outcomes of prolonged exposures. *J Electromyogr Kinesiol* 2004;14(1).

69. WARREN GL, et al. Excitation failure in eccentric contraction-induced injury of mouse soleus muscle. *J Physiol* 1993;468:487–499.

70. WARREN GL, et al. Eccentric contraction-induced injury in normal and hindlimb-suspended mouse soleus and EDL muscles. *J Appl Physiol* 1994;77(3):1421–1430.

71. WARREN GL, et al. Materials fatigue initiates eccentric contraction-induced injury in rat soleus muscle. *J Physiol* 1993;464:477–489.

72. ARMSTRONG RB, WARREN GL, WARREN JA. Mechanisms of exercise-induced muscle fibre injury. *Sports Med* 1991;12(3):184–207.

73. O'REILLY KP, et al. Eccentric exercise-induced muscle damage impairs muscle glycogen repletion. *J Appl Physiol* 1987;63(1):252–256.

74. SZOMOR ZL, APPLEYARD RC, MURRELL GA. Overexpression of nitric oxide synthases in tendon overuse. *J Orthop Res* 2006;24(1):80–86.

75. HAGG GM. Static work loads and occupational myalgia – a new explanation mode In: ANDERSON P, HOBART D, DANHOFF J, editors. Electromyographical Kinesiology. Amsterdam: Elsevier Science Publishers; 1991.

76. cSJOGAARD G, SOGAARD K. Muscle injury in repetitive motion disorders. *Clin Orthop Relat Res* 1998; (351):21–31.

77. SJOGAARD G, JENSEN B. Muscle pathology with overuse. In:RANNEY D, editor Chronic Musculoskeletal Injuries in the Workplace. Philadelphia: W.B. Saunders Company; 1997.

78. BAI YH, et al. Pathology study of rabbit calf muscles after repeated compression. *J Orthop Sci* 1998;3 (4):209–215.

79. GAFFNEY FA, SJOGAARD G, SALTIN B. Cardiovascular and metabolic responses to static contraction in man. *Acta Physiol Scand* 1990;138(3):249–258.

80. Sjogaard G. Water and electrolyte fluxes during exercise and their relation to muscle fatigue. *Acta Physiol Scand Suppl* 1986;556:129–136.

81. Sjogaard G. Muscle energy metabolism and electrolyte shifts during low-level prolonged static contraction in man. *Acta Physiol Scand* 1988;134(2): 181–187.

82. Sjogaard G. Exercise-induced muscle fatigue: the significance of potassium. *Acta Physiol Scand Suppl* 1990;593:1–63.

83. Sjogaard G, et al. Intramuscular pressure, EMG and blood flow during low-level prolonged static contraction in man. *Acta Physiol Scand* 1986;128(3):475–484.

84. Sjogaard G, Savard G, Juel C. Muscle blood flow during isometric activity and its relation to muscle fatigue. *Eur J Appl Physiol Occup Physiol* 1988;57 (3):327–335.

85. Jerome SN, Kong L, Korthuis RJ. Microvascular dysfunction in postischemic skeletal muscle. *J Invest Surg* 1994;7(1):3–16.

86. Seyama A. The role of oxygen-derived free radicals and the effect of free radical scavengers on skeletal muscle ischemia/reperfusion injury. *Surg Today* 1993;23(12):1060–1067.

87. Skjeldal S, et al. Histological studies on postischemic rat skeletal muscles. With emphasis on the time of leukocyte invasion. *Eur Surg Res* 1993;25(6):348–357.

88. Solomonow M, et al. Biomechanics and electromyography of a common idiopathic low back disorder. *Spine* 2003;28(12):1235–1248.

89. Holmes TH, Wolff HG. Life situations, emotions, and backache. *Psychosom Med* 1952;14(1):18–33.

90. Rempel D, Abrahamsson SO. The effects of reduced oxygen tension on cell proliferation and matrix synthesis in synovium and tendon explants from the rabbit carpal tunnel: an experimental study in vitro. *J Orthop Res* 2001;19(1):143–148.

91. Murthy G, et al. Forearm muscle oxygenation decreases with low levels of voluntary contraction. *J Orthop Res* 1997;15(4):507–511.

92. Murthy G, et al. Ischemia causes muscle fatigue. *J Orthop Res* 2001;19(3):436–440.

93. Cannon JG, et al. Acute phase response in exercise: interaction of age and vitamin E on neutrophils and muscle enzyme release. *Am J Physiol* 1990;259(6 Pt 2): R1214–R1419.

94. Baker BA, et al. Stereological analysis of muscle morphology following exposure to repetitive stretch-shortening cycles in a rat model. *App Physiol, Nutr Metab* 2006;31(2):167–179.

95. Baker BA, et al. Quantitative histology and MGF gene expression in rats following SSC exercise in vivo. *Med Sci Sports Exercise* 2006;38(3):463–471.

96. Cutlip RG, et al. Impact of muscle length during stretch-shortening contractions on real-time and temporal muscle performance measures in rats in vivo. *J Appl Physiol* 2004;96(2):507–516.

97. Geronilla KB, et al. Dynamic force responses of skeletal muscle during stretch-shortening cycles. *Eur J Appl Physiol* 2003;90(1–2):144–153.

98. Cutlip RG, et al. Impact of stretch-shortening cycle rest interval on in vivo muscle performance. *Med Sci Sports Exercise* 2005;37(8):1345–1355.

99. Sarno JE, Treatment for low back pain. *Scand J Rehabil Med* 1980;12(4):175–176.

100. Sarno JE. Etiology of neck and back pain. An automatic myoneuralgia? *J Nervous Mental Dis* 1981;169 (1):55–59.

101. Sarno JE. Mind Over Back Pain. New York (NY): Berkley Books; 1982. p. 124.

102. Sarno JE. Healing Back Pain. New York (NY): Warner Books; 1991. p. 193.

103. Bengtsson A, et al. Primary fibromyalgia. A clinical and laboratory study of 55 patients. *Scand J Rheumatol* 1986;15(3):340–347.

104. Bengtsson A, Henriksson KG, Larsson J. Muscle biopsy in primary fibromyalgia. Light-microscopical and histochemical findings. *Scand J Rheumatol* 1986;15(1):1–6.

105. Lund N, Bengtsson A, Thorborg P. Muscle tissue oxygen pressure in primary fibromyalgia. *Scand J Rheumatol* 1986;15(2):165–173.

106. Barr AE, Barbe M.F. Inflammation reduces physiological tissue tolerance in the development of work-related musculoskeletal disorders. *J Electromyogr Kinesiol* 2004;14(1):77–85.

107. Lundborg G, Dahlin LB. Anatomy, function, and pathophysiology of peripheral nerves and nerve compression. *Hand Clin* 1996;12(2):185–193.

108. Rempel D, Dahlin L, Lundborg G. Pathophysiology of nerve compression syndromes: response of peripheral nerves to loading. *J Bone Joint Surg Am* 1999;81 (11):1600–1610.

109. Dyck PJ, et al. Structural alterations of nerve during curff compression. in Proceedings of the National Academy of Sciences1990.

110. Mackinnon SE, et al. Chronic nerve compression—An experimental model in the rat. *Ann Plastic Surg* 1994;13(2):112–120.

111. Perusse L, et al. The human gene map for performance and health-related fitness phenotypes: the 2002 update. *Med Sci Sports and Exercise* 2003;35(8):1248–1264.

112. Gordon ES, Gordish Dressman HA, Hoffman EP. The genetics of muscle atrophy and growth: the impact and implications of polymorphisms in animals and humans. *Int J Biochem Cell Biol* 2005;37 (10):2064–2074.

113. Riechman SE, et al. Association of interleukin-15 protein and interleukin-15 receptor genetic variation with resistance exercise training responses. *J Appl Physiol* 2004;97(6):2214–2219.

114. Roth SM, et al. C174T polymorphism in the CNTF receptor gene is associated with fat-free mass in men and women. *J Appl Physiol* 2003;95(4):1425–1430.

115. Roth SM, et al. Interleukin-6 (IL6) genotype is associated with fat-free mass in men but not women. *J Gerontol. Ser A Biol Sci Med Sci* 2003;58(12):B1085–1088.

116. Clarkson PM, et al. ACTN3 genotype is associated with increases in msucle strength in response to resistance training in women. *J Appl Physiol* 2005; 99: 154–163.

117. Schrager MA, et al. Insulin-like growth factor-2 genotype, fat-free mass, and muscle perfromance across the adult life span. *J Appl Physiol* 2004;97: 2176–2183.

118. Folland J, et al. Angiotensin-converting enzyme genotype affects the response of human skeletal muscle to functional overload. *Exp Physiol* 2005;85(5):575–579.

119. Thomis MA, et al. Exploration of myostatin polymorphisms and the angiotensin-converting enzyme insertion/deletion genotype in responses of human muscle to strength training. *Eur J Appl Physiol* 2004;92(3):267–274.

120. Solovieva S, et al. Interleukin 1 polymorphisms and intervertebral disc degeneration. *Epidemiology* 2004; 15(5):626–633.

121. Solovieva S, et al. Possible association of interleukin 1 gene locus polymorphisms with low back pain. *Pain* 2004;109(1–2):8–19.

CHAPTER 6

THE ASSESSMENT OF BIOMECHANICAL FORCES ACTING ON THE LOW BACK

THE OVERALL goal of this chapter is to establish the ability of modern biomechanical models to assess muscle tensions and the resulting spine tissue loads. An understanding of how these muscle tensions and spine loads develop is essential to the understanding of low back pain causal pathways since excessive tissue load initiates the pain signal. The chapter begins with a review of how approaches to the assessment of spine tissue loading have evolved over the years. Basic biomechanical principles are presented and the discussion demonstrates how incremental improvements in model fidelity have made it possible to develop person-specific spine models making it possible to assess the activation of the causal pathways described in Chapter 5. These models enable one to identify loads occurring on specific tissues within the back structures and tissues. The chapter emphasizes that if we understand how muscles are recruited during an activity, it can be possible to partition out the influence of various physical, nonphysical, and individual factors.

It should be clear from our current understanding of pain pathways that pain perception associated with the low back is complex and can be influenced by many factors including tissue loading, cytokine upregulation, previous pain experiences, and cognitive processing that can intensify or modify the perception of pain. It is also clear that before pain perception can be shaped or mediated, some form of stimulus must be present and the ability of the stimulus to initiate pain varies widely depending on the specific conditions. The initial stimulus is often a result of tissue loading or forces being imposed on the low back. Hence, a physical stimulus is often necessary to initiate the sequence of events and activate the pathway that can eventually result in low back pain. This chapter examines how forces are imposed on the spine's pain-sensitive tissues and will review biomechanical logic associated with the prediction of spinal loads.

Biomechanics is an interdisciplinary field in which information from both the biological sciences and engineering mechanics is used to quantify the forces present on the body during work. Biomechanics assumes that, from a physics standpoint, *the body behaves according to the laws of Newtonian mechanics.* Mechanics can be defined as "the study of forces and their effects on masses" (1). The object of interest in occupational biomechanics is a quantitative assessment of mechanical loading properties occurring within the musculoskeletal system. The goal of such an assessment is to quantitatively describe the musculoskeletal loading that occurs during work so that one can derive an appreciation for the degree of risk associated with work-related tasks. This high degree of precision and quantification is the characteristic that distinguishes occupational biomechanics analyses from other types of analyses. Thus, with biomechanical techniques, we can address the issue of "how much exposure to the occupational risk factors is too much exposure?"

The approach to a biomechanical assessment is to characterize the human–work system situation through a mathematical representation or model. A model helps us understand the nature of the forces acting on a tissue that could not be easily measured by any other method. Models are simply the "glue" that hold our logic together and helps us understand how the complex subsystems within a biomechanical structure interact and ultimately stress a tissue. Albert Einstein suggested that explanations should be as simple as necessary to describe a process, but no simpler. Thus, the same holds for biomechanical modeling. While models can be complex, the goal of a model is to only make it as complex as necessary to accurately represent the process of interest. By applying these techniques to work situations, these models can help us understand the degree to which the activities we perform (e.g., work) can result in forces on a tissue that may result in the initiation of a pain response. Thus, biomechanical models allow us to assess forces acting on the spine tissues under actual exposure situations; something that would be impossible to do under real-life conditions any other way.

The advantage of representing the worker in a biomechanical model is that the model permits one to quantitatively consider the *trade-offs* associated with workplace risk factors to various parts of the body in the design of a workplace. It is difficult to accommodate all parts of the body in an ideal biomechanical work environment since improving the conditions for one body segment often make things worse for another part of the body. Therefore, the key to the proper application of biomechanical principles is to consider the appropriate biomechanical trade-offs associated with various parts of the body as a function of the work requirements and the various workplace design options and constraints. Ultimately, biomechanical analyses would be most effective in predicting workplace risk during the design stage before the physical construction of the workplace has begun. While the concept of a biomechanical model may seem complex, many workplace assessment tools are based on model predictions. Thus, it is useful to examine the degree to which these underlying models can accurately predict tissue load.

6.1   BIOMECHANICAL CONCEPTS APPLICABLE TO THE BACK

6.1.1   Load Tolerance

In biomechanical terms, loading refers to the forces that are imposed on a tissue. A fundamental concept in the application of biomechanics to the assessment of spine loading is that to quantify risk, the force or load imposed on a structure or tissue can be compared to the tolerance of the structure or tissue to estimate risk. Figure 6.1 illustrates the traditional concept of biomechanical risk (2). This figure illustrates how a loading pattern is experienced by a structure and is repeated as the work cycles recur during a job. Structure tolerance is also shown in this figure. When the magnitude of the load imposed on a structure is less than that of the tissue tolerance, then the task is considered safe and the magnitude of the difference between the load and the tolerance is considered the safety margin. Conversely, if the imposed load exceeds the tissue tolerance, then the tissue is damaged. This concept has been employed extensively in engineering and represents the way engineers design safe structures. Consider the case of a bridge. Engineers consider the heaviest load that the bridge should be able to support and then build in a structural strength several times that limit to ensure safety.

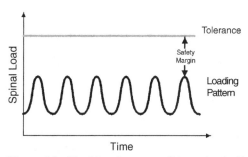

Figure 6.1   Traditional concept of biomechanically defined risk. When the forces or loads imposed on the spinal tissue are less than the level of tissue tolerance, the task is assumed to be relatively free of risk. If the load exceeds the tolerance, the tissue can experience damage. (Adapted from reference 2).

Traditionally, tissue tolerance has been defined as the ability of the tissue to withstand a load without physical disruption or damage. However, given the current understanding of proinflammatory responses, such as cytokines, this concept can be expanded to include the tolerance defined as the point at which the tissue exhibits an inflammatory reaction.

A trend in modern work is that the tasks are becoming increasingly repetitive, yet involve lighter loads. The conceptual load–tolerance model can also be adjusted to also account for this type of risk exposure. Figure 6.2 shows that occupational biomechanics logic can account for this trend by decreasing the tissue tolerance over time. This can represent how the tolerance decreases during repetitive wear and tear (cumulative trauma) (Figure 6.2a) and can also represent how cytokine upregulation may change the tissue tolerance over time (Figure 6.2b). Hence, biomechanical models and logic are moving toward systems that consider manufacturing and work trends in the workplace and attempt to represent these observations (such as cumulative trauma disorders) in the model logic.

6.1.2   Moments and Levers

Biomechanical loads are only partially defined by the magnitude of weight supported by the body. A moment (also called torque) is defined as the product of force and distance. Within the low back, the position of the weight handled (or mass of the body segment) relative to the axis of rotation (fulcrum) of the spine (typically L5/S1) defines the imposed load on the body and is referred to as a *moment*. This concept can be demonstrated through the picture of a

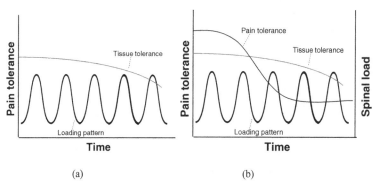

(a)   (b)

Figure 6.2   Cumulative trauma biomechanical risk defined as (**a**) the relationship between the imposed load and the tissue tolerance (that is reduced over time) and (**b**) the relationship between the tissue load and the point at which inflammatory responses occur (which can also reduce over time but at a much more rapid rate).

seesaw in Fig. 6.3a. Here we see that a small child can counterbalance a large man if the distance between the child and the seesaw's fulcrum is large compared to the distance between the large man and the fulcrum. This figure suggests that in a lever system, the magnitude of the force required to move an object is a function of both the weight of the object and the distance of the object from a fulcrum (mechanical advantage). Hence, if the back is considered as a lever system, then the load imposed on the spine is not simply a function of just the weight lifted.

As implied in the above example, moments are a function of the mechanical lever systems of the body. In biomechanics, the musculoskeletal system is represented by a system of levers and it is the lever systems that are used to describe the tissue loads with a biomechanical model. The biomechanics of the back and spine can be represented by a first-class lever. First-class levers are those that have a fulcrum placed between the imposed load (on one end of the system) and an opposing force (*internal to the body*) imposed on the opposite end of the system. In this case, the spine serves as the fulcrum. As the human lifts, a moment (*load imposed external to the body*) is imposed anterior to the spine due to the object weight times the distance of the object from the spine. This moment is counterbalanced by the activity of the back muscles; however, they are located in such a way that they are at a mechanical disadvantage since the distance between the back muscles and the spine is much less than the distance between the object lifted and the spine (Fig. 6.3b).

6.1.3   External Versus Internal Loading

The concepts of levers help demonstrate the concept of internal forces versus external forces acting on the spine. *External* loads refer to those forces that are imposed on the body as a direct result of gravity acting on an external object being manipulated by the worker. However, *internal* forces counteract these external forces or loads. Figure 6.3b shows how it is possible for an external load to have a great biomechanical advantage compared to a person's internal force during lifting. This figure demonstrates the importance of mechanical advantage in a lever system. If a small load has a much larger lever arm relative to a fulcrum compared to the lever arm on the other side of the fulcrum, then a very large force will be required to balance this small load. As shown in Fig. 6.3b, this is often the case during lifting, where very large internal forces are needed to counteract the external mechanical advantage since the back muscles are located very close to the spine relative to the location of the external load.

Figure 6.3c shows an example of how large the internal forces must be in a very simple model. Figure 6.3c shows a 222 N (about 50 lb) external load being held at a distance of 1 m from the spine. Gravity acts on this external load and creates a moment about the spine of 222 Nm (222 N × 1 m). However, to maintain equilibrium, this external force must be counteracted by an *internal* force that is generated by the back muscles. However, the internal load (muscle) acts at a distance relative to the spine (5 cm or 0.05 m) that is much closer to the fulcrum than the external load. Thus, the internal force must be supplied at a biomechanical disadvantage (because of the smaller lever arm) and must produce a force that is much larger (4440 N or 998 lbs) compared to the external load (222 N or 50 lbs) to keep the musculoskeletal system in equilibrium.

It is not unusual for the magnitude of the internal load to be much greater (often more than 10 times greater) than the external load. These muscle-generated loads become even greater when the external load is accelerated (since force equals product of mass and acceleration). Hence, the magnitude of the internal force required to move an object can be affected by dynamic motion of the object. If the external force is subject to inertia of motion, the magnitude of the internal force could either increase or decrease, depending on the

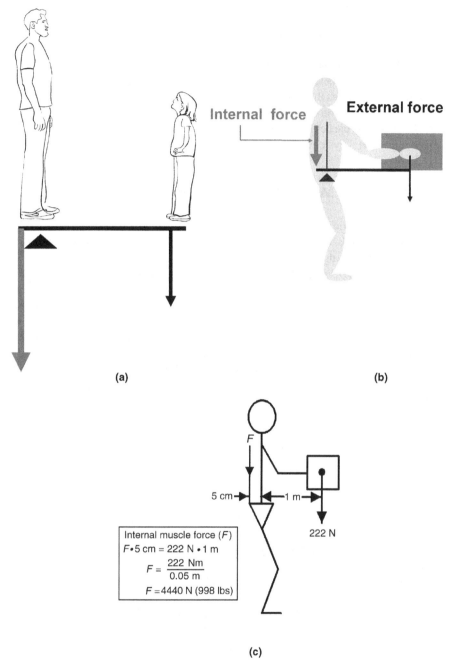

Figure 6.3 (a) The concept of mechanical advantage due to a large lever arm relative to the fulcrum, (b) the body represents a similar lever system requiring very large muscle forces to counteract the external load, and (c) an example of the large internal force (*F*) required to support an external force held at a distance of 1 m from the spine.

direction of object motion. To make matters worse, when multiple muscles are recruited (muscle cocontraction) to support the external load, joint loads increase because the muscles work against each other ("fight" each other) to maintain control.

The internal loading contributes the most to both acute and cumulative tissue loads with the musculoskeletal system during work. The net sum of the external load and the internal load defines the total loading experienced at the joint. Therefore, when evaluating the impact of work on spine loading, one must not only consider the externally applied load but must also be particularly sensitive to the magnitude of the internal forces that can load the musculoskeletal system.

6.2   HOW CAN WE MODIFY INTERNAL SPINE LOADS?

The previous section emphasized the importance of understanding the relationship between the external loads imposed on the body and the internal loads generated by the force-generating mechanisms within the body. The *key to proper work design is based on the principle of designing workplaces so that the internal loads are minimized*. Internal forces can be thought of as both the component that supports and loads the tissue and the target of overexertion. Thus, muscle strength or capacity can be considered as a tolerance measure. If the forces imposed on the muscles and tendons as a result of the task exceed the strength (tolerance) of the muscle or tendon, potential tissue damage is possible. Generally, three components of the physical work environment (biomechanical arrangement of the musculoskeletal lever system, length–strength relationships, velocity, and temporal relationships) can be manipulated to facilitate this goal and serve as the basis for many ergonomic recommendations.

6.2.1   Biomechanical Arrangement of the Musculoskeletal Lever System

The posture imposed via the design of the workplace can affect the arrangement of the body's lever system and thus can affect the magnitude of the internal load required to support the external load. The arrangement of the lever system could influence the magnitude of the external moment imposed on the body as well as dictate the magnitude of the internal forces and the subsequent risk of either acute or cumulative trauma. If one considers the biomechanical arrangement of the spine (shown in Fig. 6.3c) it is evident that the magnitude of the internal force generated within the back musculature is defined by the location of the external load relative to the spine. If the horizontal distance between the load and the spine was reduced to half (by reorienting the load location), the internal force necessary to support the external load would be *reduced* by 2220 N or nearly 500 lb. Hence, the positioning of the mechanical lever system (which can be accomplished through work design) can greatly affect the internal load transmission within the body. A task can be performed in a variety of ways, but some of these positions are much more costly than others in terms of loading of the musculoskeletal system. Thus, the simplest way to reduce loads on the spine's tissues is to simply rearrange the work so that the moment relative to the spine is reduced.

6.2.2   Length–Strength Relationship

Another important relationship that influences the load on the musculoskeletal system is the length–strength relationship of the muscles. This relationship is shown in Fig. 6.4. The active

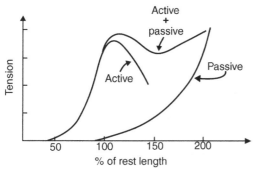

Figure 6.4 Length–tension relationship for a human muscle. (Adapted from Basmajian JV, De Luca CJ. Muscles Alive: Their Functions Revealed by Electromyography. 5th ed., Baltimore (MD): Williams and Wilkins; 1985.)

portion of this figure refers to active force generating structures such as muscles. When muscles are at their resting length (generally seen in the fetal position), they have the greatest capacity to generate force. However, when the muscle length deviates from this resting position, the muscle's capacity to generate force is greatly reduced because the crossbridges (portion of the muscle fiber capable of generating force) between the components of the muscle proteins become inefficient. When a muscle stretches or when a muscle attempts to generate force while at a short length the ability to generate force is greatly diminished. As indicated in Fig. 6.4, the passive tissues in the muscle can also generate tension when muscles are stretched. Thus, the length of a muscle during task performance can greatly influence the force available to perform work and can influence risk by altering the available internal force within the system. Therefore, what might be considered a moderate force for a muscle at the resting length can become the maximum force a muscle can produce when it is in a stretched or contracted position, thus increasing the risk of muscle strain. When this relationship is considered in combination with the mechanical load placed on the muscle and tendon (via the arrangement of the lever system), the position of the joint arrangement becomes a major factor in the design of the work environment. Typically, the length–strength relationship interacts synergistically with the lever system. The joint position can have a dramatic effect on force generation and can greatly affect the internal loading of the joint and the subsequent risk of cumulative trauma. Therefore, positioning workers with their back muscles near their resting length will minimize muscle force, fatigue, and risk of overexertion.

6.2.3   The Impact of Velocity on Muscle Force

Motion can also influence the ability of a muscle to generate force and, therefore, load the biomechanical system. Motion can be a benefit to the biomechanical system if momentum is properly employed or it can increase the load on the system if the worker is not taking advantage of momentum. This relationship between muscle velocity and force generation is shown in Fig. 6.5. The figure indicates that, in general, the faster the muscle is shortening (as when lifting), the greater the reduction in force capability of the muscle. This reduction in muscle capacity can result in the muscle strain that may occur at a lower level of external loading and a subsequent increase in the risk of cumulative trauma. Also note that Fig. 6.5 indicates that force generation can increase when a muscle lengthens (as when lowering). Since the vast majority of work involves motion, many of the contemporary biomechanical models now include the effect of dynamic motion.

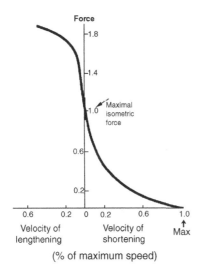

Figure 6.5 Influence of velocity on muscle force. (Adapted from The Textbook of Work Physiology. McGraw-Hill; 1977.)

6.2.4 Temporal Relationships

Strength Endurance: Strength must be considered as both an internal force as well as a tolerance. However, it is important to realize that strength is transient. A worker may generate a great amount of strength during a one-time exertion; however, if the worker is required to exert their strength either repeatedly or for a prolonged period, the amount of force that the worker can generate can be reduced dramatically, resulting in an increase in fatigue and a decrease in the strength tolerance limit. Figure 6.6 demonstrates this relationship. The dotted line in this figure indicates the maximum force generation capacity of a static exertion over time. Maximum force is only generated for a very brief period. As time advances, strength output decreases exponentially and levels off at about 20% of maximum after about 7 min. Similar trends occur during repeated dynamic conditions with different rest times between exertions as indicated in the solid lines in Fig. 6.6. If a task requires a large portion of a

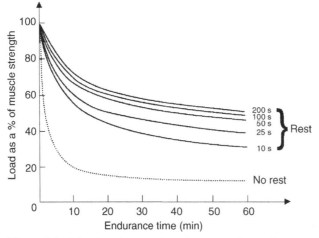

Figure 6.6 Muscle endurance times in consecutive static contractions of 2.5 s duration with varied rest periods. (Adapted from Chaffin DB, Andersson GB. Occupational Biomechanics. New York (NY): John Wiley & Sons, Inc.; 1991).

worker's strength, one must consider how long the magnitude of strength must be exerted to ensure that the work does not strain the musculoskeletal system.

Rest time: As we have already observed, the risk of cumulative trauma increases when the ability of the worker to produce force is exceeded by a task's force requirements, thus resulting in fatigue and lowering of tolerance. Another factor that may influence strength capacity (and tolerance to muscle strain) is rest time. Rest time has a profound affect on a worker's ability to exert force. Energy for a muscular contraction is regenerated during work. Adenosine triphosphate (ATP) is required to produce a power-producing muscular contraction. ATP changes into adenosine diphosphate (ADP) once a muscular contraction occurs; however, the ADP is not capable of producing a significant muscular contraction. The ADP must be converted back to ATP to enable another muscular contraction. This conversion occurs with the addition of oxygen to the system. If oxygen is not available, the system goes into oxygen debt and insufficient ATP is available for a muscular contraction. This process is discussed in an earlier chapter (Fig. 4.8) where it is indicated that oxygen is a key ingredient to maintain a high level of muscular exertion. Oxygen is delivered to the target muscles via the blood. Under static exertions, the blood flow is reduced and blood available to the muscle is subsequently reduced. This restriction of blood flow and subsequent oxygen deficit is responsible for the rapid decrease in force generation (muscle strength) over time as shown in Fig. 6.6. The solid lines in Fig. 6.6 indicate that the force-generation capacity of the muscles increases when different amounts of rest are permitted during a prolonged exertion. As more rest time is permitted, increases in force generation are achieved as more oxygen is delivered to the muscle and more ADP can be converted back to ATP. This relationship indicates that any more than about 50 s of rest, under these conditions, does not result in a significant increase in force-generation capacity of the muscle. Practically, this relationship indicates that to optimize the strength capacity of the worker and minimize the risk of muscle strain, a schedule of frequent and brief rest periods would be more beneficial than lengthy infrequent rest periods.

6.3 INCORPORATING SPINE LOAD REDUCTIONS INTO THE WORK SYSTEM

This discussion has shown that if the goal of work design is to minimize the impact of physical risk factors on the risk of low back pain, there are several principles that one can work with to accomplish this goal. Hence, by adjusting the work positions and components of the work for a person in the workplace, we are able to influence spine loading by considering the biomechanical lever system arrangement, the velocity of the motions, muscle length, and the temporal relationships inherent to the work (work–rest cycles, rest time, and exertion duration). The key to proper work design involves developing an appreciation for how these factors can influence spine loads collectively and considering the trade-offs between these factors in a work system.

6.4 LOADING OF THE LUMBAR SPINE

Forces or loads are imposed on the lumbar spine in response to events and tasks performed by the person. The summary of the various forces imposed on the spine during an activity can be represented by a singe force vector with magnitude and directional components. This summary is useful for comparing the overall loading of the spine under different work conditions. However, to assess the biomechanical *risk* of an activity, one must compare the

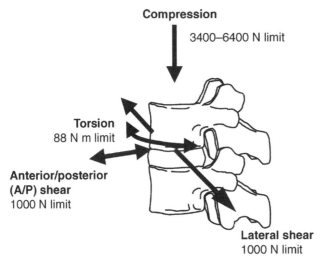

Figure 6.7 Summary of load dimensions for the lumbar spine.

forces imposed on the spine in the different dimensions of loading with the different tolerances associated with each dimension. This comparison can be done on a tissue by tissue-level comparison using the tolerance limits discussed in Chapter 5, or it can occur at a more general level where the collective tissue tolerances in each direction of loading are considered. This latter approach is more common in most work-oriented biomechanical models and will be discussed here.

The nature of spine loading can be summarized by several types of loads acting on the spine: (1) axial forces that either apply compression or tension upon the spine along its longitudinal axis; (2) lateral loads imposing shear forces on the spine from side to side; (3) anterior–posterior (A/P) shear forces that load the spine in the forward and backward direction; and (4) torsional forces that twist the spine. These forces are shown graphically in Fig. 6.7 along with the generally accepted tolerance limits for physical damage to the tissues. The spine is relatively strong in compression and thus has a fairly high tolerance limit. However, the spine can be toppled very easily when lateral (shear) forces are imposed. Hence, tolerance to shear loading is rather low. The specific tolerances to these loads in the various directions of loading are discussed in detail in Chapter 5.

6.5 SPINE LOAD ASSESSMENTS

An important component of evaluating the load–tolerance relationship and the potential risk associated with work is an accurate and realistic assessment of the loading experienced by a tissue. The tolerance literature suggests that it is important to understand the specific nature of the tissue loading including factors such as compression force, shear force in multiple dimensions, load rates, positions of the spine structures during loading, frequency of loading, and so on. Thus, *accurate and specific* information about loading is essential if one is to use this information to assess potential risk associated with occupational tasks.

Presently, it is infeasible to directly monitor the loads imposed on the spine structures and tissues while workers are performing an occupationally related task in the workplace. Instead, indirect means such as biomechanical models are typically used to estimate loading. All biomechanical models attempt to evaluate how exposure to external loads results in internal forces that may exceed tolerance limits. External forces (due to gravity or inertia) must be overcome by the worker to do work. Internal forces (e.g., muscles, ligaments, etc.) must supply counterforces to support the external load. It is this relationship that is the focus of biomechanical models of the spine. The key to accurate and realistic biomechanical models it to understand how the reaction of the internal forces behaves in response to work. Several approaches to biomechanical modeling have been used for these purposes resulting in different trade-offs between their ability to realistically assess spine loading associated with a task and ease of model use.

6.6 MODELS OF SPINE LOAD

In general, models should not be unnecessarily complex. Models must be only as complex as necessary to achieve the goals of the model. This concept has driven the development of biomechanical spine models over the years. Early models were extremely simple and assessed spine loads in a very gross manner. However, as the body of knowledge expanded and researchers discovered the complexity of the tissue tolerances of the spine, it soon became clear that more complete and accurate models of the workplace were necessary to assess the risk in the workplace.

Static models: The first models used to assess spine loading during occupational tasks were reported in the 1970s. Early models of spine loading made assumptions about which trunk muscles (internal forces) supported the external load held in the hands during a lifting task (3–5). These models are classified as single-equivalent muscle models since they assumed that a single muscle vector within the trunk could summarize the internal supporting force (and spine loading) required to counteract an external load lifted by a worker. The model assumes that a lift could be represented by a static equilibrium lifting situation and that no muscle coactivation occurs among the trunk musculature during lifting. The models often employed anthropometric regression relationships to estimate body segment lengths representative of the general population.

Two output variables were predicted with these early models that were used in a load-tolerance assessment of work exposure. The model's first output is spine compression and typically is compared to the compression limits of 3400 and 6400 N. The second model output was population static strength of six joints. L5/S1 joint strength is used to assess overexertion risk to the back. The model has evolved into a personal computer based model and is typically used for general assessments of materials handling tasks involving slow movements (where motion is insignificant) where excessive compression loads are suspected of contributing to risk. An example of the computer program is shown in Fig. 6.8. The model can be linked to field observations by videotaping a lifting task and recording the weight of the object lifted. Early risk assessments of the workplace have used this method to assess spine loads on the job (6).

During the 1980s, biomechanical models were expanded to account for the contribution of multiple internal muscles' reactions in response to the lifting of an external load. Much of the spine tolerance literature at this time was beginning to recognize the significance of three-dimensional spine loads as compared to using only compression loads in defining potential risk. This resulted in biomechanical models that predicted compression forces as well as shear forces imposed on the spine. The first functional multiple muscle system model proposed for material handling assessments (7) demonstrated how loads manipulated outside the body could impose large spinal loads due to the *coactivation* of several trunk muscles needed to counterbalance the external load (Fig. 6.9). The modeling approach represented much more realism than previous models; however, the approach resulted in

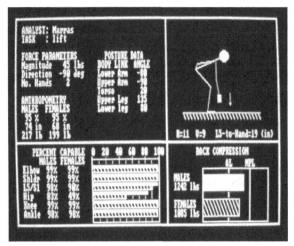

Figure 6.8 Examples of single-equivalent muscle model computer models developed by D.B. Chaffin. (a) The first biomechanical computer model was two dimensional and used to assess low back risk due to manual materials handling; later developments of the model permitted three-dimensional static loading analyses.

indeterminant (unsolvable and not unique) model solutions since there were more muscles forces represented in the model than functional relationships available to uniquely solve the problem. To overcome this problem, modeling efforts made assumptions about which muscles should be active during a task (7–9). These efforts resulted in models that worked well for static representations of a lift but not necessarily for dynamic lifting situations where greater cocontractions of the trunk muscles were common (10).

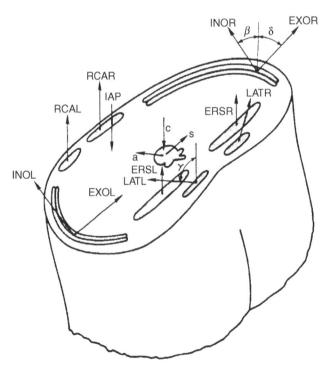

Figure 6.9 Cross-sectional view of the human trunk at the lumbrosacral junction. (Adapted from reference 7).

These early models provided reasonable approximations of muscle recruitment and the subsequent spine loads when evaluating static postures, since a steady-state static posture typically involved little muscle cocontraction. However, they did not work well for realistic tasks that involved dynamic, complex work movements since the models were unable to determine which muscles or combination of muscles were involved in the support of the changing external load (due to the indeterminacy of the model solution).

These models were unable to resolve the muscle recruitment pattern of the muscles and were unable to account for the rapid changes in muscle activity that occurred due to movement. Since understanding of trunk muscle reactions to the external environment is the key to accurate assessment of spine loading, it soon became clear that more complex, dynamic models were essential to understand how the physical aspects of work influenced low back loading in the workplace.

Dynamic models: To overcome the problem of predicting the recruitment pattern of multiple trunk muscles during a realistic, dynamic work activity, later efforts attempted to directly monitor muscle responses and use this information as input to biomechanical models. These "biologically assisted" models have the advantage of directly monitoring the activity of the internal force producing muscles in the trunk and eliminate the need to predict how the muscles would behave under complex, dynamic loading conditions. These biologically assisted models typically used electromyography (EMG) to assess muscle recruitment and this became the input to multiple muscle models. EMG eliminated the problem of indeterminacy since specific muscle activities were uniquely defined through the neural activation of each muscle. Since these biologically assisted models are unique to the response of an individual's muscles, they were not only able to accurately assess spine compression and shear loads for a specific occupationally related movements (11–19), but were also able to document differences in muscle activation patterns. These unique muscle activation differences allowed one to assess the resultant differences in spine loading between individuals performing the same task. EMG-assisted models also made it possible to assess how a worker would respond to psychological stress since the muscle's reactions were directly monitored in response to any type of physical as nonphysical stress.

Using this modeling approach, variations in loading among a population could be assessed (20–27). Validation measures suggest that these models have excellent external as well as internal validity (15,20,28). The scientific literature (29) demonstrated the importance of accounting for trunk muscle coactivation when assessing spine loading and found that not accounting for coactivation could results in miscalculation of spinal loading by up to 70%.

The advantage of biologically assisted models is that they are able to account for how the body responds to realistic dynamic complex exertions. This not only provides a much more realistic assessment of the magnitude and nature of loads experienced by the spine but also provides insight into the tension profile of each power-producing muscle surrounding the spine. By examining trunk muscle cocontractions as well as the force–time history of individual muscles, we are able to gain insight into muscle function disruption-based low back pain.

The disadvantage of biologically assisted models is that they require EMG recordings from multiple muscle sites while the worker is performing their work tasks. Because of the large amount of instrumentation needed to perform such analyses, it is often difficult or not feasible to execute these analyses at the workplace (see Fig. 6.10). Therefore, many of these studies have been performed while simulating work conditions under laboratory conditions. A number of studies have employed EMG-assisted modeling to assess specific aspects of the work that may be common to many work conditions. Several efforts used EMG-assisted models to assess three-dimensional spine loading during materials handling activities (12,26,30–33).

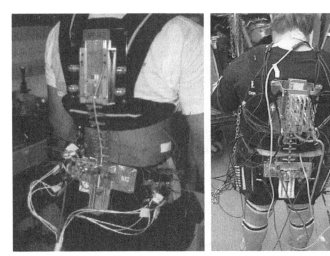

Figure 6.10 Examples of instrumentation (position sensors, muscle sensors, and lumbar motion monitors) required as input to EMG-assisted models. Such instrumentation is feasible for laboratory analyses but difficult to utilize in the work environment.

6.7 BIOLOGICALLY DRIVEN MODELING OF SPINE LOADING

Over the past 20 years, continuing efforts have refined and improved biologically assisted (EMG-assisted) biomechanical models that are capable of accurately assessing dynamic spine loading of a specific individual in response to occupational tasks (11–19,27,34–48). The model developed in the Biodynamics Laboratory at the Ohio State University has evolved into a modeling tool that is sensitive enough to distinguish differences in spine loading patterns among different individuals due to differences in body dimensions, task exertion technique, experience, back health status, and personal factors. The results of the studies using this model are reported in forthcoming chapters; however, the model logic is described here.

The model assumes that if two imaginary planes were passed horizontally through the lower lumbar spine and the upper lumbar spine, all the major power-producing muscles that support the spine and load the spine would be identifiable and would transcend these two planes (see Fig. 6.11a). The advantage of this two-plane representation is that if one is able to track the movement of these two planes relative to one another, then the model would be capable of accounting for dynamic motion including differences in torso muscle lengths. This figure indicates that if we know the force magnitude and relative locations of the muscle force vectors that connect these two planes relative to the spinal column, we can then predict the mechanical advantage that each muscle force has relative to the spine, then sum the forces in each direction of force and derive the compression, shear, and torsional forces acting on the spine.

The key to accurately predicting the force imposed on the spine lies in an accurate understanding of muscle force interpretation. The force generated from each muscle shown in Fig. 6.11 is governed by the following Equation 6.1:

$$\text{Force}_j = \text{Gain}_j \frac{\text{EMG}_j(t)}{\text{EMGmax}_j} \cdot \text{Area}_j \cdot f(\text{vel}_j) \cdot f(\text{length}_j) \tag{6.1}$$

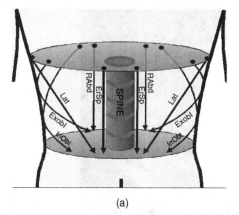

(a)

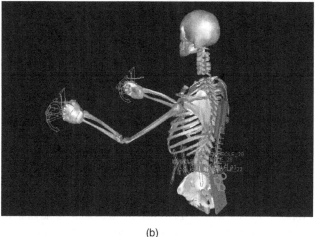

(b)

Figure 6.11   (**a**) Trunk mechanics logic underlying the OSU biodynamic EMG-assisted biomechanical model assumes that all forces acting on the lumbar spine can be identified by forces acting between the two imaginary transverse planes passed through the lumbar spine. (**b**) Measures of the external load (in this case hand forces) and trunk muscle vectors representing the internal forces imposing load on the spine. (The current model was recently embedded in the MSc. ADAMS Software environment (MSc. Software, Inc). and utilizes the lifemod (Biomechanics Research Group, Inc.) biomechanical overlay.)

This equation indicates that the force for a given muscle can be derived from the product of (1) the gain or force generation capacity of the muscle (in N/cm^2), (2) the relative (%) activity level of the muscle (EMG activity of a task relative to the maximum EMG activity possible for the muscle), (3) the cross-sectional area of the muscle, (4) the velocity of the muscle, and (5) the length of the muscle. In determining the muscle force, the product of the gain and the cross-sectional area define the upper limit of force generation possible from the muscle during muscle shortening (as in lifting). This maximum possible force is then mediated by the relative activation level of the muscle defined by the relative (%) EMG activity level, the velocity at which the muscle is moving (Fig. 6.5), and the instantaneous length of the muscle during the exertion (Fig. 6.4).

Muscle cross-sectional area was determined from MRI scans of the lumbar spine (49). MRI images are examined and traced to represent the cross-sectional area of the muscles of interest (Fig. 6.12). The cross-sectional area must be corrected for fiber angle so that the force

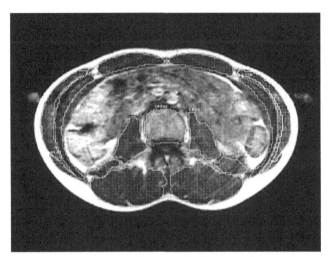

Figure 6.12   Cross-sectional representation of the torso muscles evaluated via MRI scans.

generation of the muscle is accurately represented. Male and female regression equations have also been derived on the basis of this data so that muscle cross-sectional area can be represented by easy-to-collect anthropometric data (49).

Muscle length and velocity characteristics have been derived through experimentation for extension of the torso (11,12), as well as for flexion activities (46). Muscle gain traditionally has been experimentally derived and set to a constant for a given subject. However, recent efforts have employed optimization techniques to derive different gain values for different muscles (50).

Once these muscle forces are assessed over the exertion of interest, then the instantaneous muscle force is multiplied by its respective mechanical advantage relative to the spine. Studies have employed MRI technology to precisely define the origin and insertion points of the power-producing muscles along the two imaginary planes utilized by the model (51). Figure 6.13a and b shows how the mechanical advantages of each muscle relative to the spine was derived in the sagittal and coronal planes, respectively. This study has also derived regression equations that have made possible the prediction of trunk muscle mechanical advantage from torso anthropometry.

Figure 6.14 shows the data collection portion of the model. The model simultaneously displays a video of the task of interest, trunk motion in three dimensions as measured using the lumbar motion monitor (LMM) (a tri-axial goniometer shown on the worker's back Fig. 6.10 and in the skeletal model in Fig. 6.11b to account for trunk muscle velocity and length), muscle activities, muscle forces, muscle coactivities, moments imposed on the spine

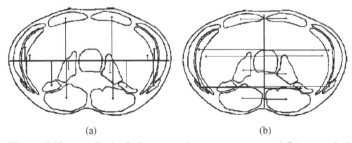

(a)   (b)

Figure 6.13   (a) Sagittal plane muscle moment arms and (b) coronal plane moment arms relative to the spine used to assess the mechanical advantage of the trunk muscles in the biomechanical model.

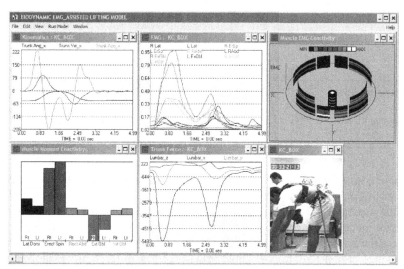

Figure 6.14   Data collection software of the EMG-assisted computer model able to simulate dynamic manual materials handling tasks.

and spinal forces. Using this Windows-based model, the influence of the dynamic task activities can be associated with the resultant spine loading and the external moments and specific muscle reactions that govern the spine loads. This model was able to assess three-dimensional spine loading at L5/S1 in response to dynamic sagittal, lateral, and torsional external loads (15).

There are no practical means to directly validate a biomechanical model in vivo since this would require load sensors to be implanted in the spine. However, models can be validated through indirect means by assessing the ability of the model to predict measures that one can feasibly record. Trunk moments have been selected as this measure. Measured and model predicted trunk moments are compared and must agree if the model is correctly simulating trunk mechanics. Statistical correlations between predicted and measured moment profiles serve as measures of model performance and indicate how well the model accounts for the variability in the dynamic moment. If the model accurately predicts applied moments about the spine, then the predicted spinal load must also be reasonable.

The biodynamic EMG-assisted biodynamic model has been tested and validated in several studies. Three studies have evaluated model sensitivity in each of the primary planes of movement. Each experiment was intended to test model robustness, independently, in each of the cardinal planes of the body. Three measures of performance and validity were used as criteria with which to evaluate model performance. First, for a model to be considered robust and accurate, it must precisely represent the *changes* in trunk and spine loading over time. The measure of performance that relates to changes in trunk loading during these trials is the correlation between predicted and measured (via the force plate) trunk moment as a function of time. The R^2 statistic indicating the relationship between measured trunk moment (via the force plate) and predicted trunk moment (via the EMG-assisted model) serves as an indication of the ability of the model to accurately assess the changes in dynamic trunk loading. This statistic is an indication of the robustness of the model and is sensitive to changes in shape of the trunk moment versus time curve generated by both the model and force plate during an experimental run. Second, a well-developed biomechanical model must accurately estimate the *magnitude* of trunk load during a lifting trial. By comparing the measured and predicted magnitude of external load imposed on the spine (moment), we can evaluate the magnitude of the error inherent in the model. The statistic employed to indicate

TABLE 6.1 Summary of Trunk Loading Conditions and Model Validity Measures in the Three Cardinal Planes of the Body

Motion plane	# Trials	Loads supported (kg)	Trunk velocity (°/s)	R^2 (Avg)	AAE (N m)	Gain N/cm^2
Forward bending (sagittal plane)	703	0, 18.2, 36.4	0,30,60,90 + free dynamic	0.89	<15	47
Lateral bending (frontal plane)	574	13.6, 27.3	0,15,30,45	0.91	6–10	64
Twisting (transverse plane)	320	Max, 50% max	0,10,20	0.80	N/A	35

this quantity was the average absolute error (*AAE*) between the measured moment and the predicted trunk moment during a lifting trial. Finally, a realistic biomechanical model should reflect biomechanical and physiological plausibility. This plausibility is often reflected by comparing model predicted parameters to the limits described in the physiological literature. Predicted muscle *gain* provides a good measure of this physiologic feasibility. The literature (52–54) suggests that muscle gain should be between 30 and 100 N/cm^2. Estimates of muscle gains above this limit would suggest an infeasible model.

Table 6.1 summarizes the experimental parameters and model validity performance measures for each of the three experiments. This summary indicates that the model has been thoroughly tested over a variety of occupationally relevant conditions (55,56). The analysis also shows that the model performance is well within acceptable performance limits for accuracy as well as biomechanical plausibility. Current model improvements have further improved performance.

Even though this analysis does not provide direct validity of the model (which never could be provided for ethical reasons), collectively, these trends provide independent assurances that at least the changes observed in model performance have relevance to observed risk in industry.

Recent model advances have significantly expanded the capabilities of this model. The model is now capable of assessing the three-dimensional loads imposed on each functional spinal unit from L1 to S1. The model represents the worker via a skeletal figure and can indicate disk forces by a vector at each lumbar disk level (see Fig. 6.15). These vector

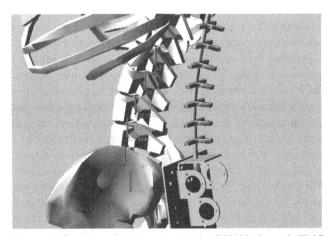

Figure 6.15 Recent improvements to the OSU biodynamic EMG-assisted biomechanical model permit assessment of tissue loading at each level of the spine from L1 to S1. (The current model was recently embedded in the MSc. ADAMS Software environment (MSc. Software, Inc.) and utilizes the lifemod (Biomechanics Research Group, Inc.) biomechanical overlay.)

representations respond instantaneously to any external load. In addition, the model can assess the load distribution of forces through the ligaments of the spine, the muscles, and the contact forces acting on the facet joints.

Once the loads imposed on the spine tissues during a task are evaluated, it is possible to predict changes in spine tolerance over time for particular spine tissues. Tissue tolerance is assessed by way of a finite-element model (FEM) embedded within the model as shown in Fig. 6.16. This model represents tissues as small triangular (tetrahedral) elements that can deform over repeated loading. In this manner, it is possible to assess the impact of continued spine loading over long periods such as months and years and determine which structures will fail and in how much time.

Hence, these models may soon be able to predict the physical change in the tissue due to cumulative trauma over the course of many years. These efforts have resulted in some of the most accurate and task-specific prediction of spine loading to date.

The most recent advances in the Ohio State University biodynamic model has permitted the import of specific worker images into the model. It is possible to import the specific anatomic images of a worker's spine into the model via CT or MRI imaging. By using the worker's specific anatomic geometry in conjunction with the worker's specific muscle activation patterns (via EMG), it is possible to uniquely build a worker-specific model for a specific individual. Figure 6.17 shows the results of such a model for a spinal segment for a specific individual. Note the difference in the geometry of the vertebral segments compared to the idealized representations shown in Fig. 6.15. This type of specificity makes it possible to evaluate loads on specific tissues such as ligaments (numbers in Fig. 6.17) and contact forces among the posterior elements of the spine (arrows in Fig. 6.17) as well as end plate stressors (light and dark structures at the top and bottom of the disk) for a particular individual. While this model is still under development, it is expected that this model will be able to account for variability in spinal loads under work conditions by accounting for the unique individual characteristics of different workers exposed to similar work conditions.

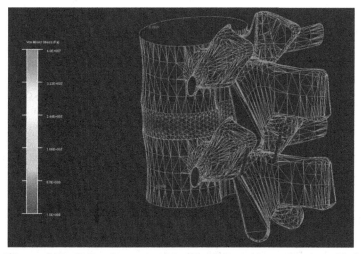

Figure 6.16   Finite-element model of the disk used in conjunction with the biodynamic EMG-assisted biomechanical model that make it possible to assess disk degeneration over time. (The model was developed using MSC. PATRAN, MSC. NASTRAN, and MSC. ADAMS (MSC. Software, Inc.))

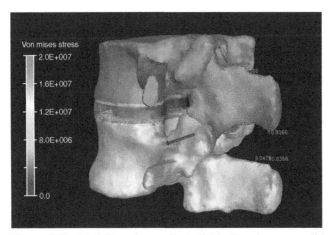

Figure 6.17   Modeling of a specific individual's spine accomplished by importing an image of a worker's spine into the EMG-assisted biomechanical model. The image shows ligament loads (represented by numbers in the figure), contact forces among the posterior elements of the spine (represented via arrows), and end plate stressors via finite-element modeling (light and dark structures at the top and bottom of the disk). (The model was developed using MSC. PATRAN, MSC. NASTRAN, and MSC. ADAMS (MSC. Software, Inc.))

6.8   STABILITY-DRIVEN SPINE LOADING MODELS

Stability refers to the ability of a system or structure to remain in balance and, therefore, minimize the chances that the structure will collapse, topple, or move in such a manner that it will damage tissue. Clinical spinal instability has been defined as "the loss of the spine's ability to maintain its patterns of displacement under physiologic loads so there is no initial or additional neurologic deficit, no major deformity, and no incapacitating pain" (57). In other words, the idea behind instability is that if the spinal column is not properly supported or stable, there is a risk that one of the vertebral bodies might become ill aligned and push against a nerve, stretch a ligament, push against a muscle, or in some way cause a disruption in the system that would stimulate nociceptors and lead to pain. In biomechanics, stability refers to the ability of the musculoskeletal control system to respond to a perturbation and reestablish a state of equilibrium of the spine after a perturbation. Spine stability is determined by the net stiffness, damping, and inertia of the torso. During instability, the mechanical balance or stability of the spine system becomes disrupted. Instability can result in spine structure displacement (e.g., unnatural vertebral movement), and this displacement may lead to damage and inflammation of pain-sensitive tissues. Such events have been documented during extreme physical exertions (58) and there is little doubt that instability is a potential mechanical pathway leading to low back pain.

Stability can be important from a biomechanical standpoint for two reasons. First, proper assessment of spine stability might be able to predict when tissues might be at risk of overload and damage due to unstable conditions. Second, it has been hypothesized that this principle might dictate the recruitment pattern of the trunk musculature during an exertion. Thus, stability measures might be able to describe how muscles are recruited and may provide muscle recruitment information to biomechanical models of the spine, thereby providing an alternative to equipment intensive EMG-assisted modeling approaches.

There are two types of stability conditions. Static stability refers to the ability of the spine to return to its original position after a perturbation. Dynamic stability refers to the ability of the system to reestablish a path of movement after a perturbation and is much more common during work. While several researchers have been able to describe static stability in the torso, none have been able to predict dynamic stability behavior (20,37,59–67). Unstable biomechanical systems can initiate tissue damage when the system is out of balance so that excessive forces are imposed on tissues or when the musculoskeletal system overcompensates for a perturbation. When the musculature cannot offer adequate support to a joint (due to improper muscle recruitment, fatigue, structure laxity, or weakness), the structure may move abnormally and create excessive forces on a tissue.

The mechanisms of the stability process within the human are generally not well understood. Figure 6.18 shows a proposed process by which some believe spine stability is achieved in the human body (68). For stability, one must monitor or perceive their position in the world (circle 1 in Fig. 6.18) and compare this with what would be required to perform a task (circle 2). Continuous adjustments are made between the muscle and tendon forces generated and achieved until the system achieves steady state (circles 3–6). For achieving stability in this manner, risk of instability must be assessed and corrective actions must be performed in an extremely short period.

Several efforts have attempted to use stability as criterion to govern detailed biomechanical models of the torso (35,37,59,62,63,65,67–71). The work performed in this area to date has been directed toward static response of the trunk as well as sudden loading responses (37,60,62,63,65,72). While it is likely that some occupational low back pain occurs as a result of instability under static loading conditions, the cocontraction associated with instability corrections can increase spine loadings and lead to cumulative loading. In addition, prolonged muscle tension (resulting from cocontraction) might result in greater risk via the muscle function disruption pathways as opposed to the acute trauma pathway that is traditionally believed to be associated with instability-related muscle problems (Fig. 5.2). Thus, there can be trade-offs associated with stability-versus overexertion-related effects of instability. It has been hypothesized that instability increases risk and should be of more concern at low levels of loading, whereas overexertion pathway may represent a higher risk at higher levels of loading (Fig. 6.19) (69). However, the nature of work in industry is changing and these acute trauma pathways are believed to be less probable. Given the industry trend toward low force, high repetition jobs, one would speculate that the majority of occupationally related low back pain is more likely related to instability leading to cumulative loading of the spinal tissues.

One way in which the body controls for instability is through coactivation of the trunk muscles (67). As the structures of the spine become less taut and increase their laxity due to a loss of disk height, muscle fatigue, movements, or other causes, the chances of increasing

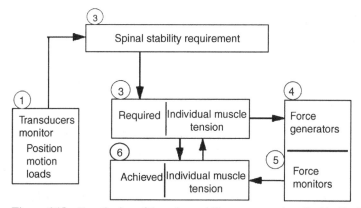

Figure 6.18 Functioning of the spine stability system as described by Panjabi. (From reference 68).

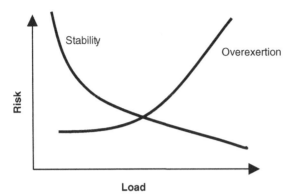

Figure 6.19 Trade-off between the ill effects of stability and overexertion as a function of load level under acute trauma conditions. (From reference 69).

instability increase and the chance of a mechanical disruption of the system increases. However, the body can naturally guard against instability by tensing the muscles surrounding the spine or cocontracting the trunk muscles. This coactive muscle tension is commonly observed in those suffering from low back pain. In addition, this coactivation pattern results in a disruption of the natural motion patterns of the spine (73,74) as well as increased spine loading (22,75).

In summary, there appear to be legitimate pathways between biomechanical loading and low back pain associated with instability. However, given the conditions of modern work, cumulative loading is more likely the mechanism of low back pain risk. Instability may play more of a role in the exacerbation of low back pain compared to the initial onset of the disorder.

6.8.1 Predictions of Muscle (Motor) Control within Torso

Since spine loading is primarily governed by the response of the internal force generators (mostly muscle activity) to the work conditions, several efforts have attempted to understand and predict how the muscles respond to particular occupational conditions. The literature has already shown how static models and stability models have difficulty predicting the role of the multiple muscles involved in dynamic activities. Therefore, much of the research has been in search of tools and techniques that would be able to accurately predict muscle activities in response to occupational conditions.

Several approaches to this objective have been attempted in the literature and include optimization, neural networks, fuzzy-neural modeling, and attempts to describe objective functions for the models. The muscle response patterns, also known as motor control, have been studied extensively over the last couple of decades and the study provide significant insight into the functioning of the back (45,76–89).

Descriptions of the trunk's motor control patterns showed how the motor patterns can change as a function of an individual's unique response patterns based on experience, personality, and so on, or it may change based on task demands. For example, Fig. 6.20 indicates the order in which trunk muscles and intra-abdominal pressure are recruited, peak in activity, and return to rest as a function of the speed of torso motion. As this figure indicates, significant differences in recruitment patterns (and the subsequent spine loading) occur as the torso motion increases in velocity.

Several attempts to use optimization to predict muscle involvement can be found in the literature (8,9,34,90–96). However, when the trunk is viewed as a realistic multiple muscle

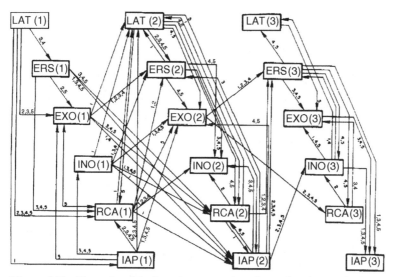

Figure 6.20 Example of the how the sequencing of muscles changes in the torso depending on the velocity requirements of the exertion. (98) (muscles: LAT = latissiums dorsi, ERS = erector spinae, EXO = external oblique, INO = internal oblique, and RCA = rectus abdominus; IAP represents intra-abdominal pressure; trunk velocities: 1 = isometric; 2 = 25%, 3 = 50%, 4 = 75%, and 5 = 100% of isokinetic capacity). (From reference 98).

system, there are more muscles involved in an exertion than functional descriptions of the forces acting on the system. This situation results in a statically indeterminate solution and suggests that there is no unique solution to the problem. Optimization has attempted to provide more constraints to the problem space; however, many of these constraints are boundary constraints that restrict the solution to above or below a certain limit. These solutions have been found to be non representative of actual trunk muscle recruitment behavior (97).

Others have attempted to describe motor control via neural networking techniques (44,45,99–102). As with the optimization approach, these techniques work reasonably well for static exertion conditions. However, they are more challenged in predicting dynamic activities of the torso.

One effort has attempted to describe muscle activities probabilistically (27). This effort developed a database that describes the muscle variability (for the major trunk muscles) in probabilistic terms for a given external force exertion (including trunk motion characteristics). Based on this database, a stochastic (probabilistic) model of trunk muscle activation was developed. The model was based on simulation of experimentally derived data and predicted the possible combination of time-dependent trunk muscle coactivities that could be expected given a set of trunk bending conditions. The simulations are then used as input to EMG-assisted biomechanical models to represent the range of spine loads that would be expected under occupational conditions. This modeling indicated that variability in trunk muscle force had little affect on spine compression but greatly influenced lateral (±90% of mean value) and anterior–posterior shear (±40% of mean value). Thus, this investigation showed that small variations in muscle forces can greatly influence shear loading of the spine and may be responsible for under-recognition of the spine during work tasks. This stochastic model of muscle force represents one method that has been able to "drive" biologically assisted models without actually monitoring EMG activity.

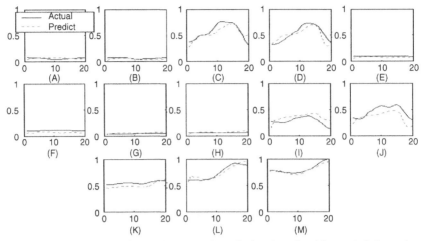

Figure 6.21 Examples of neurofuzzy EMG predictions based on kinematic information. (Courtesy of Y. Hou, J.M. Zurada, and W. Karwowski).

More recent efforts to predict multiple muscle patterns within the trunk under dynamic conditions have attempted to model muscle responses as a function of trunk kinematics using neuro-fuzzy modeling techniques (103,104). As with stochastic muscle modeling, this technique uses a database of kinematic and kinetic information as input to train an "engine" that predicts EMG activity. Figure 6.21 shows an example of how this model can generate time history of the EMG signal given dynamic trunk motion and load support information. This figure indicates that the techniques can indeed generate realistic time-dependent multiple muscle activities that match EMG activity for several diverse trunk motions. However, the engine must be offered a very large database of task activities performed in multiple dimensions of motion for it to resolve the specific activity of the various muscles. Much larger EMG databases are needed for this engine to generate the range of activities expected under the range of occupational conditions.

6.9 WHAT DRIVES MOTOR CONTROL? THE MENTAL MODEL

One of the reasons that motor control is so difficult to predict is that it represents motor control as a result of a dynamic, constantly updating, mental process that adapts and responds to the unique environmental conditions. Motor control is governed by motion control programs residing in the brain. One can think of this motion control program as a continuously updating computer program that calculates the amount of muscle force and the sequence of muscle recruitment (pattern) that is needed to successfully fulfill an exertion objective. The prediction pattern and muscle force magnitudes are estimated based on the current environmental conditions, predicted task demands based on the senses, feedback from muscles, the knowledge and experience of the person (training or pain), the timing requirements (speed requirements) of the task, and most likely several individual (genetic) factors (e.g., limits on contraction speed).

Thus, one of the reasons that muscle prediction is so difficult is that one is trying to quantitatively model the mental processing that occurs within a worker. The concept of a *mental model* has been considered by many cognitive scientists. Mental models help us understand how people build impressions of and respond to their surroundings. As stated by Don Norman (105) "…our conceptual models of the way objects work, events take place, or

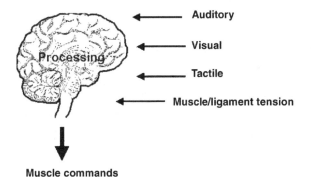

Muscle commands

Figure 6.22 Information synthesis involved in muscle recruitment. Input to the motor control processing system that results in muscle commands that increase stability through cocontraction.

people behave, result from our tendency to form explanations of things. These models are essential in helping us understand our experiences, predict the outcomes of our actions, and handle unexpected occurrences. We base our model on whatever knowledge we have, real or imaginary, naive or sophisticated." Thus, it is this mental model that dictates how we will respond to both physical and mental conditions.

The decision of which muscles to recruit and to what magnitude of muscle activity to recruit is dictated by judgment made by the motor control program based on a combination of the perception of the task requirements and the experiences of the individual from which the worker forms a mental model of the world. Figure 6.22 shows the types of information that are used by the human system to make decisions about muscle recruitment. This information involves not only tactile feedback from the extremities via Golgi tendon units in the muscles and ligaments but also visual and auditory feedback from the environment. This information is mediated by the individual's personality, experiences, and perceptions of the work. Thus, this filtered "expectation" drives muscle recruitment (muscle commands) via this mental model. It is this expectation that is optimized and satisfaction of the expectation is what drives the system. In fact, perhaps the only manner in which one can correctly model the recruitment of the muscles in such a dynamic system is to understand the person's objective of an activity at any given point in time (given the conditions). It is this cognitive objective under the given conditions that determines how and why the person will recruit their muscles in a given manner. For example, recruitment of muscles belonging to one with prior back pain would be expected to emphasize stability, whereas the recruitment pattern of an experienced worker would probably demonstrate little coactivation. Coactivation would be further governed by the intended pace of the task, the precision required, and the environmental conditions (e.g., surface conditions, noise, etc.).

Hence, one can hypothesize that knowledge of the person's condition and experiences, the work requirements, and the environment all combine to form a mental model of the situation. Through this mental model, we interpret the task objective that we are attempting to satisfy when we recruit muscles. This governing principle is known as the "satisfaction principle" and has been found to represent eye movement behavior well (106).

Given the complexity of this recruitment, it is unlikely that prediction models will reach the fidelity of biologically assisted models (i.e., EMG-assisted models) in the near future. Therefore, EMG-assisted models currently form the basis for accurate biomechanical assessments of the spine. These models help us appreciate the functioning of the musculo-skeletal system on the back until such a time as predictive models of muscle recruitment become accurate and reliable.

6.10   SUMMARY

It should be clear from this description that the central motor program or mental model acts as a filter to interpret cognitive and tactile information and respond with muscle activation signals that define the loading characteristics of the muscles and the spine structures. Any input into this mental model has the potential to alter the muscle patterns and loading pattern of the spine. Hence, the organization of this system provides clues as to how loading patterns of the spine and muscle tensions can be altered. It should be evident from this description that physical factors (that produce sensations in the muscles, ligaments, and tendons), cognitive impressions (shaped by visual and auditory information in the surroundings), former experiences, and the processing system (unique to the individual) all have the potential to define the loads experienced by the musculoskeletal system and, thus, also have the ability to mediate the loading of the musculoskeletal system. As can be seen, the mental model drives the motor control system and is the key to spine structure and trunk muscle loading. This is consistent with the logic of risk factors discussed in Chapter 1 (Fig. 1.2). Until predictions of trunk muscle recruitment become more accurate and reliable under realistic dynamic movement conditions, we must monitor the muscle recruitment patterns associated with various task performance parameters and a specific individual to understand spine loading. Since biologically assisted (EMG-assisted) biomechanical models directly assess muscle recruitment patterns, they provide a means to partition the contribution of physical work compared to personal factors and psychosocial and organizational factors via a series of controlled experiments.

KEY POINTS

- Biomechanical modeling allows one to consolidate one's logic regarding the functioning of the biomechanical system into a more understandable mechanism.
- Biomechanical models can quantify ªhow much exposure is too much exposure° to the external environment. This is performed by comparing the load imposed on a tissue to the (physical and biochemical) tolerance capacity of the tissue.
- The force-generating structures within the body (e.g., muscles) counteract the forces imposed on the body from outside the body (e.g., work).
- The response of the force-generating structures within the body (muscles) to the external environment determines the magnitude, direction, and timing of the load experienced by the spine tissues. Thus, it is extremely important to understand how the various trunk muscles behave during a task if an accurate assessment of spine forces is desired.
- Biomechanical modeling has evolved over the past 30 years. Modern models capable of measuring activity of the spectrum of trunk muscles are able to assess the response of the muscles to motion and dynamic loading and evaluate the load imposed on the various pain-initiating tissues of the spine and back structures.
- Although there have been many attempts to develop prediction models of muscle recruitment patterns within the trunk, none have been able to accurately predict muscle responses under the variety of dynamic conditions and environments to which the worker is exposed. However, probabilistic models and neuro-fuzzy models hold promise for accomplishing this goal.

- Muscle recruitment patterns and the resultant spine loading pattern are ultimately dictated by the manner in which the worker interprets the work environment. Physical and cognitive information is used to develop a ᵃmental modelᵒ of the workplace and muscle recruitment patterns (and spine loading) are a result of estimates of what is needed to achieve the goals of the work task. The mental model and resulting expectation is biased by perceptions of the work.

- Biologically assisted (EMG-assisted) models currently provide our best understanding of the functioning of the musculoskeletal control system and the loading of the spine in response to physical, organizational, and personal risk factors for back pain.

REFERENCES

1. KROEMER KHE. Biomechanics of the human body. In SALVENDY G, editor. Handbook of Human Factors. New York (NY): John Wiley & Sons, Inc.; 1987.
2. MCGILL SM. The biomechanics of low back injury: implications on current practice in industry and the clinic. J Biomech 1997;30(5):465–475.
3. CHAFFIN DB. A computerized biomechanical model: development of and use in studying gross body actions. J Biomech 1969;2:429–441.
4. CHAFFIN DB, BAKER WH. A biomechanical model for analysis of symmetric sagittal plane lifting. AIIE Trans 1970;2(1):16–27.
5. CHAFFIN DB, et al. A method for evaluating the biomechanical stresses resulting from manual materials handling jobs. Am Ind Hygiene Assoc J 1977;38 (12):662–675.
6. HERRIN GD, JARAIEDI M, ANDERSON CK. Prediction of overexertion injuries using biomechanical and psychophysical models. Am Ind Hygiene Assoc J 1986;47 (6):322–330.
7. SCHULTZ AB, ANDERSSON GB. Analysis of loads on the lumbar spine. Spine 1981;6(1):76–82.
8. BEAN JC, CHAFFIN DB, SCHULTZ AB. Biomechanical model calculation of muscle contraction forces: a double linear programming method. J Biomech 1988;21(1):59–66.
9. HUGHES RE, BEAN JC, CHAFFIN DB. Evaluating the effect of co-contraction in optimization models. J Biomech 1995;28(7):875–878.
10. MARRAS WS, KING AI, JOYNT RL. Measurement of loads on the lumbar spine under isometric and isokinetic conditions. Spine 1984;9(2):176–187.
11. GRANATA KP, MARRAS WS. An EMG-assisted model of loads on the lumbar spine during asymmetric trunk extensions. J Biomech 1993;26(12):1429–1438.
12. GRANATA KP, MARRAS WS. An EMG-assisted model of trunk loading during free-dynamic lifting. J Biomech 1995;28(11):1309–1317.
13. MARRAS WS, GRANATA KP. A biomechanical assessment and model of axial twisting in the thoracolumbar spine. Spine 1995;20(13):1440–1451.
14. MARRAS WS, GRANATA KP. Spine loading during trunk lateral bending motions. J Biomech 1997;30(7):697–703.
15. MARRAS WS, GRANATA KP. The development of an EMG-assisted model to assess spine loading during whole-body free-dynamic lifting. J Electromyogr Kinesiol 1997;7(4):259–268.
16. MARRAS WS, SOMMERICH CM. A three-dimensional motion model of loads on the lumbar spine: I. Model structure. Hum Factors 1991;33(2):123–137.
17. MARRAS WS, SOMMERICH CM. A three-dimensional motion model of loads on the lumbar spine: II. Model validation. Hum Factors 1991;33(2):139–149.
18. MCGILL SM. A myoelectrically based dynamic three-dimensional model to predict loads on lumbar spine tissues during lateral bending. J Biomech 1992;25 (4):395–414.
19. MCGILL SM, NORMAN RW. Partitioning of the L4–L5 dynamic moment into disc, ligamentous, and muscular components during lifting. Spine 1986;11(7):666–678.
20. GRANATA KP, MARRAS WS, DAVIS KG. Variation in spinal load and trunk dynamics during repeated lifting exertions. Clini Biomech (Bristol, Avon) 1999;14(6):367–375.
21. MARRAS W, et al. Spine loading as a function of lift frequency, exposure duration, and work experience. Clin. Biomech (Bristol, Avon) 2006;21(4):345–352.
22. MARRAS WS, et al. Spine loading characteristics of patients with low back pain compared with asymptomatic individuals. Spine 2001;26(23):2566–2574.
23. MARRAS WS, et al. The influence of psychosocial stress, gender, and personality on mechanical loading of the lumbar spine. Spine 2000;25(23):3045–3054.
24. MARRAS WS, DAVIS KG, JORGENSEN M. Spine loading as a function of gender. Spine 2002;27(22):2514–2520.
25. MARRAS WS, DAVIS KG, JORGENSEN M. Gender influences on spine loads during complex lifting. Spine J 2003;3(2):93–99.
26. MARRAS WS, GRANATA KP. Changes in trunk dynamics and spine loading during repeated trunk exertions. Spine 1997;22(21):2564–2570.

27. MIRKA GA, MARRAS WS. A stochastic model of trunk muscle coactivation during trunk bending. Spine 1993;18(11):1396–1409.

28. MARRAS WS, GRANTA KP, DAVIS KG. Variability in spine loading model performance. Clin Biomech (Bristol, Avon) 1999;14(8):505–514.

29. GRANATA KP, MARRAS WS. The influence of trunk muscle coactivity on dynamic spinal loads. Spine 1995;20(8):913–919.

30. DAVIS KG, MARRAS WS. Assessment of the relationship between box weight and trunk kinematics: does a reduction in box weight necessarily correspond to a decrease in spinal loading? [in process citation]. Hum Factors 2000;42(2):195–208.

31. DAVIS KG, MARRAS WS, WATERS TR. Reduction of spinal loading through the use of handles. Ergonomics 1998;41(8):1155–1168.

32. DAVIS KG, MARRAS WS, WATERS TR. The evaluation of spinal loads during lowering and lifting. Clin Biomec. (Bristol, Avon) 1998;13(3):141–152.

33. MARRAS WS, DAVIS KG. Spine loading during asymmetric lifting using one versus two hands. Ergonomics 1998;41(6):817–834.

34. CHOLEWICKI J, McGILL SM. EMG assisted optimization: a hybrid approach for estimating muscle forces in an indeterminate biomechanical model. J Biomecha 1994;27(10):1287–1289.

35. CHOLEWICKI J, McGILL SM. Mechanical stability of the in vivo lumbar spine: implications for injury and chronic low back pain. Clin Biomech (Bristol, Avon) 1996;11 (1):1–15.

36. CHOLEWICKI J, McGILL SM, NORMAN RW. Comparison of muscle forces and joint load from an optimization and EMG assisted lumbar spine model: towards development of a hybrid approach. J Biomech 1995;28 (3):321–331.

37. CHOLEWICKI J, SIMONS AP, RADEBOLD A. Effects of external trunk loads on lumbar spine stability. J Biomech 2000;33(11):1377–1385.

38. DAVIS KG. Interaction between biomechanical and psychosocial workplace stressors: implications for biomechanical responses and spinal loading, In Biodynamics Laboratory. Columbus, (OH): The Ohio State University; 2001.

39. MARRAS W, et al. Accuracy of a three dimensional lumbar motion monitor for recording dynamic trunk motion characteristics. Int J Ind Ergon 1992;9(1):75–87.

40. MARRAS WS. State-of-the-art research perspectives on musculoskeletal disorder causation and control: the need for an intergraded understanding of risk. J Electromyogr Kinesiol 2004;14(1):1–5.

41. MARRAS WS, DAVIS KG. A non-MVC EMG normalization technique for the trunk musculature: Part 1. Method development. J Electromyogr Kinesiol 2001;11(1):1–9.

42. MARRAS WS, DAVIS KG, MARONITIS AB. A non-MVC EMG normalization technique for the trunk musculature: Part 2. Validation and use to predict spinal loads. J Electromyogr Kinesiol 2001;11(1):11–18.

43. McGILL SM, NORMAN RW. Dynamically and statically determined low back moments during lifting. J Biomech 1985;18(12):877–885.

44. NUSSBAUM MA, CHAFFIN NB. Evaluation of artificial neural network modelling to predict torso muscle activity. Ergonomics 1996;39(12):1430–1444.

45. NUSSBAUM MA, MARTIN BJ, CHAFFIN DB. A neural network model for simulation of torso muscle coordination. J Biomech 1997;30(3):251–258.

46. THEADO EW. Modification of an EMG-Assisted Biomechanical Model: For Pushing and Pulling Applications. Columbus (OH): Ohio State University; 2003. p. 89.

47. THELEN DG, SCHULTZ AB, ASHTON-MILLER JA. Quantitative interpretation of lumbar muscle myoelectric signals during rapid cyclic attempted trunk flexions and extensions. J Biomech 1994;27(2):157–167.

48. THELEN DG, SCHULTZ AB, ASHTON-MILLER JA. Co-contraction of lumbar muscles during the development of time-varying triaxial moments. J Orthop Res 1995;13 (3):390–398.

49. MARRAS WS, et al. Female and male trunk geometry: size and prediction of the spine loading trunk muscles derived from MRI. Clin Biomech (Bristol, Avon) 2001;16(1):38–46.

50. PRAHBU J, MARRAS WS, MOUNT-CAMPBELL C. An investigation on the use of optimization to determine the individual muscle gains in a multiple muscle model. Clin Biomech (Bristol, Avon) 2007 (in review).

51. JORGENSEN MJ, et al. MRI-derived moment-arms of the female and male spine loading muscles. Clin Biomech (Bristol, Avon) 2001;16(3):182–193.

52. McGILL SM, NORMAN RW. Effects of an anatomically detailed erector spinae model on L4/L5 disc compression and shear. J Biomech 1987;20(6):591–600.

53. REID JG, COSTIGAN PA. Trunk muscle balance and muscular force. Spine 1987;12(8):783–786.

54. WEIS-FOGH T, ALEXANDER RM. The sustained power output from stiated muscle. In Scale Effects in Animal Locomotion. London: Academic Press; 1977. p. 511–525.

55. MARRAS WS, et al. Biomechanical risk factors for occupationally related low back disorders. Ergonomics 1995;38(2):377–410.

56. MARRAS WS, et al. The role of dynamic three-dimensional trunk motion in occupationally-related low back disorders. The effects of workplace factors, trunk position, and trunk motion characteristics on risk of injury. Spine 1993;18(5):617–628.

57. PANJABI MM. Clinical spinal instability and low back pain. J Electromyogr Kinesiol 2003;13(4): 371–379.

58. McGILL S. Low Back Disorders: Evidence-Based Prevention and Rehabilitation (Vol. XV). Champaign (IL): Human Kinetics; 2002. p. 295.

59. CHOLEWICKI J, McGILL S. Mechanical stability of the in vivo lumbar spine: implications for injury and chronic low back pain. Clin Biomech (Bristol, Avon) 1996;11 (1):1–15.

60. CHOLEWICKI J, POLZHOFER GK, RADEBOLD A. Postural control of trunk during unstable sitting. J Biomech 2000;33(12):1733–1737.

61. CHOLEWICKI J, et al. Delayed trunk muscle reflex responses increase the risk of low back injuries. Spine 2005;30(23):2614–2620.

62. CHOLEWICKI J, VANVLIET IJ. Relative contribution of trunk muscles to the stability of the lumbar spine during isometric exertions. Clin. Biomech. (Bristol, Avon) 2002;17(2):99–105.

63. GRANATA KP, ORISHIMO KF. Response of trunk muscle coactivation to changes in spinal stability. J Biomech 2001;34(9):1117–1123.

64. GRANATA KP, ROGERS E, MOORHOUSE K. Effects of static flexion–relaxation on paraspinal reflex behavior. Clin Biomech (Bristol, Avon) 2005;20(1):16–24.

65. GRANATA KP, WILSON SE. Trunk posture and spinal stability. Clin Biomech (Bristol, Avon) 2001;16 (8):650–659.

66. MCGILL S. Ultimate Back Fitness and Performance. Waterloo (Canada): Wabuno Publishers; 2004.

67. MCGILL SM, et al. Coordination of muscle activity to assure stability of the lumbar spine. J Electromyogr Kinesiol 2003;13(4):353–359.

68. PANJABI MM. The stabilizing system of the spine: Part I. Function, dysfunction, adaptation, and enhancement. J Spinal Disord 1992;5(4):383–389. discussion 397.

69. GRANATA KP, MARRAS WS. Cost-benefit of muscle cocontraction in protecting against spinal instability. Spine 2000;25(11):1398–1404.

70. PANJABI MM. The stabilizing system of the spine: Part II. Neutral zone and instability hypothesis. J Spinal Disord 1992;5(4):390–396. discussion 397.

71. SOLOMONOW M, et al. Biomechanics of increased exposure to lumbar injury caused by cyclic loading: Part 1. Loss of reflexive muscular stabilization. Spine 1999;24 (23):2426–2434.

72. GRANATA KP, ORISHIMO KF, SANFORD AH. Trunk muscle coactivation in preparation for sudden load. J Electromyogr Kinesiol 2001;11(4):247–254.

73. MARRAS WS, et al. The quantification of low back disorder using motion measures. Methodology and validation. Spine 1999;24(20):2091–2100.

74. MARRAS WS, WONGSAM PE. Flexibility and velocity of the normal and impaired lumbar spine. Arch Phys Med Rehabil 1986;67(4):213–217.

75. MARRAS WS, et al. Spine loading in patients with low back pain during asymmetric lifting exertions. Spine J 2004;4(1):64–75.

76. CALLAGHAN JP, MCGILL SM. Muscle activity and low back loads under external shear and compressive loading. Spine 1995;20(9):992–998.

77. PARNIANPOUR M, et al. 1988 Volvo award in biomechanics. The triaxial coupling of torque generation of trunk muscles during isometric exertions and the effect of fatiguing isoinertial movements on the motor output and movement patterns. Spine 1988;13(9):982–992.

78. CHANG AH, LEE WA, PATTON JL. Practice-related changes in lumbar loading during rapid voluntary pulls

79. PEREZ MA, NUSSBAUM MA. Lower torso muscle activation patterns for high-magnitude static exertions: gender differences and the effects of twisting. Spine 2002;27(12):1326–1335.

80. O'SULLIVAN PB, et al. Altered motor control strategies in subjects with sacroiliac joint pain during the active straight-leg-raise test. Spine 2002;27(1):E1–E8.

81. HODGES PW, RICHARDSON CA. Inefficient muscular stabilization of the lumbar spine associated with low back pain. A motor control evaluation of transversus abdominis. Spine 1996;21(22):2640–2650.

82. ALLISON GT, HENRY SM. The influence of fatigue on trunk muscle responses to sudden arm movements, a pilot study. Clin Biomech (Bristol, Avon) 2002;17 (5):414–417.

83. PERREAULT EJ, et al. Summation of forces from multiple motor units in the cat soleus muscle. J Neurophysiol 2003;89(2):738–744.

84. COWAN SM, et al. Simultaneous feedforward recruitment of the vasti in untrained postural tasks can be restored by physical therapy. J Orthop Res 2003;21 (3):553–558.

85. HOF AL. Muscle mechanics and neuromuscular control. J Biomech 2003;36(7):1031–1038.

86. MCGILL S, et al. Previous history of LBP with work loss is related to lingering deficits in biomechanical, physiological, personal, psychosocial and motor control characteristics. Ergonomics 2003;46(7):731–746.

87. KAVCIC N, GRENIER S, MCGILL SM. Determining the stabilizing role of individual torso muscles during rehabilitation exercises. Spine 2004;29(11):1254–1265.

88. HOWARTH SJ, et al. On the implications of interpreting the stability index: a spine example. J Biomech 2004;37 (8):1147–1154.

89. SILFIES SP, et al. Trunk muscle recruitment patterns in specific chronic low back pain populations. Clin Biomech (Bristol, Avon) 2005;20(5):465–473.

90. HUGHES RE, et al. Evaluation of muscle force prediction models of the lumbar trunk using surface electromyography. J Orthop Res 1994;12(5):689–698.

91. NUSSBAUM MA, CHAFFIN DB, RECHTIEN CJ. Muscle lines-of-action affect predicted forces in optimization-based spine muscle modeling. J Biomech 1995;28(4):401–409.

92. RASCHKE U, CHAFFIN DB. Support for a linear length–tension relation of the torso extensor muscles: an investigation of the length and velocity EMG-force relationships. J Biomech 1996;29(12):1597–1604.

93. GAGNON D, LARIVIERE C, LOISEL P. Comparative ability of EMG, optimization, and hybrid modelling approaches to predict trunk muscle forces and lumbar spine loading during dynamic sagittal plane lifting. Clin Biomech (Bristol, Avon) 2001;16(5):359–372.

94. STOKES IA, GARDNER-MORSE M. Muscle activation strategies and symmetry of spinal loading in the lumbar spine with scoliosis. Spine 2004;29(19): 2103–2107.

made while standing [in process citation]. Clin Biomech (Bristol, Avon) 2000;15(10):726–734.

95. van DIEEN JH, KINGMA I. Effects of antagonistic co-contraction on differences between electromyography based and optimization based estimates of spinal forces. Ergonomics 2005;48(4):411–426.

96. LI G, PIERCE JE, HERNDON JH. A global optimization method for prediction of muscle forces of human musculoskeletal system. J Biomech. 2006;39(3):522–529.

97. MARRAS WS. Predictions of forces acting upon the lumbar spine under isometric and isokinetic conditions: a model–experiment comparison. Int J Ind Ergon 1988;3(1):19–27.

98. MARRAS WS, REILLY CH. Networks of internal trunk-loading activities under controlled trunk-motion conditions. Spine 1988;13(6):661–667.

99. NUSSBAUM MA, CHAFFIN DB, MARTIN BJ. A back-propagation neural network model of lumbar muscle recruitment during moderate static exertions. J Biomech 1995;28(9):1015–1024.

100. ZURADA J, KARWOWSKI W, MARRAS WS. A neural network-based system for classification of industrial jobs with respect to risk of low back disorders due to workplace design. Appl Ergon 1997;28(1):49–58.

101. KINGMA I, et al. Lumbar loading during lifting: a comparative study of three measurement techniques. J Electromyogr Kinesiol 2001;11(5):337–345.

102. NUSSBAUM MA, CHAFFIN DB. Pattern classification reveals intersubject group differences in lumbar muscle recruitment during static loading. Clin Biomech. (Bristol, Avon) 1997;12(2):97–106.

103. LEE W, KARWOWSKI W, MARRAS WS. A neuro-fuzzy model for predicting EMG of trunk muscles based on lifting task variables. XIVth Triennial Congress of the International Ergonomics Association; San Diego (CA): Human Factors and Ergonomics Society; 2000.

104. LEE W, et al. A neuro-fuzzy model for estimating electromyographical activity of trunk muscles due to manual lifting. Ergonomics 2003;46(1–3): 285–309.

105. NORMAN D. The Design of Everyday Things. New York (NY): Basic Books; 1988.

106. ERLANDSON RF, FLEMING DG. Uncertainty sets associated with saccadic eye movements-basis of satisfaction control. Vision Res 1974;14(7):481–486.

CHAPTER 7

THE INFLUENCE OF PHYSICAL WORK FACTORS ON MUSCLE ACTIVITIES AND SPINE LOADS

*T*HIS CHAPTER *systematically describes how the physical components of the workplace can influence spine loading and can initiate the pain pathways described earlier. The chapter begins by reviewing the findings of several biomechanical-based industrial surveillance studies and showing how biomechanical factors increase the risk of low back pain reporting. Next, using the advanced models described in Chapter 6, the chapter reviews how the physical features of work can influence structure and tissue loading within the spine. Person-specific studies that have explored the influence of physical work factors and physical modifiers are included. These factors include load moment exposure, trunk motions, asymmetric loading, lateral and twisting motions, lift origin height, one-hand versus two-hand lifting, object lowering, cumulative exposure to loads, lift frequency, work exposure duration, experience, handle usage, lifting while leaning, team lifting, pushing, and seated work. The chapter concludes by evaluating the relationship between spine loading components and risk assessments in industrial environments.*

7.1 INTRODUCTION

This chapter describes how the physical aspects of work can impose loads on the spine and low back tissues that have the potential to activate the pain pathways described earlier. Over the past 30 years, numerous studies have attempted to define the role of physical work factors on the experience of low back pain. The physical work factors represented by these studies span the spectrum from seated work to heavy lifting. These studies have approached this issue from various perspectives, including psychophysical abilities, strength capacity, and biomechanical loading. Since the goal of this chapter is to review the influence of physical factors on the potential initiation of the pain pathway due to tissue stimulation, we will focus exclusively on quantitative biomechanical assessments that are capable of isolating load–response relationships associated with physical work tasks. Specifically, since both spine structure loading and trunk muscle forces can lead to pain, we will focus on biomechanical information that will help us assess the three-dimensional loading experienced by the spinal structures as well as the forces developed among the system of muscles that support the spine during work tasks. This is accomplished by reviewing both the industrial surveillance studies and laboratory studies.

7.2 INDUSTRIAL QUANTITATIVE SURVEILLANCE OF PHYSICAL EXPOSURE

Through quantitative industrial surveillance studies, it is possible to glean clues as to what specific biomechanical aspect of the work tend to be associated with greater reporting of low back pain. Several literature reviews based on industrial surveillance studies have reported increases in low back pain reporting when workers are exposed to the general categories of lifting or forceful movements, awkward postures, heavy physical work, and whole body vibration (1). However, these reviews are of limited utility in understanding the loading exposures to the muscles and structures of the spine since most studies do not have a high enough level of resolution to define a threshold level or zone above which low back pain becomes more prevalent in a dose–response fashion. In other words, many of the previous industrial surveillance studies have not been able to precisely describe "how much exposure is too much exposure" to risk factors.

The early literature has indicated that back health is not linearly related to exposure (2,3). As discussed previously, there appears to be a J-shaped function associated with low back pain risk and work exposure. These studies have indicated that moderate levels of tissue loading are most protective of low back pain. Extremely low levels of load exposure appear to increase risk moderately and extremely high levels of loading increase risk of low back pain by a large amount. These findings are most likely related to the change in tolerance levels or adaptation associated with loading of the spine structures. Moderate levels of loading probably initiate a training effect to increase the capacity and tolerance threshold of the individual. High levels of loading simply break down the tolerance of the individual quickly and increase risk. Low levels of load exposure most likely decrease capacity and tolerance threshold by accelerating the degeneration of the tissues. Hence, these observations indicate that there are probably ideal levels of physical exposure that, when considered along with worker conditioning, can optimize back health.

Biomechanically based industrial surveillance assessments are concerned primarily with collecting biomechanically meaningful information (exposure metrics) within occupational environments. While many assessments of occupationally related low back disorder risk have been reported in the literature, many of these assessments have not used exposure metrics that are useful in state-of-the art biomechanical assessments since they fail to properly quantify the physical risk factor exposure. This lack of quantification would mask or obscure any relationship between the physical factors and risk. For example, numerous studies (4–13) have found that lifting heavy loads are associated with an increased risk of low back pain. While these studies are useful from an epidemiologic standpoint to help establish the link between a particular class of exposures and risk, such gross categorical exposure metrics provide little insight into the causal pathway underlying the observation since the quality of the information is crude from a biomechanical standpoint. From a biomechanical perspective, a given external load can impose either large or small loads on the spine (internal forces) depending on the load's mechanical advantage relative to the spine (14). Therefore, to truly understand biomechanical loading, specific quantifiable exposure metrics that are meaningful in a biomechanical context are necessary. Only then can one address the issue of how much exposure to a biomechanical variable is too much exposure.

7.3   STRENGTH CAPACITY ASSESSMENTS OF WORK LOAD

If surveillance studies are to be useful in identifying thresholds of exposure for back health, they must increase the biomechanical resolution of the collected information by increasing the quantification of biomechanical exposure measures. Several epidemiologic or industrial surveillance studies meeting the biomechanical quality criteria have appeared in the literature and offer evidence that low back pain is related to exposure to physical work parameters on the job. One of the first studies exploring this relationship (2) involved a 1-year prospective study, where the load imposed on workers relative to the strength of the workers (called the lifting strength ratio or LSR) was assessed. This study found that "the incidence rate of low back pain (was) correlated with higher lifting strength requirements as determined by assessment of both the location and magnitude of the load lifted." These observations are consistent with overexertion based inflammatory pathways discussed in Chapters 4 and 5. The authors concluded that load lifting could be considered hazardous. It is important to note that this study suggested that not only load magnitude was significant in defining risk but load location was also important. Hence, this study indicates that the magnitude of the load as well as the orientation of the load relative to the person was a key in defining risk.

This evaluation also reported an interesting relationship between the frequency of exposure to lifts of different magnitude (relative to worker strength) and risk. They found that exposure to more often than 150 lifts per day had the highest incidence rate. The second highest incidence rate was observed for workers who lifted less frequently than 50 times a day. Finally, the lowest incidence rates were observed for workers lifting 50–150 times per day. This study reinforces the idea that load dose–response is non-linearly related to risk. The study also suggests that exposure to moderate lifting frequencies appeared to be protective, suggesting that an individual's conditioning can also play a role in risk.

Another noteworthy study involves an assessment where job demands were compared with worker's psychophysically defined strength capacity (15). The job demand definition considered load location relative to the worker, frequency of lift, and exposure time. Demands were considered for all tasks associated with a materials handling job. The jobs demands were compared to the strength capacity of the worker in a Job Severity Index (JSI). Part of the database was used for model formulation, while the other part was used for model validation. This study identified the existence of a JSI threshold above which the risk of low back injury increased. This study found that the "total direct injury expense for those working at the JSI levels above 1.5 (threshold) was about $60,000 per 100 full time employees (FTE) as compared with an injury expense of only $1000 per 100 FTE for those working at JSI levels of 1.5 or less."

In a combined retrospective–prospective epidemiologic study (16) performed over a 3-year period in five large industrial plants, 2934 material handling tasks associated with 55 jobs were assessed. They evaluated jobs using both the lifting strength ratio or LSR (that assesses strength demands compared to strength capacity) as well as estimates of absolute back compression forces. The LSR analysis revealed a positive correlation for back pain incidence rates as well as a positive relationship for other musculoskeletal disorder incidence rates. This study also employed a simple biomechanical model to estimate compressive loads on the back. They found that musculoskeletal injuries were twice as likely for predicted spine compression forces that exceeded 6800 N. The analyses also suggest that prediction of risk is best associated with the most stressful tasks (as opposed to indices that represent risk aggregation).

7.3.1   Static Analyses of Work Load

A case–control (case–referent) study of automobile assembly workers (17) evaluated all back pain cases in a facility over a 10-month period and compared these to referent employees that were randomly selected after review of medical records, interview, and examination. Job analyses were performed by analysts who were blinded to the case/referent status. This study was concerned with evaluating risk of back pain associated with nonneutral (nonupright standing) working postures. Postures associated with tasks performed by the workers who experienced back pain were compared to postures of those who did not report back pain. In addition, the study used a simple single-equivalent muscle static biomechanical model to predict spine compression of workers who reported low back pain compared with those who did not (17). Back pain was associated with those tasks that required moderate (21–45°) or severe (over 45°) forward flexion and trunk deviations in the lateral and twisting planes (of more than 20°). Figure 7.1 defines these postures. The risk of back pain increased when workers were exposed to multiple risky postures and increasing duration (more than 10% of cycle time) of these problematic postures. This indicates that risk increased as the portion of the duty cycle spent in the most severe postures increased.

No differences between those reporting back pain and back pain free workers were noted as a function of spine compression when assessed by this particular model. However, the study did note that many of the tasks required dynamic loading of the spine. Thus, this lack of biomechanical significance may simply indicate that a more sophisticated model was needed to assess spine loading under these conditions.

The predictive value of a formula that considers the combination of "easy to measure" static variables at the worksite was considered in an effort to assess risk of low back pain (18). In a surveillance study of 50 industrial jobs, the evaluation considered factors expected to be associated with spine loading, including horizontal load moment arm distance, heights of the lift, twisting angle, and lift frequency. These values defined an expected worker tolerance (identified by biomechanical, physiological, strength, or psychophysical limits) and were

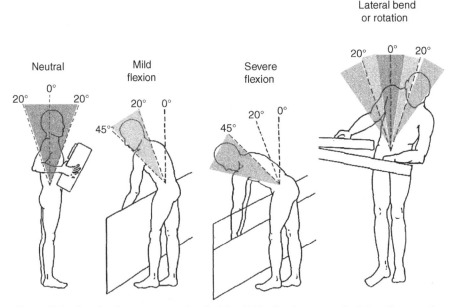

Figure 7.1   Sustained postures associated with mild (yellow) or severe (red) bending associated with more back pain reports. (Adapted from reference 17).

compared to the load lifted, defining a lifting index (LI). If the LI was found to be above 1.0, then risk was assumed to be present for at least some of the workforce. The results of this study indicated that as the LI increased the odds of back pain increased up until a LI of 3.0. However, above 3.0, the odds decreased. It should be pointed out that the number of observations for jobs having a LI above 3.0 was low (seven jobs). This study provided limited evidence that there is a relationship between load magnitude and risk up to a point (LI of 3.0). Hence, this study suggests that there is a limit to one's ability to assess low back pain risk due to the physical factors at the workplace when only using crude, non specific measures.

7.4   DYNAMIC ANALYSES OF WORK LOAD

A case–control study evaluated over 400 industrial jobs involving over 25 million worker-hours of exposure in nearly 50 different companies observed 114 workplace and worker-related variables in an effort to identify sources of low back pain risk (19,20). This study examined the characteristics of materials handling jobs that were associated with high rates of low back pain reporting ("high risk group" which averaged over one quarter of the workers reporting back pain each year) compared to materials handling jobs where workers did not report back pain ("low risk group" with zero reports per year). The differences in the exposure measures in these high risk low back pain jobs versus the low risk of low back pain jobs can be seen in Table 7.1. This table shows the complex nature of trunk motions associated with the workplace. Note that in the high risk jobs, workers generally produce much quicker trunk motions.

Exposure to load moment (load magnitude × distance of load from spine) distinguished between these two risk groups best. In fact, load moment was found to be the single most powerful predictor of low back disorder risk (Table 7.2). This study also examined trunk kinematics (movements) associated with the work tasks using a motion tracking system called the lumbar motion monitor or the LMM (Fig. 7.2) as well as traditional biomechanical variables in the workplace. This study identified 16 trunk kinematic variables resulting in statistically significant odds ratios associated with risk of low back pain in the workplace.

The results of this study indicated that risk of low back pain at work could not be characterized well by simply assessing one biomechanical variable. A multidimensional approach was needed to truly characterize risk. When load moment was considered in combination with several trunk kinematic variables associated with the task, the predictive power for low back pain increased significantly. While none of the single variables were as strong a predictor as load moment, when load moment was combined with three kinematic variables (relating to the three dimensions of trunk motion) along with an exposure frequency measure, a strong multiple logistic regression model resulted that described risk very well (odds ratio = 10.7). Thus, this study indicated that, from a biomechanical standpoint, risk was multidimensional in nature in that exposure to the combination of the five variables was needed to describe risk. Hence, for the prediction of risk, knowledge of load exposure magnitude is important, but to better understand the risk of low back pain, one needs to know how the workers were moving when they were exposed to these load moments.

The multidimensional risk information was incorporated into a multiple logistic regression risk model that could recognize the trade-off between the risk variables (described in Chapter 11). For example, a work situation that exposes a worker to low magnitude of load–moment can still represent a high risk situation if the other four variables in the model were of sufficient magnitude.

TABLE 7.1 Values of Measured Variables Associated with High and Low Risk Jobs for Low Back Pain (From Reference 20)

Factors	High risk (N = 111)				Low risk (N = 124)				
	Mean	SD	Minimum	Maximum	Mean	SD	Minimum	Maximum	
Workplace factors									
Lift rate (lifts/h)	165.89	176.71	15.30	900.00	118.83	169.09	5.40	1500.00	2.1*
Vertical load location at origin (m)	1.00	0.21	0.38	1.80	1.05	0.27	0.18	2.18	1.4
Vertical load location at destination (m)	1.04	0.22	0.55	1.79	1.15	0.26	0.25	1.88	3.2†
Vertical distance traveled by load (m)	0.23	0.17	0.00	0.76	0.25	0.22	0.00	1.04	0.8
Average weight handled (N)	84.74	79.39	0.45	423.61	29.30	48.87	0.45	280.92	6.4†
Maximum weight handled (N)	104.36	88.81	0.45	423.61	37.15	60.83	0.45	325.51	6.7†
Average horizontal distance between load and L5–S1 (m)	0.66	0.12	0.30	0.99	0.61	0.14	0.33	1.12	2.5*
Maximum horizontal distance between load and L5–S1 (m)	0.76	0.17	0.38	1.24	0.67	0.19	0.33	1.17	3.7†
Average moment (N m)	55.26	51.41	0.16	258.23	17.70	29.18	0.17	150.72	6.8†
Maximum moment (N m)	73.65	60.65	0.19	275.90	23.64	38.62	0.17	198.21	7.4†
Job satisfaction	5.96	2.26	1.00	10.00	7.28	1.95	1.00	10.00	4.7†
Trunk motion factors									
Sagittal plane									
Maximum extension position (°)	−8.30	9.10	−30.82	18.96	−10.19	10.58	−30.00	33.12	3.5†
Maximum flexion position (°)	17.85	16.63	−13.96	45.00	10.37	16.02	−25.23	45.00	1.5
Range of motion (°)	31.50	15.67	7.50	75.00	23.82	14.22	399.00	67.74	3.8†
Average velocity (°/s)	11.74	8.14	3.27	48.88	6.55	4.28	1.40	35.73	6.0†
Maximum velocity (°/s)	55.00	38.23	14.20	207.55	38.69	26.52	9.02	193.29	3.7†
Maximum acceleration (°/s²)	316.73	224.57	80.61	1341.92	226.04	173.88	59.10	1120.10	4.2†
Maximum deceleration (°/s²)	−92.45	63.55	−514.08	−18.45	−83.32	47.71	−227.12	−4.57	1.2

Lateral plane									
Maximum left bend (°)	−1.47	6.02	−16.80	24.49	−2.54	5.46	−23.80	13.96	1.4
Maximum right bend (°)	15.60	7.61	3.65	43.11	13.24	6.32	0.34	34.14	2.6*
Range of motion (°)	24.44	9.77	7.10	47.54	21.59	10.34	5.42	62.41	2.2*
Average velocity (°/s)	10.28	4.54	3.12	33.11	7.15	3.16	2.13	18.86	6.1†
Maximum velocity (°/s)	46.36	19.12	13.51	119.94	35.45	12.88	11.97	76.25	4.9†
Maximum acceleration (°/s²)	301.41	166.69	82.64	1030.29	229.29	90.90	66.72	495.88	4.1†
Maximum deceleration (°/s²)	−103.65	60.31	−376.75	0.00	−106.20	58.27	−294.83	0.00	0.3
Twisting plane									
Maximum left twist (°)	1.21	9.08	−27.56	29.54	−1.92	5.36	−30.00	11.44	3.2†
Maximum right twist (°)	13.95	8.69	−13.45	30.00	10.83	6.08	−11.20	30.00	2.2*
Range of motion (°)	20.71	10.61	3.28	53.30	17.08	8.13	1.74	38.59	2.9†
Average velocity (°/s)	8.71	6.61	1.02	34.77	5.44	3.19	0.66	17.44	3.8†
Maximum velocity (°/s)	46.36	25.61	8.06	136.72	38.04	17.51	5.93	91.97	4.7*
Maximum acceleration (°/s²)	304.55	175.31	54.48	853.93	269.49	146.65	44.17	940.27	2.9†
Maximum deceleration (°/s²)	−88.52	70.30	−428.94	−5.84	−100.32	72.40	−325.93	−2.74	1.6*

Descriptive statistics of the workplace and trunk motion factors in each of the risk groups.
*Significant at a ≤ 0.05 (two sided).
†Significant at a ≤ 0.01 (two sided).
Adapted from Marras et al. (1993).

TABLE 7.2   Odds Ratios (Indication Degree of Risk) Between High Risk for Low Back Pain and the Individual Work Factors Measured at the Worksite (From Reference 20)

Factors	Coefficients	Odds ratio	SE	95% Confidence interval
Workplace factors				
Lift rate	0.00005	1.00	0.0004	0.99–1.01
Vertical load location at origin	−0.6748	1.02	0.5636	0.98–1.07
Vertical load location at destination	−1.8747	1.23*	0.5817	1.08–1.39
Vertical distance traveled by load	−0.8702	1.03	0.6742	0.99–1.07
Average weight handled	0.0152	2.76*	0.0027	1.94–3.93
Maximum weight handled	0.0135	3.17*	0.0022	2.19–4.58
Average horizontal distance between load and L5–S1	0.7808	1.01	0.8838	0.99–1.02
Maximum horizontal distance between load and L5–S1	1.7037	1.11*	0.6770	1.02–1.20
Average moment	0.0313	4.08*	0.0050	2.62–6.34
Maximum moment	0.0254	5.17*	0.0037	3.19–8.38
Job satisfaction	−0.3502	1.56*	0.0760	1.29–1.88
Trunk motion factors				
Sagittal Plane				
Maximum extension position	0.0561	1.36*	0.0144	1.17–1.58
Maximum flexion position	0.0391	1.60*	0.0081	1.31–1.93
Range of motion	0.0405	1.48*	0.0091	1.24–1.75
Average velocity	0.1735	3.33*	0.0314	2.17–5.11
Maximum velocity	0.0204	1.73*	0.0044	1.37–2.19
Maximum acceleration	0.0036	1.70*	0.0008	1.35–2.14
Maximum deceleration	−0.0035	1.04*	0.0023	0.98–1.09
Lateral plane				
Maximum left bend	0.0099	1.00	0.0202	0.99–1.02
Maximum right bend	−0.0037	1.00	0.0186	0.99–1.01
Range of motion	0.0071	1.01	0.0118	0.98–1.03
Average velocity	0.2184	1.73*	0.0452	1.38–2.15
Maximum velocity	0.0441	1.55*	0.0098	1.28–1.87
Maximum acceleration	0.0054	1.51*	0.0013	1.24–1.84
Maximum deceleration	0.0017	1.01	0.0022	0.98–1.04
Twisting Plane				
Maximum left twist	0.0758	1.21*	0.0220	1.09–1.35
Maximum right twist	0.0523	1.13*	0.0203	1.03–1.24
Range of motion	0.0298	1.08*	0.0147	1.00–1.16
Average velocity	0.1511	1.66*	0.0324	1.34–2.05
Maximum velocity	0.0202	1.17*	0.0069	1.05–1.31
Maximum acceleration	0.0026	1.16*	0.0009	1.05–1.29
Maximum deceleration	0.0014	1.01	0.0017	0.98–1.04

*Odds ratio significantly different from 1 a ≤ 0.05; the odds ratios were computed with weight means.

This model has been validated in a prospective workplace intervention study (21). This study's results are summarized in Fig. 7.3. This prospective study evaluated work related low back reports before and after physical interventions to the workplace and compared the back pain reports to LMM risk model predictions before and after the intervention. As shown in Fig. 7.3a, the population of jobs was represented by three types of trends in terms of low back

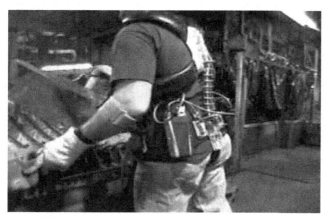

Figure 7.2   LMM used to collect information about kinematic exposure in industrial environments.

pain reports. First, in about one-third of the observed jobs the risk went from a high risk situation before the intervention to a low risk situation after the intervention. Second, another one-third of the jobs went from a high risk situation to a moderate risk (of low back pain) situation. Finally, the last one-third of the jobs showed no change in risk over the observation period. Based upon these observed low back pain risk reports, it is troubling that in two-third of the situations, changes were made to the workplace through interventions that did not result in adequate reduction in low back risk. This finding does not indicate that interventions are ineffective as much as it indicates that the wrong interventions were chosen for these specific jobs. As shown in Fig. 7.3b, the LMM risk assessment model was capable of predicting the ability of the various interventions to mediate the risk. When the risk prediction model predicted there would be a large change in risk due to the intervention, a large relative change occurred. When the risk model predicted little change would occur, little change in low back pain reporting was observed.

Hence, this study emphasizes two important points. First, the relationship between physical risk factor exposure and low back pain is multidimensional. Adjusting merely one dimension of the physical environment (such as load weight or posture) in an intervention will result in minimal improvement in risk for most dynamic work. Second, to optimize work, quantitative measures of the multidimensional risk factors are needed so that one could

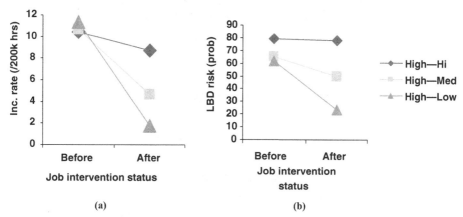

(a)   (b)

Figure 7.3   Three categories of job risk change shown as a function of (**a**) incidence rates and (**b**) low back pain risk model (LMM) predictions. The similarity in response patterns indicates validity of the multidimensional LMM risk model.

assess "how much exposure to a risk factor is too much exposure to the risk factors." Quantification of the proper risk variables can provide realistic insight into the trade-offs associated with these multiple risk factors.

When the results of this study are considered in conjunction with the previous study investigating nonneutral postures, it is clear that excessive and deviated trunk motions can increase the risk to the back. Furthermore, as the posture becomes more extreme or the trunk motion becomes more rapid, risk becomes greater. From a biomechanical perspective, these observations strongly suggest that risk of low back disorder is associated with three-dimensional dynamic loading of the spine. Thus, for the working back to be understood, it is necessary to consider the multidimensional physical risk factors that could influence the dynamic three-dimensional loading of the spine.

Another study (22) assessed cumulative loading of the spine in automotive assembly workers using a case–control methodology. Figure 7.4 shows the risk associated with the various acute and cumulative biomechanical measures. This study complements the picture provided by the previous described studies. Two points are evident from this figure. First, as shown in the previous studies (19,20), risk of low back pain was also associated with complex (multidimensional) interactions between the spine loading variables. This figure indicates that complex spine loading involving shear forces, trunk velocity, posture, and load moment were more indicative of risk than simple spine compression (a measure that has traditionally served as a tolerance measure of the spine). Second, the figure indicates that cumulative measures of load are also associated with risk at the worksite. Hence, the temporal components of biomechanical loading play an important role in low back pain reporting. The study identified four independent risk factors for low back disorder. These factors consisted of integrated load moment (over a work shift), hand forces, peak shear force on the spine, and peak trunk velocity. This study showed that workers in the top 25% of loading exposure on all risk factors were at about six times the risk of low back pain than those in the bottom 25% of loading.

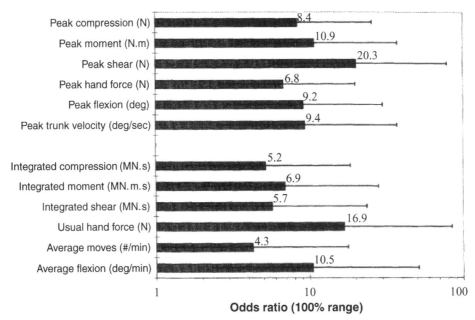

Figure 7.4 Risk estimates of acute and cumulative biomechanical measures observed by Norman and associates. (From reference 22).

Another effort (23) evaluated a database of 126 workers to precisely quantify and assess the complex trunk motions of workers associated with different degrees of low back disorder risk. They found that higher risk groups exhibited complex trunk motion patterns consisting of high magnitudes of multiplane trunk velocities, especially at extreme sagittal flexion angles, whereas the low risk groups did not exhibit any such patterns. This study demonstrated that elevated levels of complex simultaneous velocity patterns along with key workplace factors (load moment and frequency) were unique to groups with increased low back disorder risk. Once again, the *combination* of biomechanical loading factors appears to be associated closely with low back pain at work.

7.5 SURVEILLANCE CONCLUSIONS

Collectively, these industrial surveillance studies have provided insight as to which components of the physical environment are important to understanding low back pain risk. Overall, these studies suggest that when meaningful biomechanical assessments are performed at the workplace, strong associations between biomechanical factors and risk of low back disorders are observed. Several key components of biomechanical risk assessment can be derived from this review. First, risk is multidimensional in that a synergy among risk factors appears to intensify risk. However, some studies have shown that risk associations are nonmonotonic. Hence, a picture of the degree of complexity needed to properly describe low back risk in response to physical work factors emerges. Second, studies that have compared worker task demands to worker capacity have often been able to identify thresholds above which risk of low back pain increases. Thus, a load–tolerance relationship appears to be present. Third, many studies have reported that low back pain risk can be identified well when the three-dimensional location of the load relative to the body (load moment and load location) are quantified in some way. Fourth, many studies have shown that risk can be well characterized when the three-dimensional dynamic demands of the work are characterized. Fifth, many studies have shown that frequency of an activity is associated with risk, indicating a temporal or cumulative component to risk.

Jointly, these studies indicate that it is important to understand the multidimensional, dynamic, three-dimensional biomechanical exposure to physical work to characterize risk. However, to understand how these physical factors influence the pain pathways, it is necessary to understand how the internal forces of the body respond to these multidimensional conditions.

7.6 SPINE LOADING AND TASK PERFORMANCE

The field-based studies have indicated that there are multiple dimensions of the physical environment that must be considered if one is to appreciate their biomechanical role in spine loading and the potential for initiation of low back pain. We can build upon these field observations and use this information as a basis for an understanding of how spinal loading occurs under high risk conditions. Analyses that employ the EMG-assisted models described previously have the potential to offer insight into how the internal forces (muscles) react to these physical risk factors and influence spine loads. These biologically assisted techniques are used throughout this chapter to quantitatively assess the dimensions of spine loading associated with exposure to various physical work related risk factors and understand how the risk factors influence risk.

The studies described in the following sections can be broadly categorized into two dimensions: (1) those studies that evaluate biomechanical spine loads associated with physical workplace factors and (2) studies that describe the biomechanical implications associated with modification of those physical factors.

7.7 SPINE LOADING AND PRIMARY PHYSICAL WORKPLACE FACTORS

Primary physical factors relate to fundamental workplace factors that are commonly identified as potential risk factors associated with the workplace. The following sections describe how variations in exposure to these workplace factors relate to spine loading.

7.7.1 Moment Exposure

In the spine, the mechanical moment of concern is defined by the distance between an object being manipulated by the worker and the spine multiplied by the weight of the object. The industrial surveillance studies have indicated that those exposed to moments of increasing intensity as part of their jobs are more likely to experience back pain reports (19,22). From a biomechanical perspective, this makes perfect sense. The greater the magnitude of the external mechanical load, the greater the internal reaction force. However, the internal forces must increase in magnitude at a greater rate than the external forces since the internal forces are at a severe mechanical disadvantage. Figure 7.5 demonstrates how spine compression, lateral shear, and anterior–posterior shear change as the magnitude of the moment exposure increases. As shown in this figure, increases in external load result in increases in compression as well as increase in shear.

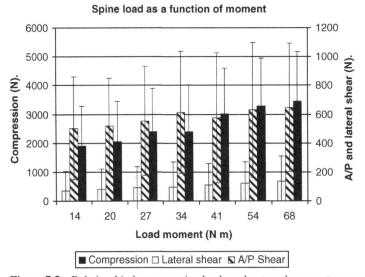

Figure 7.5 Relationship between spine loads and external moment exposure.

7.8   ROLE OF TRUNK MUSCLE COCONTRACTION IN SPINE LOADING

One of the most important principles associated with the low back pain pathways involve the sequence and magnitude of trunk muscles' activation. Since the trunk musculature provides the primary active internal support for externally generated moments, they play a key role in affecting the spine's support structure disruption pathway as well as the muscle function disruption pathway described earlier. Increasing the external load handled by the worker increases the internal loading of the spine in all dimensions as shown in Fig. 7.5. However, to respond properly to these external loads, the system of muscles within the trunk must increase their collective force generation. When the system of muscles simultaneously increases their level of contraction, the level of cocontraction is also increased to maintain stability of the spine. However, the cocontraction is also responsible for increased overall loading of the spine since the agonist (driving) and antagonist (breaking) muscles must fight each other in order to stabilize the trunk and support the external load. This increase in the structural load obviously increases the risk of damage to the spine structure tissues through acute and cumulative trauma pathways. However, an underappreciated risk also exists via the muscle function disruption pathway. Cocontraction of the trunk muscles significantly increases the tension within the supporting muscles of the trunk. As an example of this process, Fig. 7.6 shows the increase in spine compression as a result of increasing external load weight lifted. As expected, the compression increases fairly monotonically over the range of weights lifted. However, if one examines the activity of the agonist (Fig. 7.7) and antagonist (Fig. 7.8) muscles employed during these lifting tasks, one can gain insight into the nature of cocontraction of the torso muscles. While the compression of the spine increases by about 60% over the ranges of loads lifted, the agonist muscles increased their activity by about the same percent. However, the antagonist muscle activities increased by nearly 80% over the same range of external loads. This rapid increase in muscle tension could affect the functioning of the muscle via the MTrP, oxygen deprivation, and/or fiber disruption pathways described earlier.

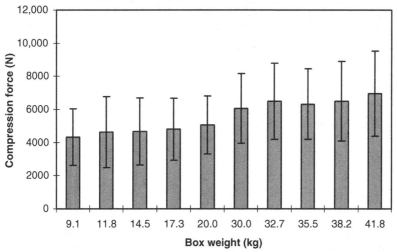

Figure 7.6   Increases in spine compression as a function of increases in load (box) weight lifted. (From reference 24).

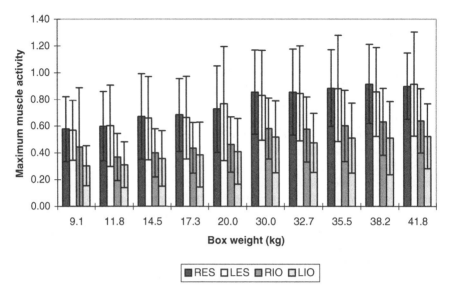

Figure 7.7   Maximum muscle activity of the (agonist) extensor muscles as a function of box weight (RES—right erector spinae, LES—left erector spinae, RIO—right internal oblique, LIO—Left internal oblique). (From reference 24).

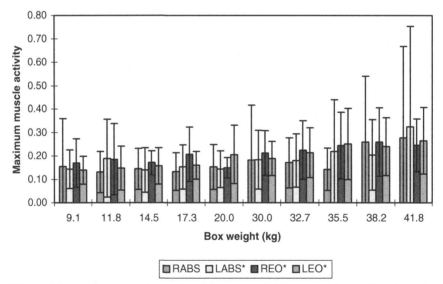

Figure 7.8   Maximum muscle activity of the (antagonist) flexor muscles as a function of box weight (RABS—right rectus abdominus, LABS—left rectus abdominus, REO—right external oblique, LEO—Left external oblique). * indicates significant effect of box weight. (From reference 24).

7.9   TRUNK MOTION

Historically, trunk motion has been underappreciated from a physical spine loading perspective. During the early development of biomechanical models, it was difficult to consider and model trunk motion because of limited computing capacity. Therefore, models were static and considered biomechanical loading as a "snapshot" of loading during an exertion. These models were unable to consider the reactions of the body's internal force generators (muscles and ligaments) to dynamic conditions. However, current data acquisition and analysis systems have more than adequate computing power to consider such influences. Industrial surveillance studies have indicated that there are certain limits to trunk motion above which there is an increased risk of low back pain reporting in industry (19,20). In addition, these studies have shown that trunk motion is part of the multidimensional picture that defines low back disorder risk in the workplace.

Several studies have evaluated the influence of trunk motion on spine loading (25–35). While motion can be beneficial or detrimental depending on how momentum is generated, generally, these studies have demonstrated that there is a biomechanical cost to trunk motion. Figure 7.9 shows the response of the right erector spinae muscle to a constant load as torso velocity increases both concentrically and eccentrically relative to an isometric (static) exertions. This figure indicates that there is a significant cost to the muscle of increasing velocity even though the external moment remains constant (36). Similar costs have been associated with trunk acceleration (37). Figure 7.10 indicates how increasing levels of acceleration can greatly increase the muscle activation level of the back extensor muscles. When the effects of increases in trunk velocity and acceleration are considered collectively on the spine, there is substantial cost in terms of increased muscle activity and increased levels of coactivation, both of which tax muscle function and can lead to disruption in muscle function and muscle-based pain. In addition, the cocontraction can be expected to lead to increased spine structure loading.

Since the cost to the musculoskeletal system of dynamic motion is significant, the ability of the trunk to support an external moment decreases dramatically as trunk motion increases. Figure 7.11 demonstrates how rapidly torso strength decreases as trunk velocity increases from static conditions (0°/s) to 90°/s. This decrease in externally applied strength is

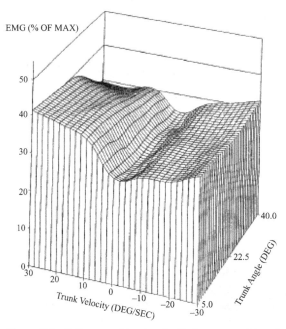

Figure 7.9   Influence of trunk velocity (—— = eccentric velocity, 0 = static, + = concentric velocity) on the activity of the right erector spinae muscle. The activity level indicates the level of EMG required to generate a constant level of force as trunk velocity changes. (From reference 36).

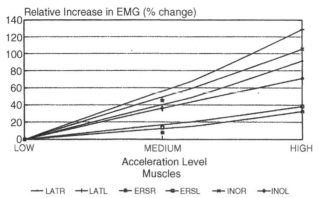

Figure 7.10 Influence of increasing trunk acceleration on right and left latissimus dorsi, erector spinae, and internal oblique muscle activities. (From reference 37).

due to the rapid increase in muscle coactivation occurring at faster speeds. The figure indicates that the presence of even slow trunk motions during work can significantly decrease the load-bearing tolerance of the back. Thus, caution must be used when assessing dynamic work situations using static models that assume that dynamic activities can be represented by quasi-static models of torso strength. These approaches can severely underappreciate the influence of motion on trunk capacity.

Even though trunk strength is decreased when back motion occurs, three-dimensional spine loading increases dramatically. Figure 7.12 demonstrates how the relative cost (defined as the increase in spine force relative to the moment supported by the spine) of spine loading increases as trunk velocity increases. This indicates that even at the lowest levels of trunk velocity, spine loading increases substantially. Specifically, compared to isometric exertions, a 30°/s exertion increases spine compression by 75%. Significant increases in lateral shear are also present as trunk motion increases.

Examination of the motor control patterns associated with increases in trunk velocity indicate that muscle coactivation increases dramatically as motion is introduced into a

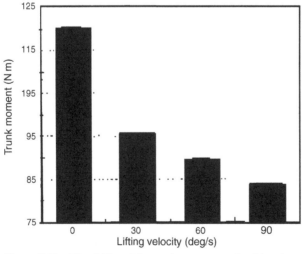

Figure 7.11 The ability of the trunk to support a load (trunk moment) decreases as the torso moves more rapidly. (From reference 25).

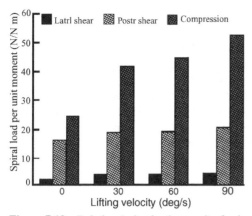

Figure 7.12   Relative (spine load per unit of spine moment supported) spine loading as a function of increasing lift (extension) velocity. Relative lateral shear force, anterior–posterior shear, and compression all increase as trunk extension velocity increases. (From reference 27).

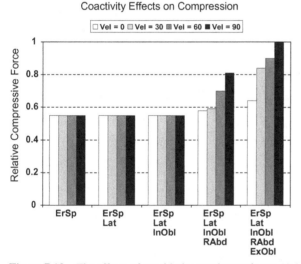

Figure 7.13   The effects of considering trunk muscle coactivity as a function of trunk velocity when estimating spine compression. Spine compression can be significantly underestimated when the influence of antagonistic coactivation is ignored. (From reference 26).

task (26). Figure 7.13 indicates how estimates of spine compression are influenced by the inclusion of muscle coactivity and the number of muscles included in the model. Antagonistic coactivation increases as trunk velocity increases and results in a sharp increase in spine loading. This increased loading is a direct result of muscle competition presumably in an attempt to maintain stability during the exertion (38) and provide guarding against small displacements of the spine.

7.10   NONSAGITTAL PLANE LOADING

Several industrial surveillance studies indicated that nonneutral or asymmetric postures and asymmetric loading of the spine during the performance of work can lead to increased reporting of low back disorders (17–20). This section examines how the spine is loaded during nonsagittal plane exertions. Several studies have reported that, because of the length–strength relationship of the trunk muscles (Fig. 6.5), activity levels increase greatly in the torso in an attempt to maintain stability and support the external load during work. As an example, Fig. 7.14 indicates how the external oblique muscle, an antagonistic muscle involved in trunk stability, responds to a constant level of external load as the trunk becomes more asymmetric at different levels of trunk angular acceleration. This figure indicates that even at very low levels of trunk acceleration, the muscle must double its activity level to support a standard external torque in asymmetric postures compared to a sagittally symmetric posture. Such responses certainly increase muscle tension and can increase the probability of activating the muscle function disruption pathway leading to low back pain.

7.10.1 Lateral Motion

We can gain insight into the musculoskeletal costs of asymmetric loading by examining the changes that occur in the musculoskeletal system during asymmetric loading and nonneutral positioning of the spine. During lateral bending movements, significant increases in coactivity within the left external oblique and latissimus dorsi muscles occur and the activity level increases monotonically as lateral trunk velocity increases (Fig. 7.15) (31). Once again, we see that these off-sagittal plane motions can increase the probability of muscle function disruption in the back.

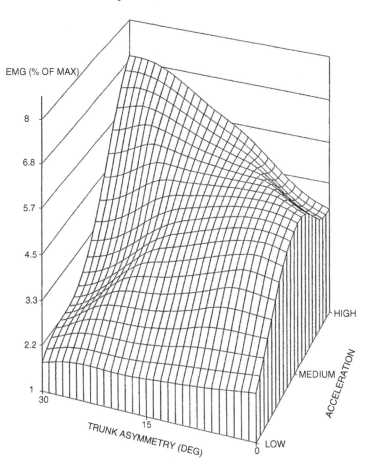

Figure 7.14 Response of the right external oblique muscle to a combination of angular trunk acceleration and trunk asymmetry. (From reference 37).

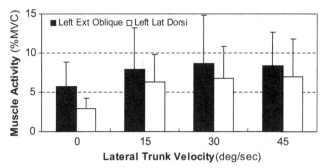

Figure 7.15 Changes in left external oblique and left latissimus dorsi activity levels as lateral trunk velocity increases. (From reference 31).

When the effects of these increases in muscle activities are considered relative to the changes in spine loading, dramatic increases in lateral shear and compression occur in the spine as indicated in Fig. 7.16. This figure indicates that exertions performed at 45°/s increase the anterior/posterior (A/P) shear by nearly 25% compared to static exertions and approach the tolerance levels of the disc for A/P shear.

It is insightful to compare the magnitude of the lateral shear force trend to those lateral velocity values that have been associated with increases in reported low back pain in industrial settings. Figure 7.16 indicates that lateral shear increases dramatically when lateral trunk velocity on the job approaches 45°/s. This is the point at which biomechanical analyses of tolerance have suggested disk damage is likely to occur (39,40). It is interesting to note that this is approximately the same (maximum) lateral velocity level at which the LMM risk data (41) suggests that high risk group membership for low back pain occurs (Table 7.1). Thus, the field surveillance observations correlate well with spine loading measurements. This agreement between different risk approaches (industrial risk observations and biomechanical risk assessments) suggests a "pattern of evidence" for the physical exposure components of low back pain and also suggests a high degree of validity.

Laboratory assessments of spine loading have also revealed that lateral bending to the right is not necessarily a mirror image of lateral bending to the left. Figure 7.17 shows the change in spine compression at L5/S1 while exerting lateral force to the right versus the left. In this study, subjects were prepositioned in either neutral, 15° left lateral bending or 15° right lateral bending static postures (31). Two observations are apparent from this figure. First, nonneutral postures increase spine compression. This finding also agrees with the field observations (17). Second, left lateral exertions are more costly than right lateral exertions from a biomechanical perspective. The reason for this discrepancy is not clear. This

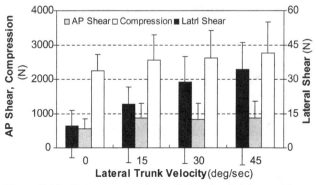

Figure 7.16 Spine compression and shear loads (along with standard deviation of load) shown as a function of trunk lateral velocity. (From reference 31).

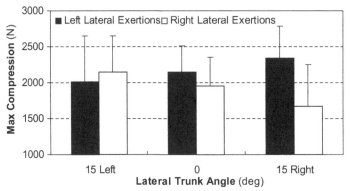

Figure 7.17   The influence of left lateral exertions versus right lateral exertions on spine compression when starting the exertion from various lateral trunk angles. (From reference 31).

difference is most likely associated with a difference in muscle mass between the right and left sides of the body that have been observed in biomechanical studies (42) and/or the increased motor patterning associated with workplaces designed for a right-handed world.

7.10.2   Twisting Motion

Twisting while exerting force also represents a work posture that has been associated with increased risk of low back pain in many studies (7,17,19,20,43–50). Field surveillance studies have indicated that even very low twisting velocities are associated with increases in low back pain reporting in industry (20). These studies have reported that average trunk twisting velocities of as low as about 9°/s, while supporting an external load, can place the worker at high risk of low back pain reporting (see Table 7.1). Biomechanical assessments of spine loading during twisting have confirmed that force exertions occurring at these trunk twisting velocities can double the relative compressive force imposed on the spine (30). Figure 7.18 shows how rapidly relative compression increases at L5/S1 once motion is

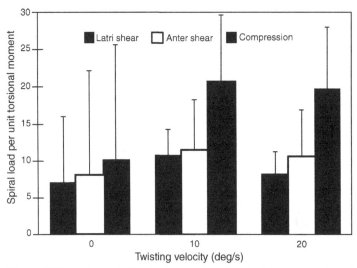

Figure 7.18   Relative 3D load increases associated with torso twisting. (From reference 30).

included in the twisting exertion. The surveillance literature and the biomechanical information once again converge on a pattern of evidence for twisting exposure.

Trunk moment generation is affected in all three planes by the position of the torso at the time twisting force application begins and the direction of twisting effort (clockwise versus counterclockwise). Figure 7.19 demonstrates that force production changes as a function of these factors. It is interesting to note that, in general, force generation is greater when bending to the right and when rotating clockwise. This trend may be explained, in part, by the fact that the latissimus dorsi muscles have about 11% greater cross-sectional area on the right side of the body compared to the left side of the body (42). Since this muscle has a relatively large mechanical advantage for twisting, this larger muscle mass results in greater force production when moving to the right.

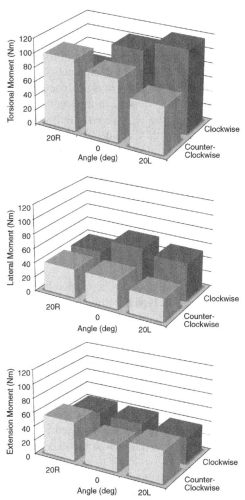

Figure 7.19   The maximum torsion moment that can be applied is influenced by the staring position as well as the direction of twist. Significant coupling of moments is also seen in twisting activities (20R or 20L). (From reference 30).

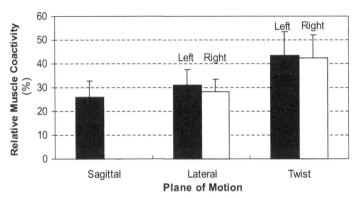

Figure 7.20   Relative trunk muscle coactivity associated with comparable exertions performed in the sagittal plane, lateral plane, and transverse (twisting) plane of the body. (From reference 31).

Increases in mechanical loading of the spine are associated with greater coactivation of the torso muscles. There is significantly greater coactivation of the trunk muscles occurring during torso twisting compared to other types of movements observed during work. Figure 7.20 indicates the relative increases in torso muscle coactivity associated with comparable exertions performed with the body loaded in the sagittal plane, lateral plane, and twisting plane of the body. Note that the relative coactivity is greatest with twisting with coactivity increasing by nearly two thirds under twisting exertion conditions compared to exertions performed in the sagittal plane. This indicates that twisting while the spine is loaded would be expected to greatly increase the muscle tension and might activate the muscle disruption pathway to low back pain. This dramatic increase in internal force coactivity also translates into the dramatic increases in spine loading observed at L5/S1.

7.10.3   Task Asymmetry

Under occupational conditions, exertions are typically not performed purely in the lateral or twisting plane. Most occupational tasks require some type of combination of exertions in the three cardinal planes of the body. These work-related postures are usually referred to as asymmetric work conditions. Figure 7.21 shows how spine loads can change when performing lifting tasks under sagittally symmetric conditions compared to asymmetric lifting angles of only 30° (lifting while the trunk is twisted 30°). This figure indicates that compression, lateral shear, and A/P shear all increase significantly as asymmetry increases. These asymmetric postures are typical of the vast majority of industrial work and should be viewed as the norm rather than the exception when evaluating risk of low back pain during work (20). Due to the degree of trunk muscle cocontraction associated with asymmetric exertions, three-dimensional spine loading greatly increases when workers are exposed to asymmetric lifting conditions.

One study examined the ability of simple two-dimensional biomechanical models to assess spine loading under asymmetric lifting conditions (51). This study identified large errors in load prediction when employing two-dimensional biomechanical models. Moment exposure was under predicted by 20% when assessing asymmetric lifts of 30° using two-dimensional models. Under predictions of 61% were reported when assessing lifts performed under 90° asymmetric lifting conditions.

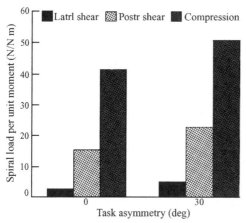

Figure 7.21   Spine load (per unit of extension moment) shown as a function of asymmetric lift origin position. Relative lateral shear, anterior–posterior shear, and compression increase significantly with asymmetry. (From reference 27).

7.10.4   Lift Height

Several investigations have provided insight into the influence of load height during lifting (52–54). Given the strong influence of the length–strength relationship (Fig. 6.5) one would expect that load vertical location would have a profound effect on muscle recruitment. In one study, subjects were asked to lift to and from different positions without moving their feet, in an attempt to understand the role of load height on loading of the spine (52). Figure 7.22

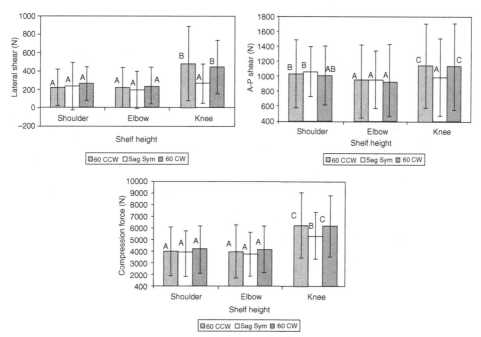

Figure 7.22   Influence of load lift origin asymmetric and height origin on the peak three-dimensional spine loads experience by the spine. Different superscript alphanumeric characters indicate a statistically significant difference between conditions (52) (A–P = anterior–posterior, 60 CCW = 60° counter clockwise, Sag Sym = sagitally symmetric, 60 CW = 60° clockwise). (From reference 52).

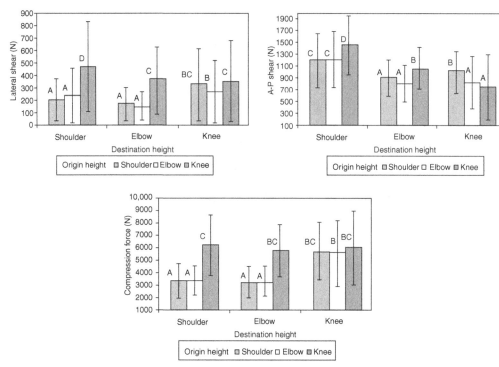

Figure 7.23   Influence of relative load height of lift origin and destination positions on the peak three-dimensional spine loads. Different superscript alphanumeric characters indicate a statistically significant difference between conditions (from reference 52). (A–P = anterior–posterior).

shows how spine compression, lateral shear, and A/P shear change as a function of a load's vertical height location at the start (origin) of a lift as well as the lift origin asymmetry. This study indicated that vertical location of the load origin was indeed a strong factor in determining spine load. In all three dimensions of loading, it was apparent that the lowest load origin (knee height) increased compression by the greatest amount regardless of task asymmetry. Lateral and A/P shear were also generally greater at the lowest lift height origin. Asymmetry increased loading significantly compared to symmetric lifting in all dimensions of spine loading. When the effect of load destination is considered in combination with load origin, the height is once again observed to play a significant role in spine loading with greater differences in height relating to the largest three-dimensional peak loadings of the spine (Fig. 7.23).

Figure 7.24 indicates the relative changes in compression, lateral shear, and A/P shear as a function of the path of load travel during a lift (52). This figure indicates that compared to the most neutral lift (defined as lifting from elbow height in a sagittally symmetric position), spine loads can change dramatically. Compared to the most neutral lift, lateral shear can increase by 1200%, A/P shear can increase by 200%, and compression can increase by 180% when lifting through longer pathways. Hence, this study indicates that lifting position and path have a very large influence on spine load.

These previously described trends involved experiments where body postures were controlled. In comparison, a study where workers were permitted to move their feet to perform lifting tasks was performed using experienced workers as subjects. Very similar trends in loading occurred (54). In this study, distribution center workers were asked to lift

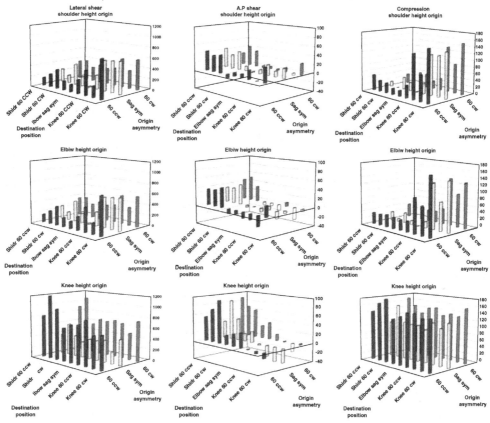

Figure 7.24 Peak three-dimensional spine loads as a function of pathway (lift origin and destination location). Note the different spine load scales for each dimension of spine load (A–P = anterior–posterior, 60 CCW = 60° counter clockwise, Sag Sym = sagitally symmetric, 60 CW = 60° clockwise). (From reference 52).

loads that varied in weight from 18.2 to 27.3 kg. Figure 7.25a and b indicates that the load location origin had a greater influence on spine compression and A/P shear than did the weight of the load lifted. Factors discussed in the previous chapter, such as the length–strength relationship of the muscles and the force–velocity relationship influence spine loadings under these conditions. Hence, *it is not sufficient to simply control the weight of the object while lifting if one is to optimize work conditions. These studies suggest that it is extremely important to understand the load origin position and travel path.*

The contributions of the various workplace layout characteristics to the different dimensions of spine loading are shown in Fig. 7.26 for an experiment where workplace characteristics were systematically varied over a series of lifts. This figure shows the relative variance that is explained by load height origin, load destination origin, and load asymmetry at the origin and destination for spine compression, lateral shear, and A/P shear. The figure indicates that origin height is the strongest contributor to defining both lateral shear and compression. This was also a major contributor to lateral shear, although other workplace factors also had a significant influence on this dimension of loading. On the basis of this study (52), Table 7.3 presents a means to predict relative spine loading changes that can be expected based on the load height and asymmetry in terms of both origin and destination.

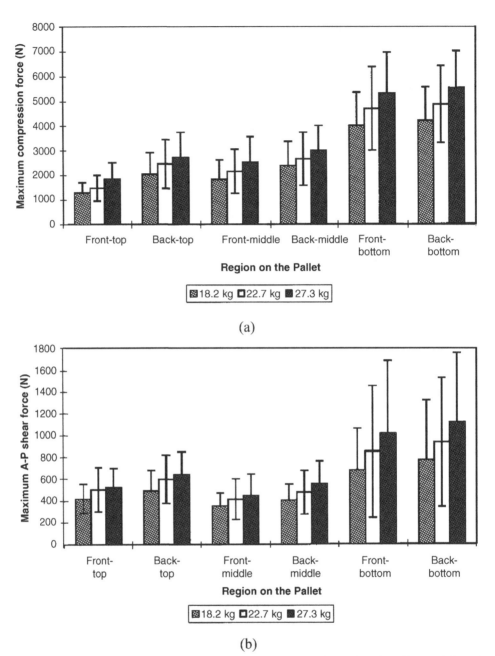

Figure 7.25 Spine compression (**a**) and anterior–posterior shear (**b**) as a function of load weight and the origin and destination of the load. (From reference 54).

7.10.5 One-Handed Versus Two-Handed Lifting

Nearly all laboratory investigations exploring the biomechanical costs associated with lifting as well as all lifting guidelines have addressed lifting activities as a two-handed activity. However, it is common, under industrial conditions, to observe employees performing lifts with one hand. One-handed lifting is particularly common in the workplace when lifting from asymmetric positions. One study (55) investigated differences in predicted

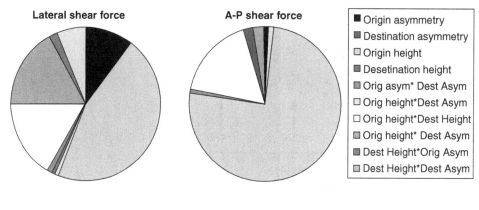

Figure 7.26   Relative contribution of the workplace layout characteristics for each of the peak three-dimensional spine loads (as predicted by the partial r^2). A–P = anterior–posterior shear. (From reference 52).

TABLE 7.3   Regression Equation That Can be Used to Predict Peak Three-Dimensional Spine Loads (newtons) Based upon Workplace Characteristics

Spine load	Equation
Lateral shear	$166.46 - 0.873*OA + 0.172*DA + 2.448*OH + 5.141*DH - 0.00315*OA*DA$ $+ 0.00846*DA*OH - 0.09578*OH*DH + 0.0121*OA*OH + 0.0059*OA*DH$ $- 0.00576*DA*DH - 0.00000079*OH*OA*DH*DA$
Anterior–Posterior shear	$7.32 + 0.063*OA - 0.412*DA + 9.481*OH + 18.721*DH - 0.01006^*OA*DA$ $+ 0.00946*DA*OH - 0.18386*OH*DH - 0.00617*OA*OH + 0.00763*OA$ $*DH - 0.00019*DA*DH - 0.0000015*OH*OA*DH*DA$
Compression	$4709.39 - 1.181*OA + 2.281*DA + 25.905*OH + 34.684*DH - 0.03*OA*DA$ $+ 0.03782*DA*OH - 1.06245*OH*DH + 0.03972*OA*OH - 0.00112*OA$ $*DH - 0.004816*DA*DH0.00000549*OH*DA*DH*DA$

Origin height (OH), destination height (DH), destination asymmetry (DA), and interactions between these characteristics. Origin and destination heights are represented by the percent of the worker's stature (from reference 52).

risk when lifting a load using one hand compared to two-handed lifts. Figure 7.27 shows that, over three different load lifting levels ranging from 3.4 to 10.2 kg, the one-handed lift increased the probability of high risk group membership (via the LMM risk model (20)) significantly. In addition, this study also found that asymmetric lifting significantly increased risk for both one-handed and two handed lifting.

This study also explored the trunk kinematic changes that occur with one-handed versus two-handed lifting and concluded that one-handed lifting resulted in significantly

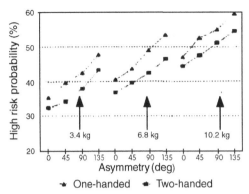

Figure 7.27   Probability of high risk group membership [as defined by Marras et al. (20)] as a function of one-handed versus two handed lifting, asymmetry of the lift, and the magnitude of the weight lifted. (From reference 55).

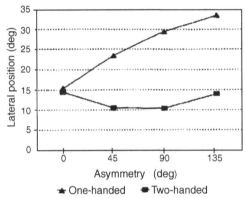

Figure 7.28   Lateral trunk position resulting from one-handed lifts compared to two-handed lifts shown as a function of task lifting asymmetry. (From reference 55).

greater lateral torso deviations compared with two-handed lifting (Fig. 7.28). Figure 7.28 shows how lateral trunk position changes little as task asymmetry increases for two-handed lifting but increased dramatically as asymmetry increases under one-handed lifting conditions. Hence, one-handed lifts have the potential for significant risk.

Several laboratory studies have also explored the biomechanical loading of the spine during one-handed versus two-handed lifting. One laboratory study investigated three-dimensional spine loads associated with one-handed versus two-handed lifting combined with lifting from sagittally symmetric positions as well as asymmetric lift origins that varied according to two (30° and 60°) clockwise and counterclockwise positions (56). Lateral shear, anterior–posterior shear, and compression were all affected by the task asymmetry as well as the combination of asymmetry and number of hands used during the lift, whether the right or left hand was used to perform the lift. In addition, spine compression was affected by the number of hands used in the lift. Figure 7.29a–c shows how these spinal forces change according to these conditions. Two-handed lifts often resulted in the greatest compression on the spine regardless of asymmetry. Another biomechanical study has reported similar spine loading trends as observed here and have concluded that one-handed lifting results in about 10% less moment exposure (external load) compared to two-handed lifts, and 30% less moment exposure when performing one-handed lifts while supporting the body with the

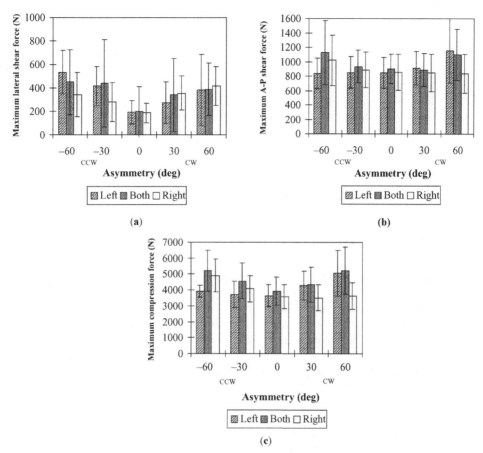

Figure 7.29 Maximum lateral shear (**a**), A/P shear (**b**), and compression (**c**) at L5/S1 resulting from one- and two-handed lifts performed with the right and left hand over five symmetric and symmetric lift origins. (From reference 56).

other hand (57). However, Fig. 7.29c indicates that lifts performed with the right hand are not just mirror images of lifts performed with the left hand in terms of spine compression. Lifts performed with the left hand while lifting from clockwise lift origins generally impose more compression on the spine than lifts performed with the right hand from counterclockwise lift origins (56). In depth analyses indicated that these differences were due to differences in trunk muscle cocontraction levels when lifting to these different origins. It is also interesting to note that when lifting from sagittally symmetric origins, spine compression was least when lifting with either hand compared to both hands. This trend was tracked to the reduced sagittal bending that occurred during one-handed lifting, which translated into a lesser trunk moment imposed by the torso during these lifts. Thus, there are some significant subtleties that dictate loading of the spine under torsional lifting conditions.

There also appear to be some trade-offs associated with the direction of spine loading associated with one-handed versus two-handed lifting. Lateral shear was slightly greater for two-handed lifts when lifting from sagittally symmetric conditions as was the case for compression. Lateral shear increased significantly as the lift origin became more asymmetric. For example, lifting with the left hand at the 60° clockwise (to the right) asymmetry origin, lateral shear increased by 58% relative to the sagittally symmetric condition. Lifting from origins located to the left (CCW) of the sagittal plane resulted in even greater lateral shear loading. Again, suggesting that right-handed lifts were not mirror images of left-handed lifts while lifting in different directions.

Asymmetric load origins generally had more of an impact on A/P shear loading than did the number of hands involved in the lift. As can be seen in Fig. 7.29b, A/P shear was greatest in the sagittally symmetric condition when using two hands. Lifting using either hand played a minor role in the reduction of A/P shear as the lift origin became more asymmetric compared to this sagittally symmetric condition.

Considering the fact that moment exposure is reduced in one-handed lifting, yet there can still be significant spinal loads associated with these conditions, it is obvious that the relative load on the spine per unit of external load supported can be generally greater during one-handed lifts compared to two-handed lifts. Thus, one must be particularly vigilant when evaluating work involving one-handed lifting.

7.11 LIFTING VERSUS LOWERING

Several studies have explored lumbar trunk muscle activities during lifting activities compared to lowering activities (58). In general, these studies have found that lowering strength (eccentric muscle activity) was greater than lifting strength due to the effect of the involvement of passive tissue during the lowering task. Thus, lowering requires less electromyographic muscle activity than lifting. However, eccentric muscle activity has also been implicated in muscle disorder causality (59,60). One laboratory-based study (61) predicted the three-dimensional loads occurring on the lumbar spine under lifting and lowering of different weight cases. As expected, the three-dimensional spine loads increased under both lifting and lowering conditions as case weight increased. However, a trade-off between the nature of spine loading was reported as a function of lift type. Lowering a weight resulted in greater compression on the lumbar spine compared to lifting; however, less A–P shear was observed during lowering (Fig. 7.30). When considering the risk of lowering, one must also keep in mind the risks associated with eccentric loading of the muscles and the increased probability of muscle function disruption discussed in Chapter 5.

The difference in magnitude between compression and shear loading on the spine also appears to vary according to velocity of the torso during the lift or lower. Figure 7.31 shows how A/P shear increases as the torso velocity increases during lifting, whereas Fig. 7.32 indicates how spine compression increases as the torso velocity increases during lowering. As with many of the conditions that lead to increased spine loading, increases in spine loads during greater trunk velocity conditions were linked to increased trunk muscle coactivity. However, the increases in coactivity appeared to be much more sensitive to the velocity of concentric (lifting) loading compared to the velocity of eccentric (lowering) loading.

An earlier study examining the differences in lifting and lowering on the trunk activities suggests that the peak torque to which people are exposed during lowering is slightly less due to changes in trunk acceleration patterns (58). This study found similar intermuscular coordination patterns between lifting and lowering, yet about 30% less EMG activity during lowering. Even though less active muscle force is employed in lowering, greater passive forces are involved that place similar loads on the muscle during lifting and lowering activities. This study speculated that greater risk of muscle-related back pain is present during lifting because the muscle force is distributed over a smaller muscle cross-sectional area, resulting in greater force per unit area of muscle and a greater risk of damage via the mechanisms articulated in Chapter 5.

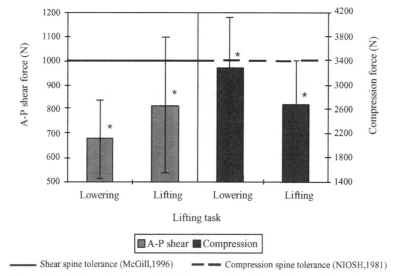

Figure 7.30   Compression and A/P shear resulting from lifting and lowering. (From reference 61).

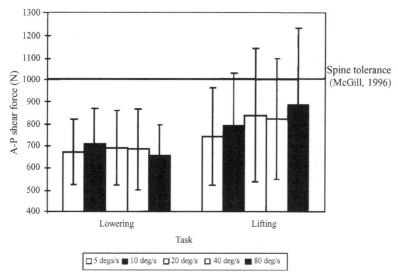

Figure 7.31   A/P shear forces as a function of trunk angular velocity and type of activity (lift versus lower). (From reference 61).

7.11.1 Cumulative Exposure

Many researchers suspect that the risks associated with physical exertions and work are related to the cumulative effects of tissue loading. While this concept is appealing from a biomechanical perspective, only a limited number of studies have been able to explore the role of cumulative biomechanical exposure from a low back risk perspective.

The surveillance literature reports two studies that have explored the relationship between cumulative load exposure and risk. One study found that self reports among institutional aids was greater among those who were exposed to greater cumulative

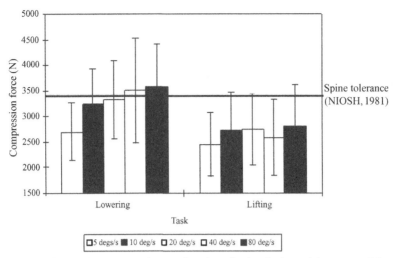

Figure 7.32 Spine compression as a function of task velocity and the nature of the task (lifting versus lowering). (From reference 61).

compressive loading as assessed by a two-dimensional static model (62). Another study evaluated the EMG activities and spine compression loads of aids in an intermediate-care facility and found that those with greater cumulative loading had more lost time (63). Since cumulative exposure is not easy to measure in the workplace, several studies have also explored the most efficient means to assess cumulative exposure on the job (64,65).

The biomechanical mechanisms involved in cumulative exposure have also been explored more quantitatively under laboratory conditions. A study investigating the systematic effects of cumulative loading has found spinal shrinkage was associated with cumulative exposure (66). However, the structures that appear to be most affected by cumulative exposure appear to be the ligaments of the spine. Repetitive or prolonged load exposure appears to alter the viscoelastic properties of the ligaments by affecting their ability to return to their original length and strength. Many of these studies have also shown a corresponding muscle reaction to compensate for this system laxity that often manifests itself in increased muscle spasms (23,67–73).

7.12 DURATION OF EXPOSURE TO LIFTING TASKS

Spine loading has also been observed to vary as a function of time of exposure to occupational tasks. In a study of spine loading during paced lifting throughout an 8-h workday, spine compression loading increased by about 5% after the first 2 h of exposure and then remained relatively constant through the following 6 h of task exposure (74). Figure 7.33 shows this trend. It can also be seen that spine compression increased over the last 2 h of task exposure; however, this increase was not found to be statistically significant.

Another study examined changes in spine loading when experienced workers palletized and depalletized loads over a 5-h work period (75). At the beginning and end points of each pallet, the workers were asked to perform a standard lift under controlled conditions. Figure 7.34a and b summarizes the findings of this study. Over the course of the lifting period, compression decreased by approximately 10%, whereas spine A/P shear increased by approximately 35%. These changes in spine loading were accompanied by changes in trunk and hip kinematics, most likely resulting from fatigue. Over the course of the study, workers

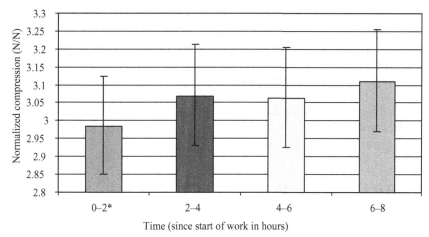

Figure 7.33 The effect of time of day on compressive spine loading (∗ indicates significantly different from other time blocks) (N/N represents normalized to body weight). (From reference 74).

reduced their trunk bending and increased their hip motion. These kinematic changes resulted in a gradual reduction of moment exposure over the 5-h work period.

Both of these studies found a change in the recruitment pattern of the trunk musculature over the duration of the task exposure period. Hence, spine loading is a transient effect. As workers are exposed to a task over long periods of time, they change the recruitment pattern of the trunk muscles. These changes in recruitment result in trade-offs in spine loading. It is also apparent that the most dramatic changes occur in the first 2-h of task exposure.

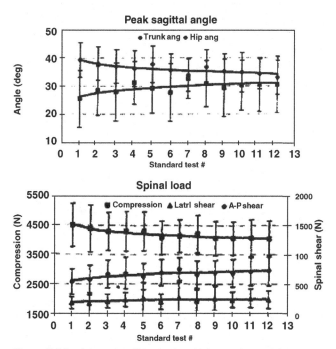

Figure 7.34 (a) Trade-off in trunk and hip angular position throughout a 5-h lifting task and (b) the corresponding trade-off between spine compression and A/P shear (standard test # is an indication of time). (From reference 75).

The impact on muscle function must also be considered during exposure to repetitive work. Figure 7.35 shows the oxygen saturation of the lumbar spine's (right and left) erector spinae muscles over an 8-h work period (76). As indicated in this figure, the oxygen demands during repetitive lifting are rather large and the average demand can increase by more than 30% throughout an 8-h workday. This increased oxygen demand is related to both increased spine loading and increased cocontraction within the trunk muscles. The oxygen demand increases rapidly at the beginning of the workday and also increases dramatically over the last 2 h of work. These times of rapid oxygen demand changes increase the potential for oxygen deprivation leading to muscle function disruption.

7.13 WORKER EXPERIENCE, TASK FREQUENCY, AND MOMENT EXPOSURE

Work experience plays a significant role in spine loading during an occupational task. A common theme among the physical tasks components that increase spine loading is that, in all cases, spine loading is increased by way of an increase in trunk muscle coactivation. Similarly, experience in performing a task can effect trunk muscle coactivation and subsequent spine loading.

In a study of the effects of experience on spine loading while performing a specific paced lifting task, experienced workers exhibited 13% less compressive load on their spines compared to inexperienced workers (77). However, spine compression was also dependent on the magnitude of the moment exposure. Figure 7.36 indicates that only the lowest load moment exposure (8 N m) condition resulted in statistically significant differences in spine compression between experience groups. It is also interesting to note that regardless of load moment exposure, novice subjects experienced similar compressive loads on the spine, whereas experienced subjects responded as expected by increasing spinal compression when the moment demands increased. Even though average novice spine compression increased with moment exposure, the effect was not statistically significant. The difference in spine compression at the 8 N m moment level was a result of increased trunk muscle antagonistic coactivation within the novice group. The experienced group, by comparison, only recruited

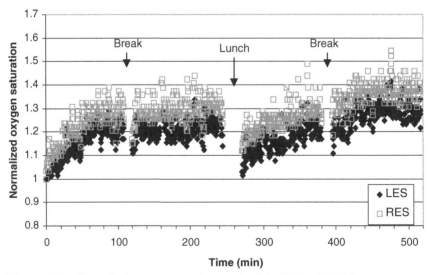

Figure 7.35 Normalized oxygen saturation trends of the LES and RES from a representative subject's data (load = 1.1 kg, lift frequency = 8 lifts/min) over the 8-h workday. (From reference 76).

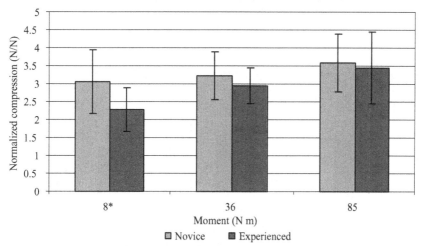

Figure 7.36   Interactive effect of moment and experience on spine compressive loading ([*] indicates significant difference between novice and experienced subjects) (N/N represents normalized to body weight). (From reference 74).

the muscles that were necessary to counteract the external load. When the load moment increased, all subjects increased their trunk muscle coactivity apparently in an effort to increase spine stability. Thus, this study suggests that worker experience during physical exertions is characterized by a minimalistic, yet appropriate recruitment of the trunk muscles. One could hypothesize that experienced subjects have fine tuned their muscle recruitment patterns to the point where they could relax their need for trunk stability and this was accomplished through a reduction of trunk muscle coactivation.

One study examined spine loading and changes in worker stature (due to cumulative exposure to lifting) during brick-laying tasks (78). As expected, spine loading increased when workers lifted heavier loads. Over the course of a 47-min lifting period, stature decreased by 2.0–3.6 mm indicating cumulative loading of the spine. However, a trade-off between frequency and load occurred with workers increasing their work pace when lighter loads were lifted. Yet, this did not appear to alter the spine loading pattern.

Lateral shear force also changes as a function of worker experience, again, due to differences in coactivity patterns between the novice and experienced workers (79). Figure 7.37 indicates that this increase in lateral shear at the eight lifts per minute (lpm) condition was dominated by the novice subjects' response where their normalized shear was nearly twice that of the experienced subjects. Novice subjects also exhibited significantly greater lateral shear loads under the 10 lpm condition compared to experienced subjects. However, at the highest lift frequency, 12 lpm, both novice and experienced subjects exhibited relatively low normalized lateral shear.

Figure 7.38 demonstrates the highly interactive and complex nature of the relationship between worker experience and physical work conditions through the interaction between experience, frequency, and moment upon lateral shear force in the spine. Of particular interest are the relatively high lateral shear forces experienced by the novice subjects in response to lift frequencies at or above 8 lpm. It is also interesting to note that at each lift frequency (except for the 8 lpm condition), the highest and lowest moment exposures produced the greatest lateral shear with the moderate moment exposure producing the lowest shear. A very different pattern was exhibited by the experienced subjects. The peak lateral shear value for the experienced group was 28% less than the peak value for the novice group. The lift frequencies at 6 lpm and below yielded the greatest lateral shear forces on the spine.

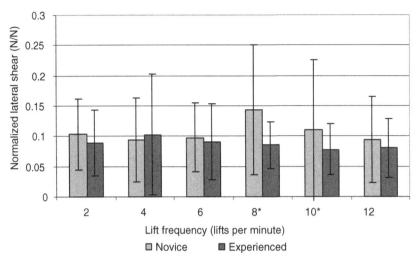

Figure 7.37 Interactive effect of experience and lift frequency on lateral shear (* indicates significant difference between novice and experienced subjects) (N/N represents normalized to body weight). (From reference 74).

In addition, at the 4 and 6 lpm frequencies, the 36 N m condition yielded the greatest lateral shears. However, for frequencies of 8 lpm and greater, the lateral shear increased monotonically with moment exposure as would be expected.

These findings suggest that the factors that influence biomechanical spine loading are not simply the physical workplace factors. One would expect that lift frequency would dominate the spinal loading patterns with greater spine loading occurring with greater lift frequencies and greater moment exposure. However, spine loading did not increase in such an orderly pattern. While compression did increase with increasing moment exposure, frequency affected complex spine loading in an unexpected manner. Furthermore, work experience played a large role in spine load determination. In-depth analyses of muscle coactivity (agonist compared to antagonist muscle activity) confirmed that many of the observed trends in spine loading were a result of statistically significant changes in the muscle coactivity (80).

Frequency of task exposure increases spine loading, through an increase in muscle coactivity, when subjects are exposed to conditions to which they are unaccustomed. Experienced workers increased trunk muscle coactivity and their subsequent spine loading when they were forced to work at slower rates of lifts, whereas inexperienced workers increased their spine loads when they were forced to lift at faster paces. We can hypothesize that experienced workers were accustomed to working faster, whereas novices were accustomed to slower paces. It appears that increased trunk muscle coactivity (and increased spine loading) was associated with exposure to unaccustomed task frequency.

When load magnitude was considered, load magnitude interacted in an unexpected manner with frequency and experience. Experienced workers responded as expected with increasing spine loading occurring at greater load moment exposures, but only at greater lifting rates. Inexperienced subjects behaved in a very unpredictable manner with the lowest load moment often imposing greater than expected spinal load (again when exposed to repetitive conditions to which they were unaccustomed).

The nonmonotonic spinal loading responses to lift frequency suggest that motor control programs are selected on the basis of the subject's perception of the task and from past experiences. It is hypothesized that the subjects may have been more apt to utilize motor programs that correspond with those lift frequencies that they commonly encountered. One

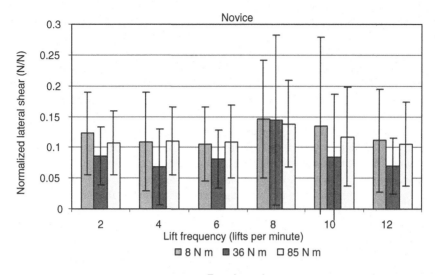

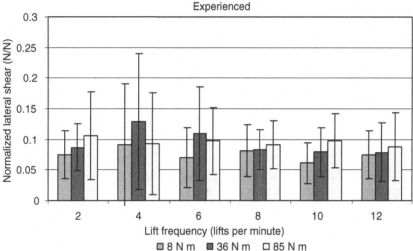

Figure 7.38   Interactive effect of frequency and moment on novice and experienced subjects' lateral shears (N/N represents normalized to body weight). (From reference 74).

study (80) found that as experience is gained in a lifting task, spinal loading decreases because the pattern of muscle activation shifts from simultaneous to sequential contraction. It was found that novices had lower loading while lifting at the low frequencies (2, 4, and 6 lpm) and that experienced subjects had lower loading while lifting at the high frequencies (8, 10, and 12 lpm), thus giving an indication of the lift rates to which both populations were typically exposed. Novices may have responded with lower spinal loads to the low lift rates simply because these frequencies are associated with the daily activities of lifting. Similarly, experienced subjects may be exposed to higher lift rates at work and may therefore be able to adapt to these levels by selecting appropriate motor programs to minimize coactivity and, therefore, spinal loading levels. On the contrary, if the subject uses a previously developed motor program for another lift frequency, the neuromuscular response of muscle coactivity may be affected. These motor control programs are not always suited for the lift frequency and the muscles are recruited to levels that are either too high or that are activated at inappropriate times, yielding high levels of coactivity and, in turn, resulting in unnecessarily high spinal loads.

Collectively, these trends point to a trend where spine loads increased when subjects were faced with lifting situations that were not compatible with their preferred or "ingrained" motor recruitment patterns. For example, experienced workers are most likely used to lifting at greater frequency rates and have most likely optimized their muscle recruitment patterns so that they minimize cocontraction and the subsequent loading. Exposing these workers to slower lift rates could require them to recruit their muscles in a manner that is unnatural for them.

Inexperienced workers, however, have not developed a very sophisticated muscle recruitment model for themselves. Therefore, they cocontract under circumstances where one would expect minimal loading (i.e., low moment exposures). These observations might help explain the "survivor" effect that has been noted in the epidemiologic literature. The survivor effect refers to potential bias in a study due to the fact that only those workers who are not susceptible to a risk factor remain on the job. Other (more vulnerable) workers quit or change jobs. This might help explain the high injury and turnover rate often observed in new workers.

These findings suggest that the most important factor in determining muscle recruitment and subsequent spinal loading might be matching the motor control program that the worker has developed for himself. This concept is consistent with the expectations of a theory (81) that suggested motor control is driven by a satisfaction principle (discussed in the previous chapter), where the match or mismatch between one's expectations of how one should recruit the muscles and what is actually required to perform a task determines the degree of cocontraction developed during a task.

Practically, these concepts point to a need to establish motor patterns through planned experiential activities. Many of the martial arts use this concept as the basis for training.

7.14 SPINE LOADING ASSOCIATED WITH MODIFICATION OF PHYSICAL WORKPLACE FACTORS

The following sections explore how biomechanical spine loads can be mediated through modification of physical workplace factors. For example, instead of lifting one may be able to change the task into a pushing task or may alter the spine loading via team lifting.

7.14.1 Handles

Proper use of handles (or coupling with a load) can have a profound influence on the three-dimensional loads experienced by the lumbar spine (54,82–84). While one early study suggested that the inclusion of handles increase spine loading (83), later studies using modern EMG-assisted modeling techniques have concluded that handles are beneficial from a spine loading standpoint. In a study of distribution center work, handles were found to significantly reduce complex loading of the spine. Maximum spine compression was reduced by 6.8%, and A/P shear was reduced by about 6% when handles were available in the cases being lifted by the workers (82). Figure 7.39 shows how handles influenced the three-dimensional loads experienced by the spine under these conditions.

The influence of handles on loading of the spine is also a function of the lift origin. Figure 7.40a and b shows how spine compression varies as a function of handle availability and the lift origin on a pallet. Figure 7.40a defines the different regions of a pallet from which workers lifted. Figure 7.40b indicates that spine compression was unaffected by

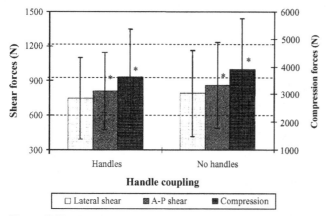

Figure 7.39 Maximum spinal loads experienced by the lumbar spine during order selecting work when using handles versus no handle conditions ([*] indicates significantly different loads between handle conditions). (From reference 82).

handle availability at the highest pallet origin positions. However, significant differences were noted as the lift origin became lower to the ground with handles decreasing spine compression. In this study, case weights between 18.2 and 27.3 kg were lifted. On average, the inclusion of handles had an affect on the spine loading similar to reducing the case weight by 4.5 kg (54).

In-depth analyses of these findings indicated that handle coupling did not influence the trunk moments to which the workers were exposed. Thus, lifting techniques were not influenced much by the presence or absence of handles. However, these analyses also indicated that antagonistic muscle coactivity was greater when lifting in the lower regions of the pallet without handles. Figure 7.41 indicates that the abdominal muscles, external oblique and internal oblique muscles, increased their activities when handles were not present. This increased trunk muscle activity was most likely necessary to stabilize the load and the torso during lifting. The NIOSH Revised Lifting Equation (85) has included a coupling multiplier for assessing the lifting risk. The results from this study indicate that the Revised Lifting Equation multiplier is appropriate for lifts performed at higher vertical lift origins but need to be more protective for lower vertical lift origins.

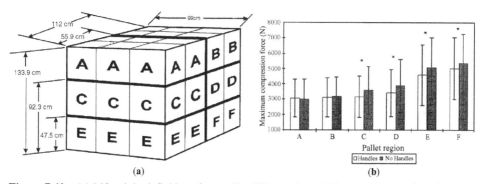

Figure 7.40 (**a**) Lift origin definitions for a pallet lifting task and (**b**) spine compression observed while lifting with and without handles when lifting from the various lift origin regions as defined by (**a**). (From reference 82).

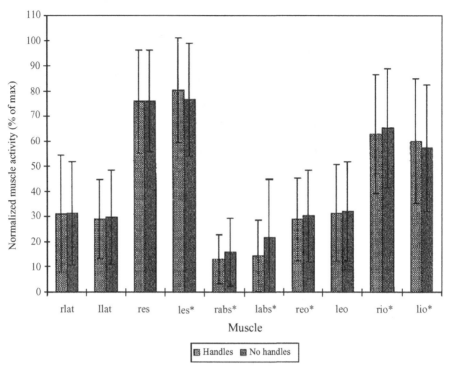

Figure 7.41   Normalized trunk muscle activities observed when lifting with handles versus without handles (r and l indicate right or left side muscle, lat = latissimus dorsi, es = erector spinae, abs = rectus abdominus, eo = external oblique, and io = internal oblique). (From reference 82).

7.15   LIFTING WHILE SUPPORTING THE BODY

Most traditional biomechanical assessments of lifting assume that the worker lifts with two hands and body support comes solely from the feet in contact with the ground. However, a common occurrence in occupational materials handling is lifting performed while the worker is unbalanced, supporting one's self on the side of a bin, and often standing on one leg while using the other leg as a counterbalance. Few quantitative biomechanical assessments can be found in the literature that explore the affect of these "realistic" job modifiers on spine loading. However, one such study found that spine loads were influenced by the number of feet in contact with the floor, the number of hands used to lift the object, and the origin of the lift (86). Figure 7.42 summarizes the influence of the number of hands used in the lift, the number of feet used for support, and the origin "region" of the lift (defined as the quadrants of a bin placed directly in front of the worker) on lateral shear forces experienced at L5/S1. This figure indicates that one-handed lifts performed while supporting the body with one leg, always imposed the highest lateral shear forces on the spine. These forces were also highest when lifting from low levels of vertical origin. The figure also shows that lifting with two hands while supporting the body with two feet always produced the lowest level of lateral force on the spine.

Leaning or supporting the body on the side of a bin significantly reduced compressive forces on the spine. Figures 7.43 and 7.44 indicate the average peak compression and A/P shear, respectively, experienced by the lumbar spine while lifting from regions of a bin while supporting the body (by using one hand to support the body against the bin). Both compression and A/P shear were greatest under all bin region conditions when lifting

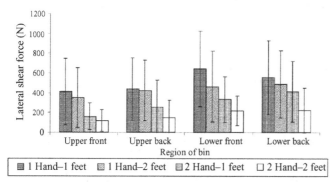

Figure 7.42 Lateral shear at L5/S1 shown as a function of the number of hands used to lift, the number of feet in contact with the ground, and the lift origin within in a bin. (From reference 86).

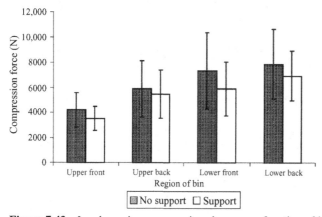

Figure 7.43 Lumbar spine compression shown as a function of load origin (bin region) and the presence of body support against the side of the bin. (From reference 86).

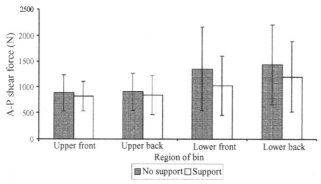

Figure 7.44 Lumbar spine A/P shear shown as a function of load origin (bin region) and the presence of body support against the side of the bin. (From reference 86).

without support compared to supporting the body by holding on to the edge of the bin. In addition, the benefits of support were much greater when lifting from low vertical lift origins. These findings suggest that bins should be designed to accommodate support by adding hand holds or contact points for the workers.

7.16   TEAM LIFTING

Two-person or team lifting is a popular method for handling materials when the capacity of one individual is expected to be exceeded by a lifting task. Many situations occur in occupations such as the construction industry, patient handling and health care, furniture handling, and retail sales where it would be difficult to provide a mechanical lifting device due to the variety of lifting situations encountered. While numerous guidelines and standards address lifting limits for individual lifting situations, there are no such limits for team lifting. In addition, a review of the literature indicates that we have a poor biomechanical understanding of these lifts.

The literature associated with team lifting offers some interesting paradoxes. Early studies reported that the sum of individual isometric and isokinetic lifting strengths was greater than the lifting capacity of the two-person team (87,88). One study (89) reported that mixed-gender teams lifted 80% of the individual's lifting capacity sum, whereas same-gender teams lifted over 90% of this sum. Regression equations that explained 90% of the variability in team lifting have indicated that the lifting capacity of the team is dictated by the weaker of the two team members (90). Another study (91) reported that during both team lifting and carrying, subjects were willing to lift weights that were greater than the sum of the individuals acceptable weights. It is also interesting to note that this study was the only one that stated they matched subjects for height and was the only study that found an increase in team lifting capacity. Hence, coordination between lifters can play an important role in team lifting.

This brief review indicates some mixed results when considering team lifting from a strength and psychophysical perspective. However, none of these studies have considered how changes between one-person lifts and team lifts might affect the spine loading and the subsequent risk of low back disorder. It is likely that changes in lifting kinematics or lifting kinetics may be a result of changing from a one-person lift to a team lift.

A more recent study has used a biologically assisted biomechanical model to assess spine loading characteristics of one-person and two-person lifting teams while workers lifted under sagittally symmetric and asymmetric conditions (92). Significant differences occurred in spine compression, lateral shear, and A–P shear as a function of the degree of asymmetry associated with a lifting condition regardless of whether one or two persons were performing the lift. The trend indicated that under team-lifting conditions, the sagittally symmetric lift produced the least amount of compression, lateral shear, and A–P shear on the spine. In general, all three components of spine loading were greatest when the lift involved an asymmetric origin and destination. Spine compression was lower for two-person lifts for a given weight, but only while lifting in sagittally symmetric conditions (Fig. 7.45). Lateral shear became much greater for two-person lifts under the asymmetric lifting conditions (Fig. 7.46). The study has linked these changes to differences in trunk kinematic patterns adopted during one-person versus two-person lifting.

The major change in muscle recruitment patterns observed under these conditions involved an increase in the activity of the oblique muscles when asymmetric load destinations were part of a lifting a condition. The oblique muscle activity increased by an average of 25% under these asymmetric destination conditions. Such increases would be of concern in terms of increasing the potential to activate the muscle function disruption pathway to back pain. It is also significant to note that lateral shear force increases to a level near the disc tolerance limit under asymmetric lifting conditions.

Finally, lift coordination or synchronization was studied to assess the potential for team training to serve as an intervention for spine loading. In this study, synchronization was accomplished by providing a verbal "count" to coordinate the actions of the two team

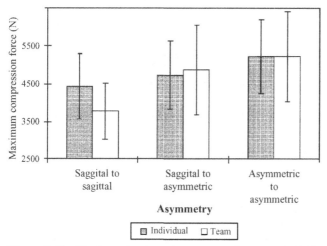

Figure 7.45 Maximum lumbar spine compression on an individual worker shown as a function of team lifting versus individual lifting of a standard amount of weight and as a function of the lift origin and destination asymmetry conditions. (From reference 92).

members. When the spine loading was evaluated under these synchronized conditions, the spine compression differences between asymmetries as a function of the number of workers involved in the lift (interaction) were no longer different. The only statistically significant difference in asymmetry as a function of the number of team members involved lateral shear force (Fig. 7.47). Under the asymmetric team-lifting conditions, the maximum lateral shear force was reduced by an average of 190 N when synchronization was included. Little difference in spinal shear occurred under the symmetric lifts under these conditions. When the kinetic and kinematic data were examined for these conditions, it was found that both the lateral and sagittal trunk moments were reduced during synchronized lifting. This reduction was particularly relevant since the shear forces were reduced to a level below what is considered risky. Maximum shear and compression were reduced by 140 and 300 N, respectively, when lifts were performed synchronously.

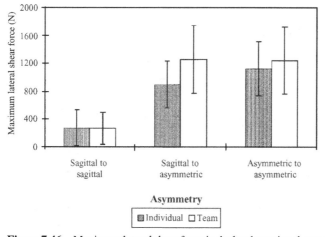

Figure 7.46 Maximum lateral shear force in the lumbar spine shown as a function of individual versus team lifting as well as task origin and destination asymmetry conditions. (From reference 92).

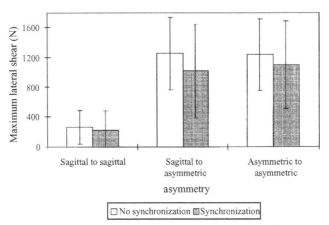

Figure 7.47 Maximum lateral shear force as a function of lift synchronization and asymmetry. (From reference 92).

These findings indicate that one means to mediate the increased risk associated with team lifting under the most problematic asymmetric lifting conditions would be to train the team members to lift in synchrony. The effect of this training appears to minimize the differences in the kinematic and kinetic trunk movement variables between the asymmetric lifting conditions.

These results indicate that there are significant trade-offs associated with one-person vs. two-person lifting. This study found that the preferable number of team members involved in lifting depends on many factors. In general, single-person lifting is beneficial when lifting under symmetric lifting conditions as long as the load lifted is not excessive. In addition, lateral shear forces may become problematic when two-person teams place a load in a specific asymmetric location compared to allowing a one-person lifter to place a load in an asymmetric "nonprecise" location. Thus, precision of placement is a variable that must be considered when lifting. However, the detrimental effects of two-person lifting can be significantly mediated, especially at asymmetric destinations, by training the lifting team to lift synchronously.

7.17 PUSHING AND PULLING

Early quantitative assessments of pushing have focused on the loading developed about L5/S1 during the exertion. EMG-assisted models have reported that compressive forces on the spine were lowest when pushing carts of low weight (85 kg) using one hand placed on handles at shoulder height (compared to hip height) (93). However, few pushing conditions resulted in spine compression at L5/S1 that exceeded the levels of force that would result in vertebral end plate damage, even when pushing the heaviest load (320 kg). Thus, early assessments of pushing and pulling activities had difficulty explaining, from a biomechanical standpoint, how push–pull activities could result in low back pain.

The EMG-assisted modeling approach has recently been adapted to account for the lumbar spine bending and curvature changes that occur during pushing exertion. Trunk movement information can be monitored using a goniometer such as the LMM during the exertion to estimate spinal curvature according to published methods (94–96). This allows the partitioning of spinal forces along the length of the lumbar spine. During pushing activities, spine compression is rather moderate; however, dramatic differences in shear loading are observed at different levels of the lumbar spine. Figure 7.48 shows the trade-off in spine load at the different level of the lumbar spine during pushing activities (97). This analysis indicated that significant biomechanical risk (in A/P shear) occurs at the higher lumbar levels (L3 through L1) where the tolerance to shear is only about 750–1000 N (98–101), whereas previous studies have only examined the load-tolerance risk at lower levels of the lumbar spine where shear forces are significantly lower. Thus, this evaluation indicates that, unlike lifting, pushing increases the loads at the upper levels of the lumbar spine compared to maximum loading occurring at L5/S1 during lifting.

Spine loading of male and female participants were evaluated as they pushed on instrumented handles at three handle heights (50%, 65%, and 80% of stature) and three hand forces levels (20%, 30%, and 40% of body weight) under free-dynamic conditions. The results were able to identify the conditions under which spinal loads increased. Significant differences in spine load were found as a function of lumbar level for compression and A/P shear overall (Fig. 7.48), hand force for compression and shear (A/P shear shown in Fig. 7.49), handle height and A/P shear (Fig. 7.50), their interaction (Fig. 7.51b) and gender (Fig. 7.52). The effects of hand force were not unexpected as it is logical to assume that greater hand force would result in greater spine load. However, for the first time, this study was able to describe how much hand force is too much hand force (relative to spine loading).

A/P shear was found to reach damaging levels as a result of handle placement. Conventional wisdom dictates that the vector of handle force application should pass through L5/S1 to minimize the torque imposed on the spine (102). This conventional wisdom would suggest placing handles at lower levels (e.g., 50% of body stature). However, the analyses indicated that A/P shear force was minimized by placing the handles at higher levels (65–80% of body stature). In-depth analyses of the hand transducer data (from this

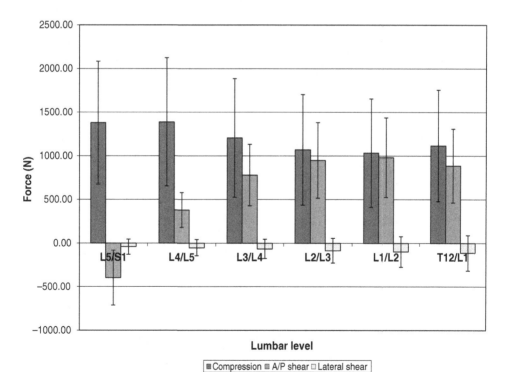

Figure 7.48   Predictions of spine loads over the five levels of the lumbar spine. Note that A/P shear dramatically changes direction and magnitude over the various lumbar levels.

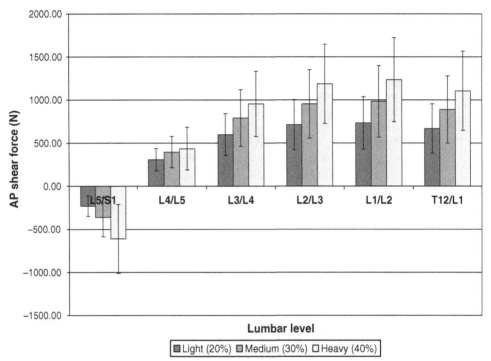

Figure 7.49 Pushing A/P shear loads by hand force level at each lumbar level.

experiment) indicated that when handles were placed at low levels, the subjects actually lifted up on the handles when pulling and pulled down on the handles when pulling from higher levels, which increased the torque around L5/S1 beyond what was expected (Fig. 7.51a). This action increased trunk muscle coactivity and the resulting spine loading.

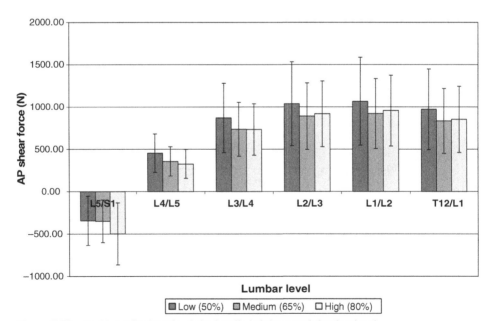

Figure 7.50 Pushing A/P shear loads by handle height at each lumbar level.

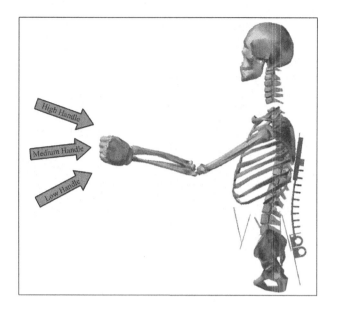

(a)

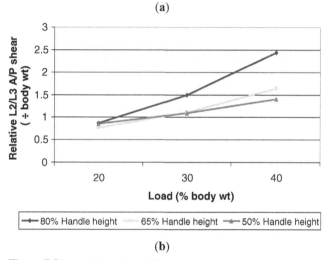

(b)

Figure 7.51   (**a**) Direction of force imposed on a handle while pulling on handles at different height levels, (The current model was recently embedded in the MSC. ADAMS Software environment (MSC. Software, Inc.) and utilizes the LifeMod (Biomechanics Research Group, Inc.) biomechanical overlay.) and (**b**) A–P shear imposed on the spine when pulling on handles of different heights at different height levels and different pull forces.

However, when subjects pushed at higher handle heights, the handle force applications were directed slightly downward, minimizing the torque about L5/S1 and the subsequent A/P shear force experienced by the spine.

Finally, dramatic differences in A/P shear occurred as a function of gender (Fig. 7.52). These differences are primarily a function of the different insertion and origin points of the trunk musculature (defining lever arm distances) that result in different muscle recruitment patterns and spine loads in males compared to females. This demonstrates how an EMG-assisted model is able to account for spine loads resulting from individual differences compared to work factors. Such analyses can be valuable in explaining how special populations of workers are affected by work conditions.

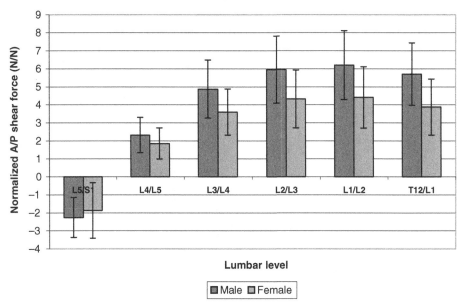

Figure 7.52 Pushing A/P shear loads by gender at each lumbar level.

7.18 SEATED AND CONSTRAINED WORK POSTURES

Seated workplaces have become more prominent with modern work, especially with the aging of the workforce and the introduction of service-oriented and data processing jobs. It has been documented that loads on the lumbar spine are greater when a worker is seated compared to standing (103). This is true since the posterior (bony) elements of the spine (facets) form an active load path when one is standing. However, when seated, these elements are disengaged and more of the load passes through the intervertebral disk. Thus, work performed in a seated position puts the worker at greater relative risk of spine loading and, therefore, greater risk of damaging the disk. Given this mechanism of spine loading, it is important to consider the design features of a chair since it may be possible to influence disc loading through chair design. Figure 7.53 shows the results of a study involving pressure measurements taken within the intervetebral disc of individuals as the back angle of the chair and magnitude of lumbar support were varied (103). It is infeasible to directly measure the forces in the spine in vivo. Therefore, disc pressure measures have traditionally been used as a rough approximation of loads imposed on the spine. This figure indicates that both the seat back angle and lumbar support features have a significant impact on disc pressure. Disc pressure decreases as the *back rest* angle is increased. However, increasing the backrest angle in the workplace is often not practical since it can also move the worker farther away from the work and thereby increasing external moment. Figure 7.53 also indicates that increasing lumbar support can significantly reduce disc pressure. This reduction in disc pressure is due to the fact that as lumbar curvature (lordosis) is reestablished (with lumbar support), the posterior elements play more of a role in providing an alternative load path as is the case when standing in the upright position.

It should also be noted that a more recent study has been unable to support these relative relationships between sitting and standing (104). While this more recent study used more up-to-date transducers to measure spine load, only one subject was observed; thus, it is premature to extrapolate these findings to a larger population.

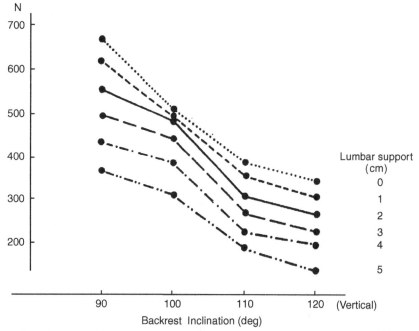

Figure 7.53 Disk pressures measured with different backrest inclinations (from vertical (90°) and different size lumbar supports). (From reference 14).

One study has compared several spine loading measures when performing physically demanding tasks while seated compared to performing the same tasks in kneeling postures (105). This study indicated that while back muscle fatigue, spine length changes, and estimates of discomfort were all improved in seated conditions compared to kneeling, the seated conditions still resulted in significant discomfort. Other studies have examined physically demanding tasks preformed while in restricted postures (106–110). These studies indicate significantly greater spine loading in postures that restrict the posture of the worker as well as more demands on the musculoskeletal system. Posture restriction appears to increase the level of trunk muscle coactivity needed to maintain the posture and support the external load compared to unrestricted postures. These findings are consistent with industrial surveillance studies that have identified greater risk associated with nonneutral trunk postures (17,19,22,111).

The risk associated with low level exertions (i.e., typing) over prolonged periods of time while sitting (as is done while interacting with a computer keyboard) has been difficult to explain from a biomechanical loading perspective. However, two recent studies suggest that sustained work under these conditions can activate one of the muscle disruption pathways described earlier (112,113). These studies are particularly fascinating in that they demonstrate that TrPTs can develop in the upper back and shoulders as a result of prolonged exposure to poor posture exposure *or* as a result of worker interaction with poor visual quality displays (Fig. 7.54).

Less is known about risk to the low back relative to prolonged standing. The trunk muscles may experience low level static exertion conditions and may be subject to static overload through the muscle static fatigue process described in Chapter 5. Muscle fatigue can result in lowered muscle force generation capacity and can, thus, initiate the cumulative trauma sequence of events. The fatigue and cumulative trauma sequence can be minimized through two actions. First, foot rests can provide a mechanism to allow relaxation of the large back muscles and thus increased blood flow to the muscle. This reduces the static load and

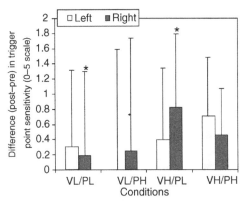

Figure 7.54 Observed myofascial trigger point (TrPT) sensitivity indicating a response to low level exertions as a function of exposure to combinations of low (VL) or high (VH) visual stress and low (PL) or high (PH) postural stress for the right and left trapezius muscles (* indicates statistically significant differences). (Adapted from reference 113).

subsequent fatigue in the muscle by the process described earlier in Chapter 5 (Fig. 5.3). When a leg is rested on the foot rest, the large back muscles are relaxed on one side of the body and the muscle can be supplied with oxygen. Alternating legs placed on the foot rest provides a mechanism to minimize back muscle fatigue throughout the day. Second, floor mats can decrease the fatigue in the back muscles provided that the mats have proper compression characteristics (114). Floor mats are believed to facilitate body sway, which enhances the pumping of blood through back muscles thereby minimizing fatigue.

Knowledge of when standing workplaces are preferable to seated workplaces is dictated mainly by work performance criteria. In general, *standing* workplaces are preferred when (1) the task requires a high degree of mobility (reaching and monitoring in positions that exceed the employee's reach envelope or when performing tasks at different heights or different locations), (2) precise manual control actions are not required, (3) leg room is not available (when leg room is not available the moment arm distance between the external load and the back is increased and thus greater internal back muscle force and spinal load result), and (4) heavy weights are handled or large forces are applied. When jobs must accommodate both sitting and standing postures, it is important to ensure that the positions and orientations of the body (especially the upper extremity) are in the same relative location under both standing and sitting conditions.

7.19 PHYSICAL WORK FACTOR SUMMARY

Table 7.4 summarizes the effects that physical work factors and their modifications have on spine loading. As shown here, most workplace physical factors explored are associated with increases in spine loads. Many of these increases in loading are associated with increases in trunk muscle coactivation. This table also shows that some of the physical factor modifications can decrease spine loading and some may increase spine loading.

Traditionally, it has been assumed that there is a direct relationship between spine loading and risk of occupation-related low back pain. However, of late, some have questioned the relationship, and little conclusive evidence is available that makes it possible to either prove or disprove the hypothesis.

One problematic aspect of such an analysis involves the accuracy and resolution of spine loading. Historically, many of the biomechanical models employed to assess biomechanical

TABLE 7.4 Relationship Between Spine Loading and Observed Risk of Low Back Pain

	Increase in factor leads to increase in LBP risk	Increase in compression, A/P and Lateral Shear	Decrease (or no change) in compression, A/P and Lateral shear	Increase in muscle coactivation
Physical workplace factor				
Moment exposure	X	X		
Role of trunk muscle cocontraction in spine loading				
When muscles simulataneously increase level of contraction				
Trunk motion	X	X		X
Asymmetric loading	X			X
Lateral motion		X		X
Twisting motion	X	X		X
Task asymmetry		X		X
Lift height		X		
One-hand vs. two-hand lifting		X		
Asymmetric lifting with either hand	X			
Lifting vs. lowering		X		
As load weight increases		X		
Lifting	X			X
Cumulative exposure	X			
Duration of exposure to lifting tasks		X		X
Worker experience, task frequency, and moment exposure				
Unexperienced workers and All when load moment increased				X
Modification to physical workplace factor				
Handles			X	
No handles				X
Lifting while supporting the body			X	
Supporting body on edge of a bin				
Team lifting				
Team lifting with asymmetric origin and destination		X		
Pushing			X	
Seated and constrained work postures	X	X		

loading (especially at the workplace) may have been too rudimentary and not able to assess occupational stress with fine enough resolution to properly identify risk. In addition, as discussed earlier, many of the epidemiologic methodologies treat spine load as a discrete variable that is either above or below a given level and that level may have been chosen arbitrarily with no realistic biomechanical value. Hence, there are several problems with assessing the strength of the relationship between spine loading and occupational risk of low back pain.

One effort has compared spine loading patterns as assessed by models of varying resolution and sophistication with estimates of risk based on historical observations (115). Historical risk was evaluated for jobs performed over an extended period of continuous palletizing activities using the lumbar motion monitor risk model for high risk group membership (discussed earlier) (41). In this study, experienced workers palletized 12 pallets of cases. Based on the data collected during the lifting activities, several biomechanical models were used to assess spine loading for all lifts monitored during the study. These biomechanical models varied from two-dimensional spine compression models that assessed compression alone to three-dimensional dynamic spine models that assessed compression and shear based on an EMG-assisted biomechanical model prediction (27,30,116). Static biomechanical analyses consisted of assessments based on a two-dimensional planar model with no coactivity consideration (14). For the dynamic estimates of spine load, both dynamic load and load rate were considered.

Table 7.5 displays the degree of association between the peak spine loads (defined by the various biomechanical models) and the probability of high risk group membership. The R^2 values represent the percent of variability accounted for by the linear relationship between the two variables in a cell. The table indicates that static estimates of spine compression account for about 13.5% of the variability in low risk group membership, whereas dynamic estimates of compression account for over three times the variability in high risk group membership. It is interesting to note that the differences between these values also agrees with the difference in risk predictability (odds ratio) between statically based field surveillance tools and dynamic surveillance tools (117).

In addition, a significant association between lateral and A/P shear load rates were observed to identify historical risk well. Table 7.6 indicates the relationship between spinal ligament strain or strain rate (as predicted via the dynamic biomechanical model) and the probability of high risk group membership. Note that the amount of variability accounted for in the model approaches 50% when ligament strain is included.

Table 7.7 indicates the degree of association between historically defined low back pain risk and spine loads when combinations of biomechanical spine loading measures are considered. This table indicates the importance of considering multiple dimensions of spine loading when considering historically observed risk for low back pain. Note that when intertransverse ligament strain rate (a measure of axial loading) is combined with compression, lateral shear, or supraspinous strain rate, the association with historically observed risk increases to over 50%. In addition, the more multidimensional the model, the more the

TABLE 7.5 Squared Correlation Coefficients (R^2) Express the Degree of Association Between Peak Spine Loads and the Probability of High Risk Group Membership (From Reference 115)

	Lateral Shear	A/P Shear	Compression
Static load	–	–	0.135
Dynamic load	0.191	0.195	0.441
Loud rate	0.343	0.345	0.428

Dynamic estimates of spine compression were the strongest individual correlation with probability of high risk group membership (115). R^2 differing by >0.09 represent statistically different model performance.

TABLE 7.6   Squared Correlation Coefficients (R^2) Express the Degree of Association Between Strain or Strain Rate in the Spinal Ligaments and the Probability of High Risk Group Membership (From Reference 115)

	InterTransv	SuperSpin
Strain	0.477	0.474
Strain late	0.004	0.002

TABLE 7.7   Relationship Between Combinations of Biomechanical Factors and Task Probability of High Risk Group Membership for Low Back Pain (From Reference 115)

Regression Models	R^2
Two-factor models	
$S_I + F_z$	0.514
$S_I + F_x$	0.542
$S_s + LR_x$	0.546
Three-factor models	
$F_x + F_z + S_I$	0.547
$S_I + S_s + F_x$	0.561
$S_s + SR_I + LR_x$	0.562
Four-factor models	
$F_x + F_y + F_z + S_I$	0.557
$S_I + S_s + F_x + LR_x$	0.567
$S_I + S_s + F_x + SR_I$	0.573

F_x, lateral shear force; F_y, A/P shear force; F_z, compressive force; S_I, InterTransv lig. strain; S_s, SuperSpin lig. strain; LR_x, lateral load rate; LR_y, AP load rate; LR_z, Compr. load rate; SR_I, InterTransv strain rate; SR_s, SuperSpin strain rate.

biomechanical factors correlated with observed risk. Given the difficulty studies have in defining LBP, these correlations represent reasonable predictions.

Collectively, these findings indicate that high risk surveillance measures derived from industry correlate well with three-dimensional dynamic biomechanical load. Thus, the more dynamic and multidimensional the biomechanical assessment of the task, the better the association with observed risk. This observation further supports that pattern of evidence associated with work-related risk of low back pain and provides yet another form of validity to this relationship.

7.20   SUMMARY

Collectively, these findings demonstrate that spine loading is governed by a complex mixture of work related factors that affect the spine in multiple dimensions of loading. These workplace features influence the degree to which trunk muscles are recruited and the pattern by which trunk muscles are recruited. Hence, the common feature among the conditions that increase spine loading is the increase in muscle coactivation. This increase in coactivation increases muscle tension and increases the likelihood of muscle function disruption pathways to low back pain. Increased coactivation also results in increased spine loading. When the stability benefits of the cocontraction are outweighed by the negative effects of loading, the support structure disruption pathway to low back pain is likely to be engaged. It is also obvious from these results that spine loading is also influenced by the worker's experience in that motor programs are selected based on experience with duration of lifting, frequency of lifting, and load weight also influencing muscle recruitment profiles. Thus, this complex mix of influences must be considered to properly assess the contribution of physical work factors to low back pain risk.

KEY POINTS

- Surveillance studies suggest that physical factor related low back pain risk at work are multidimensional in that a synergy among risk factors appears to intensify risk.

- Physical workplace risk factors include excessive moment exposure, asymmetric loading, increased dynamic motion, sustained postures that need not be of high force, repeated loading, and poor timing or coordination of the effort.

- Many of the back pain pathways associated with physical exposure cause an increase in coactivation of the trunk muscles thereby increasing spine loading.

- Industrial surveillance observations of back pain risk are consistent with biomechanical logic, but only if the effects of three-dimensional, dynamic loading are considered using biologically assisted modeling techniques.

REFERENCES

1. NIOSH. Musculoskeletal disorders and workplace factors: a critical review of epidemiologic evidence for work-related musculoskeletal disorders of the neck, upper extremity, and low back. BERNARD BP. editor. Cincinnati, OH: Department of Health and Human Services (DHHS), Public Health Service, Centers for Disease Control, National Institute for Occupational Safety and Health (NIOSH); 1997.
2. CHAFFIN DB, PARK KS. A longitudinal study of low-back pain as associated with occupational weight lifting factors. Am Ind Hygiene Assoc J 1973;34(12):513–525.
3. VIDEMAN T, NURMINEN M, TROUP JD. 1990 Volvo Award in clinical sciences. Lumbar spinal pathology in cadaveric material in relation to history of back pain, occupation, and physical loading. Spine 1990;15(8):728–740.
4. BERNARD BP. Musculoskeletal disorders and workplace factors: a critical review of epidemiologic evidence for work-related musculoskeletal disorders of the neck, upper extremity, and low back. Publication No. 97-141,Cincinnati (OH): National Institute for Occupational Safety and Health, U.S. Department of Health and Human Services (DHHS); 1997.
5. ANDERSSON GB. The epidemiology of spinal disorders. In FRYMOYER JW. editor. The Adult Spine: Principles and Practice. Philadelphia: Lippincott-Raven Publishers; 1997. p.93–141.
6. BIGOS SJ., et al. A longitudinal, prospective study of industrial back injury reporting. Clin Orthop 1992; (279):21–34.
7. BURDORF A, GOVAERT G, ELDERS L. Postural load and back pain of workers in the manufacturing of prefabricated concrete elements. Ergonomics 1991;34(7):909–918.
8. RIIHIMAKI H., et al. Low-back pain and occupation. A cross-sectional questionnaire study of men in machine operating, dynamic physical work, and sedentary work. Spine 1989;14(2):204–209.
9. BATTIE MC., et al. Isometric lifting strength as a predictor of industrial back pain reports. Spine 1989;14(8):851–856.
10. BIGOS SJ., et al. Back injuries in industry: a retrospective study: III. Employee-related factors. Spine 1986;11(3):252–256.
11. KELSEY JL., et al. An epidemiologic study of lifting and twisting on the job and risk for acute prolapsed lumbar intervetebral disc. J Orthop Res 1984;2(1):61–66.
12. VIDEMAN T., et al. Low-back pain in nurses and some loading factors of work. Spine 1984;9(4):400–404.

13. SPENGLER DM., et al. Back injuries in industry: a retrospective study: I. Overview and cost analysis. Spine 1986;11(3):241–245.

14. CHAFFIN DB, ANDERSSON GBJ, MARTIN BJ. Occupational Biomechanics. 3rd ed. New York: John Wiley & Sons, Inc.; 1999. p. 579.

15. LILES DH., et al. A job severity index for the evaluation and control of lifting injury. Hum Factors 1984;26(6):683–693.

16. HERRIN GD, JARAIEDI M, ANDERSON CK. Prediction of overexertion injuries using biomechanical and psychophysical models. Am Ind Hygiene Assoc J 1986;47(6):322–330.

17. PUNNETT L., et al. Back disorders and nonneutral trunk postures of automobile assembly workers. Scand J Work Environ Health 1991;17(5):337–346.

18. WATERS TR., et al. Evaluation of the revised NIOSH lifting equation. A cross-sectional epidemiologic study. Spine 1999;24(4):386–394; discussion 395.

19. MARRAS WS., et al. Biomechanical risk factors for occupationally related low back disorders. Ergonomics 1995;38(2):377–410.

20. MARRAS WS., et al. The role of dynamic three-dimensional trunk motion in occupationally-related low back disorders. The effects of workplace factors, trunk position, and trunk motion characteristics on risk of injury. Spine 1993;18(5):617–628.

21. MARRAS WS., et al. Prospective validation of a low-back disorder risk model and assessment of ergonomic interventions associated with manual materials handling tasks [in process citation]. Ergonomics 2000;43(11):1866–1886.

22. NORMAN R., et al. A comparison of peak vs cumulative physical work exposure risk factors for the reporting of low back pain in the automotive industry. Clin Biomech (Bristol, Avon) 1998;13(8):561–573.

23. FATHALLAH FA, MARRAS WS, PARNIANPOUR M. The role of complex, simultaneous trunk motions in the risk of occupation-related low back disorders. Spine 1998;23(9):1035–1042.

24. DAVIS KG, MARRAS WS. Assessment of the relationship between box weight and trunk kinematics: does a reduction in box weight necessarily correspond to a decrease in spinal loading? [in process citation]. Hum Factors 2000;42(2):195–208.

25. GRANATA KP, MARRAS WS. An EMG-assisted model of loads on the lumbar spine during asymmetric trunk extensions. J Biomech 1993;26(12):1429–1438.

26. GRANATA KP, MARRAS WS. The influence of trunk muscle coactivity on dynamic spinal loads. Spine 1995;20(8):913–919.

27. GRANATA KP, MARRAS WS. An EMG-assisted model of trunk loading during free-dynamic lifting. J Biomech 1995;28(11):1309–1317.

28. MARRAS WS. Toward an understanding of dynamic variables in ergonomics. Occup Med 1992;7(4):655–677.

29. MARRAS WS., et al. Spine loads in low back patients during complex lifts. Spine 2002. In review.

30. MARRAS WS, GRANATA KP. A biomechanical assessment and model of axial twisting in the thoracolumbar spine. Spine 1995;20(13):1440–1451.

31. MARRAS WS, GRANATA KP. Spine loading during trunk lateral bending motions. J Biomech 1997;30(7):697–703.

32. MARRAS WS, RANGARAJULU SL, WONGSAM PE. Trunk force development during static and dynamic lifts. Hum Factors 1987;29(1):19–29.

33. MARRAS WS, SOMMERICH CM. A three-dimensional motion model of loads on the lumbar spine: II. Model validation. Hum Factors 1991;33(2):139–149.

34. McGILL SM. Kinetic potential of the lumbar trunk musculature about three orthogonal orthopaedic axes in extreme postures. Spine 1991;16(7):809–815.

35. McGILL SM. A myoelectrically based dynamic three-dimensional model to predict loads on lumbar spine tissues during lateral bending. J Biomech 1992;25(4):395–414.

36. MARRAS, WS, MIRKA, GA. A comprehensive evaluation of trunk response to asymmetric trunk motion. Spine 1992;17(3):318–326.

37. MARRAS WS, MIRKA GA. Muscle activities during asymmetric trunk angular accelerations. J Orthop Res 1990;8(6):824–832.

38. GRANATA KP, MARRAS WS. Cost-benefit of muscle cocontraction in protecting against spinal instability. Spine 2000;25(11):1398–1404.

39. BROBERG KB. On the mechanical behaviour of intervertebral discs. Spine 1983;8(2):151–165.

40. SHIRAZI-ADL A. Finite-element evaluation of contact loads on facets of an L2–L3 lumbar segment in complex loads. Spine 1991;16(5):533–541.

41. MARRAS WS., et al. The role of dynamic three-dimensional trunk motion in occupationally-related low back disorders. The effects of workplace factors, trunk position, and trunk motion characteristics on risk of injury. Spine 1993;18(5):617–628.

42. MARRAS WS., et al. Female and male trunk geometry: size and prediction of the spine loading trunk muscles derived from MRI. Clin Biomech (Bristol Avon) 2001;16(1):38–46.

43. HOOGENDOORN WE., et al. Physical load during work and leisure time as risk factors for back pain [see comments]. Scand J Work Environ Health 1999;25(5):387–403.

44. BURDORF A, SOROCK G. Positive and negative evidence of risk factors for back disorders. Scand J Work, Environ Health 1997;23(4):243–256.

45. DAMKOT DK., et al. The relationship between work history, work environment and low-back pain in men. Spine 1984;9(4):395–399.

46. MUNDT DJ., et al. An epidemiologic study of non-occupational lifting as a risk factor for herniated lumbar intervertebral disc. The Northeast Collaborative Group on Low Back Pain. Spine 1993;18(5):595–602.

47. MIRANDA H., et al. Individual factors, occupational loading, and physical exercise as predictors of sciatic pain. Spine 2002;27(10):1102–1109.

48. MIRK P., et al. Frequency of musculoskeletal symptoms in diagnostic medical sonographers. Results of a pilot survey. Radiol Med (Torino) 1999;98(4):236–241.

49. ELLIOTT BC. Back injuries and the fast bowler in cricket. J Sports Sci 2000;18(12):983–991.

50. FRYMOYER JW., et al. Epidemiologic studies of low-back pain. Spine 1980;5(5):419–423.

51. KINGMA I., et al. When is a lifting movement too asymmetric to identify low-back loading by 2-D analysis? Ergonomics 1998;41(10):1453–1461.

52. DAVIS K, MARRAS W. Load spatial pathway and spine loading: how does lift origin and destination influence low back response?. Ergonomics 2005;48(8):1031–1046.

53. MARRAS W., et al. Spine loading and probability of low back disorder risk as a function of box location on a pallet. Int J Hum Factors Manufactur 1997;7(4): 323–336.

54. MARRAS WS., et al. Effects of box features on spine loading during warehouse order selecting. Ergonomics 1999;42(7):980–996.

55. ALLREAD WG, MARRAS WS, PARNIANPOUR M. Trunk kinematics of one-handed lifting, and the effects of asymmetry and load weight. Ergonomics 1996;39(2): 322–334.

56. MARRAS WS, DAVIS KG. Spine loading during asymmetric lifting using one versus two hands. Ergonomics 1998;41(6):817–834.

57. KINGMA I, van DIEEN JH. Lifting over an obstacle: effects of one-handed lifting and hand support on trunk kinematics and low back loading. J Biomech 2004;37(2): 249–255.

58. de LOOZE MP., et al. Joint moments and muscle activity in the lower extremities and lower back in lifting and lowering tasks. J Biomech 1993;26(9):1067–1076.

59. CLARKSON PM, HUBAL MJ. Exercise-induced muscle damage in humans. Am J Phys Med Rehabil 2002;81 (11 Suppl):S52–S69.

60. SIMONS DG. Review of enigmatic MTrPs as a common cause of enigmatic musculoskeletal pain and dysfunction. J Electromyogr Kinesiol 2004;14 (1): 95–107.

61. DAVIS KG, MARRAS WS, WATERS TR. The evaluation of spinal loads during lowering and lifting. Clin Biomech (Bristol, Avon) 1998;13(3):141–152.

62. KUMAR S. Cumulative load as a risk factor for back pain. Spine 1990;15(12):1311–1316.

63. VILLAGE J., et al. Electromyography as a measure of peak and cumulative workload in intermediate care and its relationship to musculoskeletal injury: an exploratory ergonomic study. Appl Ergon 2005;36(5):609–618.

64. ANDREWS DM, CALLAGHAN JP. Determining the minimum sampling rate needed to accurately quantify cumulative spine loading from digitized video. Appl Ergon 2003;34(6):589–595.

65. CALLAGHAN JP, SALEWYTSCH AJ, ANDREWS DM. An evaluation of predictive methods for estimating cumulative spinal loading. Ergonomics 2001;44(9):825–837.

66. MCGILL SM., et al. Studies of spinal shrinkage to evaluate low-back loading in the workplace. Ergonomics 1996; 39(1):92–102.

67. COURVILLE A., et al. Short rest periods after static lumbar flexion are a risk factor for cumulative low back disorder. J Electromyogr Kinesiol 2005;15(1):37–52.

68. LABRY R., et al. Longer static flexion duration elicits a neuromuscular disorder in the lumbar spine. J Appl Physiol 2004;96(5):2005–2015.

69. LU D., et al. Frequency-dependent changes in neuromuscular responses to cyclic lumbar flexion. J Biomech 2004;37(6):845–855.

70. SBRICCOLI P., et al. Static load repetition is a risk factor in the development of lumbar cumulative musculoskeletal disorder. Spine 2004;29(23):2643–2653.

71. SOLOMONOW M., et al. Muscular dysfunction elicited by creep of lumbar viscoelastic tissue. J Electromyogr Kinesiol 2003;13(4):381–396.

72. SOLOMONOW M., et al. Biomechanics and electromyography of a common idiopathic low back disorder. Spine 2003;28(12):1235–1248.

73. SOLOMONOW M., et al. Biomechanics of increased exposure to lumbar injury caused by cyclic loading: Part 1. Loss of reflexive muscular stabilization. Spine 1999;24(23):2426–2434.

74. MARRAS WS., et al. Spine loading as a function of lift frequency, exposure duration, and work experience. Clin Biomech (Bristol, Avon) 2006;21(4):345–352.

75. MARRAS WS, GRANATA KP. Changes in trunk dynamics and spine loading during repeated trunk exertions. Spine 1997;22(21):2564–2570.

76. YANG G., et al. The effects of work experience, lift frequency and exposure duration on low back muscle oxygenation. Clin Biomech (Bristol, Avon) 2007; 22(1):21–27.

77. CHANY A-M., et al. Changes in Spine loading patterns throughout the workday as a function of experience, lift frequency, and personality. The spine journal 2006;6:296–305.

78. de LOOZE MP., et al. Weight and frequency effect on spinal loading in a bricklaying task. J Biomech 1996; 29(11):1425–1433.

79. MARRAS W. Three-Dimensional Spine Loading as a Function of Lift Frequency and Duration of Exposure. Columbus (OH): The Ohio State University; 2005.

80. PARAKKAT J. Effect of Experience on Motor Control During Repetitive Lifting Exertions. Columbus: (OH) Department of Industrial and Systems Engineering, The Ohio State University; 2005.

81. ERLANDSON R, FLEMING D. Uncertainty sets associated with saccadic eye movements-basis of satisfaction control. Vision Res 1974;14:481–486.

82. DAVIS KG, MARRAS WS, WATERS TR. Reduction of spinal loading through the use of handles. Ergonomics 1998; 41(8):1155–1168.

83. FREIVALDS A., et al. A dynamic biomechanical evaluation of lifting maximum acceptable loads. J Biomech 1984;17(4):251–262.

84. ALMEIDA GL, CORCOS DM, LATASH ML. Practice and transfer effects during fast single-joint elbow movements in individuals with Down syndrome. Phys Ther 1994;74(11):1000–1012; discussion 1012–1016.

85. Waters TR., et al. Revised NIOSH equation for the design and evaluation of manual lifting tasks. Ergonomics 1993;36(7):749–776.

86. Ferguson SA., et al. Spinal loading when lifting from industrial storage bins. Ergonomics 2002;45(6):399–414.

87. Karwowski W, Mital A. Isometric and isokinetic testing of lifting strength of males in teamwork. Ergonomics 1986;29(7):869–878.

88. Karwowski W, Pongpatanasuegsa N. Testing of isometric and isokinetic lifting strengths of untrained females in teamwork. Ergonomics 1988;31(3):291–301.

89. Sharp M., et al. Maximum acceptable load for lifting and carrying in two-person teams. Human Factors and Ergonomics Society 39th Annual Meeting; Human Factors and Ergonomics Society;1995.

90. Rice V., et al. Predictions of two-person team lifting capacity.Human Factors and Erongomics Society 39th Annual Meeting; Human Factors and Ergonomics Society;1995.

91. Johnson S, Lewis D. A psychophysical study of two-person manual materials handling tasks. Human Factors Society 32nd Annual Meeting; Human Factors Society;1989.

92. Marras WS., et al. Spine loading and trunk kinematics during team lifting. Ergonomics 1999;42(10):1258–1273.

93. Hoozemans M., et al. Mechanical loading of the low back and shoulders during pushing and pulling activities. Ergonomics 2004;47(1):1–18.

94. Sicard C, Gagnon M. A geometric model of the lumbar spine in the sagittal plane. Spine 1993;18(5): 646–658.

95. Splittstoesser RE. A Simple Method for Predicting Dynamic Lumbar Motion Segment Angles Using Measures of Trunk Angle and Subject Anthropometry. Columbus: Ohio Ohio State University; 2001. p.63.

96. Splittstoesser RE. Prediction of lumbar motion segment angles using trunk angle and anthropometry. Human Factor and Ergonomics Society 50th Annual Meeting; San Francisco (CA): HFES;2006.

97. Knapik G.A three-dimensional, EMG-assisted, push–pull model for assessing dynamic loads at each level of the lumbar spine. Mechanical Engineering Columbus, OH: The Ohio State University; 2005; p. 117.

98. Begeman PC., et al. Viscoelastic shear responses of the cadaver and hybrid III lumbar response.38th Stapp Car Crash Conference; Ft. Lauderdale (FL);1994.

99. Iatridis JC, Ap Gwynn I. Mechanisms for mechanical damage in the intervertebral disc annulus fibrosus. J Biomech 2004;37(8):1165–1175.

100. Yingling VR, McGill SM. Anterior shear of spinal motion segments. Kinematics, kinetics, and resultant injuries observed in a porcine model. Spine 1999; 24(18):1882–1889.

101. Yingling VR, McGill SM. Mechanical properties and failure mechanics of the spine under posterior shear load: observations from a porcine model. J Spinal Disord; 1999; 12(6):501–508.

102. McGill S. Low Back disorders: evidence-based prevention and Rehabilitation. Vol. XV. Champaign, (IL): Human Kinetics; 2002; p.295.

103. Andersson BJ., et al. The sitting posture: an electromyographic and discometric study. Orthop Clin North Am 1975;6(1):105–120.

104. Wilke HJ., et al. New in vivo measurements of pressures in the intervertebral disc in daily life. Spine 1999;24(8):755–762.

105. van Dieen JH, Jansen SM, Housheer AF. Differences in low back load between kneeling and seated working at ground level. Appl Ergon 1997;28(5–6): 355–363.

106. Gallagher S., et al. Dynamic biomechanical modelling of symmetric and asymmetric lifting tasks in restricted postures. Ergonomics 1994;37(8): 1289–1310.

107. Gallagher S., et al. Effects of posture on dynamic back loading during a cable lifting task. Ergonomics 2002;45(5):380–398.

108. Gallagher S. Physical limitations and musculoskeletal complaints associated with work in unusual or restricted postures: a literature review. J Saf Res 2005;36(1):51–61.

109. Gallagher S, Hamrick CA. Acceptable workloads for three common mining materials. Ergonomics 1992;35 (9):1013–1031.

110. Splittstoesser, RE, et al. Spinal loading during manual materials handling in a kneeling posture. Journal of Electromyogr Kinesiol 2006. Forthcoming.

111. American Academy of Orthopaedic Surgeons Back Pain and Back Problems. 2005 [cited] .

112. Hoyle JA. Effects of Postural and Visual Stressors on Trigger Point Development, Muscle Activity, Blink rate, and Discomfort During Computer Work.Columbus: The Ohio State University; 2006. p. 171.

113. Treaster D., et al. Myofascial trigger point development from visual and postural stressors during computer work. J Electromyogr Kinesiol 2006;16 (2):115–124.

114. Kim J, Stuart-Buttle C, Marras WS. The effects of mats on back and leg fatigue. Appl Ergon 1994; 25(1):29–34.

115. Granata KP, Marras WS. Relation between spinal load factors and the high-risk probability of occupational low-back disorder. Ergonomics 1999;42 (9):1187–1199.

116. Marras WS, Granata KP. The development of an EMG-assisted model to assess spine loading during whole-body free-dynamic lifting. J Electromyogr and Kinesiol 1997;7(4):259–268.

117. Marras WS., et al. The effectiveness of commonly used lifting assessment methods to identify industrial jobs associated with elevated risk of low-back disorders. Ergonomics 1999;42(1):229–245.

CHAPTER 8

PSYCHOSOCIAL AND ORGANIZATIONAL FACTOR INFLUENCE ON SPINE LOADING

A LIMITED *number of studies have evaluated psychosocial factors and organizational factors using person-specific biomechanical models. These studies are reviewed and the ability of these nonphysical factors to activate the low back pain pathways (discussed in Chapter 5) is discussed.*

8.1 INTRODUCTION

This chapter is unique because it explores how psychosocial and organizational factors might increase spine tissue loads and thereby serve as a stimulus for a pain pathway initiation. While this body of literature relating psychosocial and organizational factors to increased tissue loading is sparse, this literature may fill an important logical void in that it suggests how psychosocial factors might be able to lead to low back pain.

The literature typically refers to psychosocial and organizational factors collectively and interchangeably. While there has been some debate about the differences between psychosocial factors and organizational factors, the vast majority to the literature does not distinguish between the two. For the most part, psychosocial factors and organizational factors refer to the same factors; those associated with the social aspects of work.

Psychosocial factors can relate to either individual psychosocial factors, such as anxiety and pain behavior, or work-related psychosocial factors due to the attitudes inherent in the work environment. In many contexts, psychosocial factors are also referred to in the literature as psychological factors such as psychological distress or personality. However, in the context of the conceptual model described early in this book (Fig. 1.2), we consider this to be an individual factor. This chapter focuses exclusively on work-related psychosocial influences and how they impact the musculoskeletal system. There are very few studies that have investigated the reaction of the musculoskeletal system in this manner. Therefore, these results must be interpreted with caution. However, the few studies that have been published in this area do provide findings that appear to fit the pattern of evidence of how organizational and psychosocial factors may initiate low back pain pathways discussed previously.

Work-related psychosocial factors collectively refer to the worker's subjective impressions of the social and organizational aspects of the work environment. These impressions are a function of how the work is organized, supervised, and carried out. Organizational and psychosocial factors can also interact with the temporal aspects of the physical work environment since they can directly influence work pacing.

Psychosocial responses to the work environment are rooted in the emotional state of the worker. As discussed in Chapter 6, workers develop mental models of how to recruit their muscles given their expectations of the work environment. Up until this point, we have been concerned with how a worker's mental model can influence muscle recruitment patterns and subsequent spine loading in response to physical work parameters. Given that the worker's mental model is influenced by the entirety of the environment and their experiences, it is reasonable to expect that emotionally based issues, such as psychosocial components of the workplace, could also influence the worker's mental model, resulting in changes in muscle recruitment patterns and influencing the resultant spine loading characteristics. Therefore, if we wish to understand all the factors that can influence spine loading and the subsequent risk of low back pain, we must consider nonphysical influences (such as psychosocial influences) as well as the traditional physical factors influences.

This chapter reviews the available information that shows how work-related organizational and psychosocial factors can influence the recruitment pattern of muscles and the subsequent forces imposed on the spinal tissues.

8.2   PSYCHOSOCIAL AND ORGANIZATIONAL INTERACTIONS

Several studies have suggested that psychosocial factors are correlated with the frequency of low back pain in the workplace (1–8). Researchers have suspected that reactions to the psychosocial environment might explain the relationship between work and low back pain. In particular, a growing number of investigations have linked psychosocial risk factors to the occurrence of low back pain. Back pain has been associated with monotonous work, high perceived workload, and time pressure (9–13). These factors are thought to result in mental stress (14) that would somehow increase the risk of low back pain. Epidemiologic studies support a relationship between psychosocial stress (e.g., tension, nervousness, feeling uptight, worried, and mental strain) and low back disorders (12,15–17). Job dissatisfaction (also related to mental stress) has been associated with LBD in several epidemiologic studies (2,18–23). However, based on these studies, it is unclear whether these indicators of mental stress are independent of physical loading (3,5,24). It could be the case that poor physical work conditions can influence worker attitudes and result in a poor psychosocial environment. Thus, even though the physical environment is an initiator of the problem, the situation could be also interpreted as a psychosocial problem. Several authors have found a significant correlation between biomechanical factors and psychosocial work characteristics (13,25–27), but few studies have controlled for the effect of biomechanical factors when exploring the role of psychosocial factors on low back disorders. Hence, there appears to be a complex interactive relationship between psychosocial work factors and job demands. Yet, until recently, no study has investigated the mechanism by which psychosocial stress might interact with biomechanical loading to increase risk of low back pain.

The contribution of psychosocial factors to low back pain has been discussed in relation to the epidemiology findings in Chapter 2. Since the current discussion is concerned with factors that can act through the low back pain causal pathways, the focus of this chapter will be on the studies that have been able to indicate how the work environment can influence muscle activity and, therefore, potentially activate the pain pathways. Hence, this discussion will be limited to only the biomechanical loading implications of psychosocial and organizational factors.

8.3 BIOMECHANICAL RESPONSES TO PSYCHOSOCIAL ENVIRONMENT

Recently, two studies have reported a link between psychosocial stress and changes in spine loading. The first study assessed spine loads, social interactions, and personality (28). In this study, participants were asked to perform controlled lifts under psychosocially stressful as well as nonstressful (from a psychosocial standpoint) conditions. Under the psychosocially nonstressful conditions, the experimenter was engaging with the participant and tried to make the person feel at ease. Conscious attempts were made to make eye contact, chat with the subject, verbally encourage the subject, and play background music that the subject would enjoy. While the worker was exposed to this nonstressful environment, they were asked to perform several standard lifts while they were fully instrumented with measurement equipment that enabled the assessment of spine loading by way of the EMG-assisted model described in Chapter 6.

After the first set of test lifts was completed (where spine loads were assessed), the experiment was interrupted and an argument between the experimenters was feigned. Following this interruption, the psychosocially stressful condition was initiated. The physical loading conditions to which the person was exposed were identical to the psychosocially nonstressful conditions; however, the experimenter no longer tried to make the subject feel at ease. After the feigned argument, no eye contact was made, the music ceased, no unnecessary conversations occurred, and negative comments were made about the participant's performance.

Figure 8.1 shows the lumbar spine compression load responses of the participants to the stressful compared to the nonstressful conditions. Note that some of the subjects responded dramatically to the psychosocially stressful conditions, while other subjects demonstrated little reactions to the stress.

Further analyses revealed that the change in spine loading, when exposed to the psychosocially stressful conditions compared to the psychosocially nonstressful conditions, was linked to personality profiles. In this study, the Myers–Briggs personality inventory was used to classify personality of the participants (29). This personality inventory assesses personality along four dimensions. An individual's specific personality is typically assessed

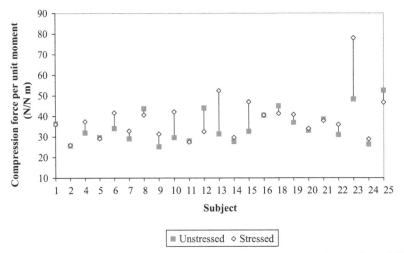

Figure 8.1 Spine compression loading of subjects in response to the psychosocially stressful and nonstressful conditions. (From reference 28).

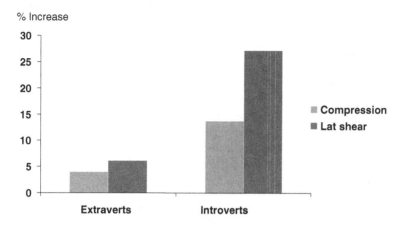

Figure 8.2 Changes in spine compression and lateral shear in response to the introduction of psychosocial stress as a function of extroversion and introversion personality traits. (From reference 28).

along a continuum along each dimension with extreme descriptors describing each personality trait. However, for summation purposes, personalities are typically judged at either dimension extreme. The first personality trait judges one as an extrovert or introvert. Extroverts tend to talk without thinking about what they are going to say, whereas introverts think through their comments prior to voicing them. The second personality trait describes one as a sensor or intuitor. Sensors prefer to concentrate on one task at a time, whereas intuitors think about several things simultaneously. The third personality trait evaluates one as a thinker or feeler. Thinkers tend to think objectively as opposed to emotionally, whereas feelers are more concerned about others' feelings. Finally, judgers versus perceivers make up the final trait dimensions of the Myers–Briggs personality inventory. Judgers see the world as orderly and do not like surprises, whereas perceivers prefer to explore the unknown.

Figures 8.2 and 8.3 show how the participants responded in terms of changes in compression and lateral shear to the experimental conditions as a function of extrovert versus introvert and to the intuitor vesus sensor personality traits, respectively. Note how vigorously the musculoskeletal system responds to stressful conditions depending on the preferences or

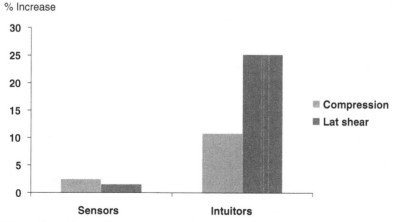

Figure 8.3 Changes in spine compression and lateral shear in response to the introduction of psychosocial stress as a function of the sensor versus intuitor personality traits. (From reference 28).

dislikes of a personality type. These responses were a result of more intense antagonistic muscle coactivations that caused the torso muscles to "fight against" one another when subjects were exposed to psychosocial conditions that were not compatible with their personality type. This amplified muscle tension increases the potential for low back pain via the muscle function disruption pathway described in Chapter 5. Thus, this study shows that psychosocial factors, by themselves, do not dramatically influence spine loading. However, when psychosocial factors were considered collectively along with personality factors, strong interaction can occur that influence trunk muscle and spine loading. These findings amplify the importance of considering the human–workplace system collectively as opposed to only considering individual categories of risk factors when assessing low back pain risk due to the workplace.

8.4 BIOMECHANICAL RESPONSES TO MENTAL STRESS AT WORK

As society advances, there have been shifts in the nature of work in many cultures. Heavy labor is more commonly done by machines that can increase the speed or pace of work. Thus, we have seen a proliferation of more repetitive yet more complex jobs that can only be performed by humans (30). Many jobs now demand high levels of mental concentration as well as rapid work pace. These factors have been implicated as organizationally related psychosocial workplace risk factors for low back pain.

Among these organizationally related risk factors, mental concentration demands have been identified as a risk factor in numerous studies (9,13,16,26,31,32); however, an almost equal number of studies report no association (25,33–37) with low back problems. This discrepancy might indicate the presence of an interaction with some other variable(s). For example, it is known that mental concentration is dependent on the complexity of the task (38). Factors such as the number of alternative actions, insufficient or contradictory data, uncertainty about consequences of actions, scarcity of time, and probability of failure have been identified as issues that may impact the perceptions of mental workload (39). In this context, mental concentration risk is a function of mental processing demands that depend on the balance between the mental reserves and the demand requirements. Thus, mental demand is a function of the intensity and complexity of the task at hand. It is reasonable to assume that task intensity and the subsequent mental demands can be influenced by the timing of task demands. For example, mental processing may have limited consequence when it occurs *prior* to physical job requirements, whereas concurrent mental processing and physical task demands may interact to exacerbate stress resulting in increased biomechanical loading of the musculoskeletal system.

In a similar fashion, rapid job pacing may also draw on the mental reserves of the worker by demanding a conscious effort of keeping up with the pace demand. Increased job pacing may have the potential to impact biomechanical loading for two reasons. First, studies have identified increased lift rate as a risk factor for low back pain (11,40–44) and laboratory studies have shown how spine loading can increase under these conditions (45–48). Second, forced pacing may also influence the individual through psychosocial mechanisms. The interaction between high mental demands and lack of job control has been associated with higher rates of musculoskeletal disorders and represents mental strain (49) (a psychosocial risk factor). Forced pacing may lead to cognitive dissonance (the mismatching of expectations with a social situation) and the creation of a monotonous work environment, which has been shown to be a risk factor of low back pain (11,12,50,51). It is hypothesized that cognitive dissonance may amplify the biomechanical response to the other workplace factors through increased coactivation of the torso musculature. The previously mentioned study demonstrated that biomechanical responses to one type of psychosocial stress support this contention (28).

This review of the available literature indicates that little is known about how psychosocial conditions might influence spine loading. However, a recent study has shed some light on how mental stress components of psychosocial stress might influence trunk muscle recruitment and spine loading (52). This study explored the interaction between the psychosocial variables of mental processing and forced pacing as well as the potential modifying influences of personality and gender on biomechanical loading of the spine during a lifting task. The physical workplace characteristics were held constant since their influence on spine loading is well understood. Only mental processing factors and pacing requirements of the work were manipulated. Spine loadings were observed as a function of these variables as well as personality and gender. The physical task required subjects to lift items weighing 6.8 and 11.4 kg from a conveyor (sagittally symmetric) to an asymmetric shelf that was either 90° clockwise (CW) or 90° counter clockwise (CCW) as determined by a mental processing task.

Mental processing was tested at two levels plus two secondary levels. The primary levels were (1) *serial mental processing* required mental processing decisions to occur prior to the act of lifting, whereas (2) *simultaneous mental processing* required any mental processing decision to occur concurrently with the lift. The secondary levels consisted of *simple* and *complex* demand levels under the serial and simultaneous conditions. These tasks were similar to tasks that might be required in a box-sorting operation. Such operations can be associated with greater risk of low back pain reporting. Under the serial mental processing condition, the simple demand level consisted of verbal commands instructing the subject to deliver a box traveling down a conveyor to a position that was either CW or CCW to the worker. The complex demand task within the serial mental processing condition required the subject to read and interpret an eight-digit number off the top of the box, enter the number into a computer, and decide whether to place it in the CW or CCW destination. An eight-digit number was adopted to ensure a relatively difficult mental processing task. Under the simultaneous mental processing condition, the simple demand level consisted of allowing the subject to place the box in the general vicinity of the destination upon a shelf. The complex demand level under the simultaneous mental processing condition required the subject to place the box precisely within a precise destination target (within a 1.3 cm tolerance) on a shelf thus requiring continuous vigilance and motor control. An electrical circuit was used to monitor this tolerance. The forced pacing factor was set at two levels for the lifts (1) slow, occurring at two lifts/min and (2) fast, occurring at eight lifts/min. Subjects performed all combinations of conditions resulting in eight unique combinatorial conditions. Each condition was repeated twice and presented in a random order.

The influence of the interaction between mental processing and task pacing on spine compression are shown in Fig. 8.4. These results show that at a slow pace there is no effect of serial mental processing on spine load. Under the more rapid paced conditions, spine compression increases moderately and becomes slightly greater under the complex serial processing condition. However, under the complex simultaneous mental processing conditions, both the simple and complex serial processing demands increase the antagonistic cocontraction and results in an increase in the A–P shear spine loading as shown in Fig. 8.5.

Table 8.1 shows how muscle activities differed as a function of the two levels of mental processing as well as the differences in lifting pace. Notice the dramatic differences between simple and complex processing under the simultaneous mental processing task. All muscles increased their activation under the complex conditions compared to the simple conditions indicating a large degree of muscle coactivation. The increase in lifting pacing had similar increases in antagonistic coactivation. By contrast, the difference in simple versus complex

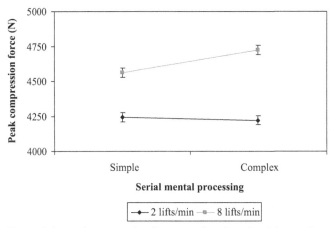

Figure 8.4 Peak compression forces as a function of serial mental processing and pacing (means and standard errors are displayed in the figure). (From reference 52).

mental processing under the serial mental processing task only affected 3 of the 10 muscles observed and then by only an average of 1–2% change in activation level.

The relative differences in spine loading under these different mental demand conditions are shown in Fig. 8.6. Note that complex mental processing can increase lateral shear by up to 70% under simultaneous, complex, mental processing conditions compared to simple, serial mental processing conditions. In addition, the amplified task complexity as well as increased task pacing accentuates the level of muscle loading through cocontraction that could enhance the probability of muscle function disruption.

This study provides an initial evaluation of the role of work-related mental processing on the effects of spine loading. This study simply scratches the surface of potential issues, in that, there are still many potential psychosocial and individual interactions left to explore that may impact biomechanical loading of the spine. However, it does demonstrate the potential influence of psychosocial issues and shows how they can influence muscle recruitment and spine tissue loading. Issues such as the relative contributions of these factors and whether thresholds exist that initiate their influence still need to be explored. This study emphasizes how interactions of non physical risk factors have a large influence on physical spine loading and potentially cumulative trauma of the spine tissues.

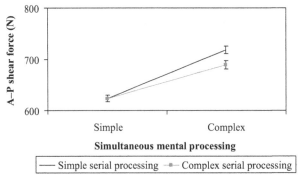

Figure 8.5 Peak A–P shear forces as a function of serial and simultaneous mental processing (means and standard errors are displayed in the figure). (From reference 52).

TABLE 8.1 Statistical Significant Summary and Data: Mean (SD) of the Muscle Activities (in Percent of Maximum (1.0) Activity) of the 10 Trunk Muscles as a Function of Serial Mental Processing, Simultaneous Mental Processing, and Pacing (From Reference 52)

	Left lat. dorsi	Right lat. dorsi	Left erect. spinae	Right erect. spinae	Left rectus abdom.	Right rectus abdom.	Left external oblique	Right ext. oblique	Left int. oblique	Right int. oblique
Serial mental processing	$P = 0.91$	$P = 0.09$	$P = 0.33$	$P = 0.01$	$P = 0.43$	$P = 0.60$	$P = 0.12$	$P = 0.82$	$P = 0.003$	$P = 0.0001$
Simple	0.34 (0.28)	0.32 (0.25)	0.73 (0.34)	0.70 (0.26)	0.16 (0.15)	0.14 (0.14)	0.28 (0.19)	0.27 (0.17)	0.55 (0.26)	0.49 (0.23)
Complex	0.34 (0.27)	0.33 (0.25)	0.74 (0.34)	0.71 (0.27)	0.15 (0.14)	0.14 (0.14)	0.28 (0.19)	0.27 (0.17)	0.57 (0.27)	0.50 (0.25)
Simultaneous mental processing	$P = 0.0001$	$P = 0.0001$	$P = 0.0001$	$P = 0.0001$	$P = 0.0001$	$P = 0.0001$	$P = 0.0001$	$P = 0.0001$	$P = 0.0001$	$P = 0.0001$
Simple	0.31 (0.24)	0.29 (0.22)	0.71 (0.32)	0.69 (0.25)	0.14 (0.13)	0.13 (0.14)	0.25 (0.17)	0.24 (0.16)	0.54 (0.26)	0.47 (0.24)
Complex	0.38 (0.31)	0.36 (0.28)	0.76 (0.35)	0.73 (0.27)	0.17 (0.16)	0.15 (0.14)	0.31 (0.20)	0.29 (0.18)	0.58 (0.27)	0.51 (0.24)
Pacing	$P = 0.0001$	$P = 0.0001$	$P = 0.0001$	$P = 0.0001$	$P = 0.12$	$P = 0.01$	$P = 0.0001$	$P = 0.0001$	$P = 0.0001$	$P = 0.0001$
Slow (2 lifts/min)	0.33 (0.27)	0.31 (0.24)	0.71 (0.33)	0.68 (0.26)	0.15 (0.15)	0.14 (0.14)	0.27 (0.18)	0.26 (0.16)	0.53 (0.25)	0.47 (0.23)
Fast (8 lifts/min)	0.35 (0.28)	0.34 (0.26)	0.76 (0.35)	0.73 (0.27)	0.16 (0.15)	0.15 (0.14)	0.29 (0.20)	0.27 (0.17)	0.59 (0.27)	0.52 (0.25)

P-values are reported for analysis of variance procedures with bolded values being significant at 0.05.

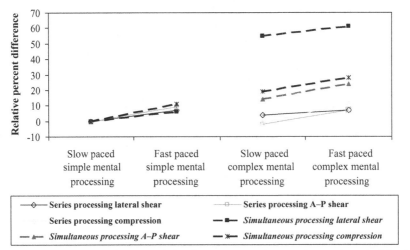

Figure 8.6 Impact of series and simultaneous mental processing on the spinal loads (values are relative to the simple mental demanding task at the slow rate). (From reference 52).

This study has found that mental stress appears to act through time pressure limits and results in the overreaction of the musculoskeletal system. This overreaction manifests itself through less controlled trunk motions and increases in torso muscle coactivation, resulting in increases in three-dimensional spine loading. Hence, these results suggest a potential mechanism by which psychosocial stress may increase lumbar spine load as a result of modern work demands and may help explain the potential biomechanical mechanisms behind some types of occupational risk.

8.5 EXPECTATION

The findings related to mental processing and psychosocial responses to exertion conditions show that a common element of the biomechanical response under the less than ideal exertion conditions is that excessive trunk muscle cocontraction that occurs under the more "stressful" conditions. We have also suggested in the chapter describing biomechanical behavior of the back (Chapter 6) that satisfaction can be a common optimization goal of the musculoskeletal control system. It appears that when the physical environment and psychosocial or organizational conditions do not match the capabilities of the worker, cocontraction of the trunk muscles occurs with a resulting increase in muscle tension and a substantial increase in spine loading. Thus, one would expect that expectation would play a significant role in the satisfaction criteria.

Several studies have investigated the role of expectation in motor recruitment patterns. Early studies of trunk muscle activities compared muscle activities when people were allowed to watch an object dropped into the hands compared to a condition where the same object was dropped from the same height, except the subject was blindfolded (unexpected condition). Muscle activities were found to be up to two and a half times greater in the unexpected condition compared to that in the expected condition and the duration of the muscle activities was also found to be longer in the unexpected conditions (53).

Later similar investigations varied the preview time provided to the subject as a load was dropped into the hands. The results indicated a linear relationship between preview times and peak muscle activity, preview times and mean muscle activity, and preview times and muscle response delays (54).

More recently, a study examined the trunk muscle responses when subjects lifted boxes of known or unknown weight magnitudes (55). Compared to the previous studies, this study was unique in that the timing of the load introduction was not in question, only the exact magnitude of the load lifted was unknown. In this case, back muscle activities increased by 10–16% depending on load magnitude, but no increases in trunk muscle coactivation were observed. Hence, a very different (less dramatic) response occurred with this more subtle form of "expectation."

Studies have also examined the "adjustment" occurring in the trunk musculature as loads are added to an object being lifted (56). The adjustments of the trunk to these perturbations were rapid and did not drastically alter the lifting motion provided the loads were of low magnitude. Thus, there appears to be a threshold above which unexpected loads disturb the musculoskeletal response of the trunk.

Collectively, these "expectation" studies indicate that there are two different forms of expectation that can influence the trunk's musculoskeletal control system. Expectation involving the temporal aspects of spine loading appears to be more important to the development of antagonistic muscle coactivation and greater spine forces than expectation involving load magnitude, where the timing of the load delivery is not in question. These studies are consistent with the notion that the musculoskeletal system is "guided" by the setting of task goals or expectations and matching the response of the musculoskeletal system to achieving those goals. These concepts certainly have the potential to explain how psychological factors such as psychosocial factors and organization factors can influence loading of the spine.

8.6 CONCLUSIONS

Collectively, these studies have demonstrated that psychosocial and organizational factors can interact with personality factors to amplify the impact of biomechanical responses to physical work factors. This review has demonstrated that increases in spine loading (capable of activating the low back pain pathways) occurs in a similar manner in response to organizational and psychosocial risk factors as it does in response to physical risk factor exposure. The biomechanical response involves an increase in muscle coactivation and a subsequent increase in spine loading with both of these reactions increasing the risk of low back pain according to the pathways described in Fig. 5.2.

One needs to reemphasize that the studies noted in this chapter simply scratch the surface of what may be knowable about the potential links between psychosocial factors and the low back experience. While there are very few studies that have explored these links, they do provide a potentially feasible pathway between this work factor and low back pain. However, many more studies are needed to truly understand this relationship.

KEY POINTS

- Psychosocial and organizational occupational risk factors have been widely reported in the epidemiology literature as being associated with low back disorder risk. However, the mechanism by which these factors increase risk has not been well understood.

- Recent studies have hypothesized that psychosocial factors can increase risk by increasing trunk muscle coactivation under stressful situations and, thereby, increase spine loading.

- One study has shown that muscle coactivation does indeed increase along with spine loading when subjects were immersed in a psychosocially uncomfortable situation. However, significant increases in spine loading only occurred in subjects with particular personality traits.

- Similar increases in muscle coactivation and spine loading occurred in those performing lifts while simultaneously performing complex mental tasks (as is done during a package sorting task), and when subjects were exposed to faster paced tasks.

- These studies are consistent with the notion that the musculoskeletal system is "guided" by the setting of task goals or expectations and the musculoskeletal system attempts to match those goals. This may explain why the system behaves as it does.

REFERENCES

1. ANDERSEN JH, et al. Physical, psychosocial, and individual risk factors for neck/shoulder pain with pressure tenderness in the muscles among workers performing monotonous, repetitive work. Spine 2002;27(6):660–667.

2. BIGOS SJ, et al. A prospective study of work perceptions and psychosocial factors affecting the report of back injury [published erratum appears in Spine 1991 Jun;16(6): 688]. Spine 1991;16(1):1–6.

3. BONGERS PM, et al. Psychosocial factors at work and musculoskeletal disease. Scand J Work Environ Health 1993;19(5):297–312.

4. BURTON AK, et al. Psychosocial predictors of outcome in acute and subchronic low back trouble. Spine 1995;20(6):722–728.

5. DAVIS KG, HEANEY CA. The relationship between psychosocial work characteristics and low back pain: underlying methodological issues. Clin Biomech (Bristol, Avon) 2000;15(6):389–406.

6. HOOGENDOORN WE, et al. Psychosocial work characteristics and psychological strain in relation to low-back pain. Scand J Work, Environ Health 2001;27(4):258–267.

7. KRAUSE N, et al. Psychosocial job factors, physical workload, and incidence of work-related spinal injury: a 5-year prospective study of urban transit operators. Spine 1998;23(23):2507–2516.

8. THORBJORNSSON CB, et al. Physical and psychosocial factors related to low back pain during a 24-year period. A nested case–control analysis. Spine 2000;25(3):369–374; discussion 375.

9. AHLBERG-HULTEN GK, THEORELL T, SIGALA F. Social support, job strain and musculoskeletal pain among female health care personnel. Scand J Work Environ Health 1995;21(6):435–439.

10. FRANK JW, et al. Disability resulting from occupational low back pain: Part I. What do we know about primary prevention? A review of the scientific evidence on prevention before disability begins. Spine 1996;21(24):2908–2917.

11. HOUTMAN IL, et al. Psychosocial stressors at work and musculoskeletal problems. Scand J Work Environ Health 1994;20(2):139–145.

12. SVENSSON HO, ANDERSSON GB. Low-back pain in 40- to 47-year-old men: work history and work environment factors. Spine 1983;8(3):272–276.

13. THEORELL T, et al. Psychosocial job factors and symptoms from the locomotor system—a multicausal analysis. Scand J Rehabil Med 1991;23(3):165–173.

14. MARSHAL J, COOPER C. Work experiences of middle and senior managers: the pressure and satisfaction. Int Manag Rev 1979;19:81–96.

15. JOHANSSON JA. Work-related and non-work-related musculoskeletal symptoms. Appl Ergon 1994;25(4):248–251.

16. JOHANSSON JA, RUBENOWITZ S. Risk indicators in the psychosocial and physical work environment for work-related neck, shoulder and low back symptoms: a study among blue- and white-collar workers in eight companies. Scand J Rehabil Med 1994;26(3):131–142.

17. WICKSTROM GJ, PENTTI J. Occupational factors affecting sick leave attributed to low-back pain. Scand J Work Environ Health 1998;24(2):145–152.

18. BIGOS SJ, et al. A longitudinal, prospective study of industrial back injury reporting. Clin Orthop Relat Res 1992;(279), 21–34.

19. BOOS N, et al. Natural history of individuals with asymptomatic disc abnormalities in magnetic resonance imaging: predictors of low back pain-related medical consultation and work incapacity. Spine 2000;25(12):1484–1492.

20. HOLMSTROM EB, LINDELL J, MORITZ U. Low back and neck/shoulder pain in construction workers: occupational workload and psychosocial risk factors. Part 2. Relationship to neck and shoulder pain. Spine 1992;17(6):672–677.

21. MAGORA A. Investigation of the relation between low back pain and occupation. V. Psychological aspects. Scand J Rehabil Med 1973;5(4):191–196.

22. PAPAGEORGIOU AC, et al. Psychosocial factors in the workplace—do they predict new episodes of low back pain? Evidence from the South Manchester Back Pain Study. Spine 1997;22(10):1137–1142.

23. VAN POPPEL MN, et al. Risk factors for back pain incidence in industry: a prospective study. Pain 1998;77(1):81–86.

24. FERGUSON SA, MARRAS WS. A literature review of low back disorder surveillance measures and risk factors. Clin Biomech (Bristol, Avon) 1997;12(4):211–226.

25. JOSEPHSON M, HAGBERG M, HJELM EW. Self-reported physical exertion in geriatric care. A risk indicator for low back symptoms? Spine 1996;21(23):2781–2785.

26. LEINO PI, HANNINEN V. Psychosocial factors at work in relation to back and limb disorders. Scand J Work Environ Health 1995;21(2):134–142.

27. TOOMINGAS A, et al. Associations between self-rated psychosocial work conditions and musculoskeletal symptoms and signs. Stockholm MUSIC I Study Group. Scand J Work Environ Health 1997;23(2):130–139.

28. MARRAS WS, et al. The influence of psychosocial stress, gender, and personality on mechanical loading of the lumbar spine. Spine 2000;25(23):3045–3054.

29. MYERS P, MYERS K, Myers–Briggs Type Indicator, Palo Alto (CA): Consulting Psychologists Press; 1998.

30. NRC. Musculoskeletal disorders and the workplace: low back and upper extremity, ed. P.o.M.D.a.t. Workplace.Washington (DC): National Academy of Sciences, National Research Council, National Academy Press; 2001. p. 492.

31. HAGEN KB, MAGNUS P, VETLESEN K. Neck/shoulder and low-back disorders in the forestry industry: relationship to work tasks and perceived psychosocial job stress. Ergonomics 1998;41(10):1510–1518.

32. HOLMSTROM EB, LINDELL J, MORITZ U. Low back and neck/shoulder pain in construction workers: occupational workload and psychosocial risk factors. Part 1. Relationship to low back pain. Spine 1992;17(6):663–671.

33. ASTRAND NE. Medical, psychological, and social factors associated with back abnormalities and self reported back pain: a cross sectional study of male employees in a Swedish pulp and paper industry. Br J Ind Med 1987;44(5):327–336.

34. BARNEKOW-BERGKVIST M, et al. Determinants of self-reported neck–shoulder and low back symptoms in a general population. Spine 1998;23(2):235–243.

35. DRURY CG, et al. Symmetric and asymmetric manual materials handling: Part 2. Biomechanics. Ergonomics 1989;32(6):565–583.

36. JOSEPHSON M, VINGARD E. Workplace factors and care seeking for low-back pain among female nursing personnel. MUSIC-Norrtalje Study Group. Scand J Work Environ Health 1998;24(6):465–472.

37. THORBJORNSSON CO, et al. Psychosocial and physical risk factors associated with low back pain: a 24 year follow up among women and men in a broad range of occupations. Occup Environ Med 1998;55(2):84–90.

38. BORG G. Subjective effort and physical abilities. Scand J Rehabil Med Suppl 1978;6:105–113.

39. HANCOCK P. The effect of gender and time of day upon the subjective estimate of mental workload during the performance of a simple task. In HANDOCK P, MESHKATI N, editors. Human Mental Workload North Holland: New York (NY);1998. p.239–251.

40. CHAFFIN DB, PARK KS. A longitudinal study of low-back pain as associated with occupational weight lifting factors. Am Ind Hygiene Assoc J 1973;34 (12):513–525.

41. HOOGENDOORN WE, et al. Flexion and rotation of the trunk and lifting at work are risk factors for low back pain: results of a prospective cohort study. Spine 2000;25(23):3087–3092.

42. MARRAS WS, et al. Biomechanical risk factors for occupationally related low back disorders. Ergonomics 1995;38(2):377–410.

43. MARRAS WS, et al. The role of dynamic three-dimensional trunk motion in occupationally-related low back disorders. The effects of workplace factors, trunk position, and trunk motion characteristics on risk of injury. Spine 1993;18(5):617–628.

44. NORMAN R, et al. A comparison of peak vs cumulative physical work exposure risk factors for the reporting of low back pain in the automotive industry. Clin Biomech (Bristol, Avon) 1998;13(8):561–573.

45. DAVIS KG, MARRAS WS. The effects of motion on trunk biomechanics [in process citation]. Clin Biomech (Bristol, Avon) 2000;15(10):703–717.

46. DAVIS KG, MARRAS WS, WATERS TR. The evaluation of spinal loads during lowering and lifting. Clin Biomech (Bristol, Avon) 1998;13(3):141–152.

47. HALL SJ. Effect of attempted lifting speed on forces and torque exerted on the lumbar spine. Med Sci Sports Exercise 1985;17(4):440–444.

48. LINDBECK L, ARBORELIUS UP. Inertial effects from single body segments in dynamic analysis of lifting. Ergonomics 1991;34(4):421–433.

49. KARASEK R et al. The Job Content Questionnaire (JCQ): an instrument for internationally comparative assessments of psychosocial job characteristics. J Occup Health Psychol 1998;3(4):322–355.

50. SARASTE H, HULTMAN G. Life conditions of persons with and without low-back pain. Scand J Rehabil Med 1987;19(3):109–113.

51. SVENSSON HO, et al.. A retrospective study of low-back pain in 38- to 64-year-old women. Frequency of occurrence and impact on medical services. Spine 1988;13(5):548–552.

52. DAVIS KG, et al. The impact of mental processing and pacing on spine loading: 2002 Volvo Award in biomechanics. Spine 2002;27(23):2645–2653.

53. MARRAS WS, RANGARAJULU SL, LAVENDER SA. Trunk loading and expectation. Ergonomics 1987;30(3): 551–562.

54. LAVENDER SA, et al. The effects of preview and task symmetry on trunk muscle response to sudden loading. Human Factors 1989;31(1):101–115.

55. DE LOOZE MP, et al. Trunk muscle activation and low back loading in lifting in the absence of load knowledge. Ergonomics 2000;43(3):333–344.

56. VAN DER BURG JC, VAN DIEEN JH. The effect of timing of a perturbation on the execution of a lifting movement. Hum Movement Sci 2001;20(3):243–255.

CHAPTER *9*

INDIVIDUAL FACTORS ROLE IN SPINE LOADING

THIS CHAPTER discusses how factors unique to the individual such as gender, personality, and experience can influence the biomechanical loading of the spine structures and tissues capable of initiating the pain pathways. To maintain consistency with previous assessments, this discussion is limited to studies that have been able to assess individual factors using person-specific assessment techniques.

9.1 INTRODUCTION

Individual characteristics may also play a role in the trunk muscle responses to the work environment as well as the behavior of the internal force producing structures of the spine and, thereby, influence the probability that the various causal pathways to back pain are activated during work. It appears that, under many circumstances, individual factors respond uniquely, through biomechanical coactivation patterns of the trunk muscles, to physical work factors. They can interact with other categories of risk factors, such as psychosocial factors, and have the ability to reconcile or exacerbate the body's biomechanical reaction. For example, studies have suggested that crude personality measures can be associated with biomechanical responses to influence an individual's response to psychosocial stress (1). Similarly, personality may further influence the biomechanical reaction to mental processing when combined with pacing via a modifying role (2). Thus, while individual characteristics are the focus of this chapter, one should keep in mind that these factors are often more compelling when one considers the complex nature of the interactions between workplace design, psychosocial factors, individual factors, and their potential biomechanical response that may play a significant role in spine loading and the potential for low back pain.

9.2 GENDER

Gender is an obvious individual difference that is believed to influence the nature of biomechanical loadings as a function of work. While several differences in anthropometry have been extensively described in the literature (3), the affect of gender on biomechanical loading of the spine involves more than just considering a woman to be a small man. The differences in relative back strength have been well documented between males and females (4–9). However, gender differences in muscle cross-sectional area that indicate large differences in maximum muscle force potential have also been reported in the literature

(10–12). A recent study (10) used MRI technology to study the differences in muscle cross-sectional area of a population of males and females. The area associated with the various power-producing muscles vital in defining spine loading via modern EMG-assisted models were documented and corrected for muscle fiber angles at each level of the lumbar spine. Table 9.1 shows the results of this study and indicates the differences in muscle cross-sectional area between males and females at each level of the spine from T8 to S1. Note that in nearly all cases, the males' anatomical cross-sectional area (ACSA) (and the associated force capacity) of the muscle are always greater than those of the females participants. This study also showed that these cross-sectional areas can be predicted well with proper anthropometric measures used in a regression equation.

Another important aspect of spine loading assessment involves the correct assessment of the line of action of the torso muscles. Muscles that have greater moment arms exert more influence on spine loads according to the logic of the EMG-assisted model that is used to assess spine forces as described in Chapter 6. Several studies have used CT or MRI imaging systems to estimate the mechanical advantage of the various power-producing muscle groups in the torso relative to the spine (11–13). Figure 9.1a and b demonstrates how the mechanical advantage of the trunk muscles are assessed, based on MRI scans in the coronal (lateral) and sagittal planes of the body, respectively. Tables 9.2 and 9.3 show the moment arms of these muscles for males and females. Note that in both planes of the body, males have greater mechanical advantage (relative to the spine) associated with their torso muscles than do the females for nearly all muscles.

These differences in muscle cross-sectional area and moment arm length suggest that it is extremely important to understand the specific motor recruitment pattern of the muscles when performing a task to understand the spine loading associated with tasks performed by males and females. One study of spine loadings using an EMG-assisted model to consider the influence of differences in recruitment patterns between males and females have indicated that spine loading differences are dependent on the nature of the task performed (14).

Some of the differences in spine loading between genders occur simply due to differences in body size and mass. To account for these differences, the data were *normalized* relative to the external moment supported by the participants. Figure 9.2 indicates that normalized compressive forces were greater for females during trunk motions of up to 45° per second of dynamic lifting motion. Females also exhibited about 20% greater normalized lateral shear under these conditions. These results indicate that once differences in body size are accounted for, differences in spine loading between genders still remain. Furthermore, these differences are uniquely associated with differences in the degree of control required and the specific task requirements.

It is evident from these results that, biomechanically, females are not simply proportionally scaled down versions of males. The magnitude of the difference in spine loadings between genders depends on the magnitude of the external moment supported by the subject (reflecting differences in body mass between genders). Differences in internal loading occur as a function of different internal moment arms between genders. However, changes in loading independent of size are related to the degree of control required and also influence biomechanical response as a function of gender.

Under whole body free-dynamic conditions, significant differences in spine loading between genders is evident and the nature of the relationship between spine loads and trunk moment is somewhat complex. It has been observed that normalized spine compression was greater for females during the slower conditions (e.g., 30° per second and 45° per second) while males experienced higher normalized loads for the fast lifting condition (e.g., 60° per second). Differences remained when the compressive loads were normalized to body mass

TABLE 9.1 Mean (SD) Fiber Angle Corrected ACSAs (cm^2) for Each Muscle and Gender (From Reference 10)

Muscle	Gender	T_8	T_9	T_{10}	T_{11}	T_{12}	L_1	L_2	L_3	L_4	L_5	S_1
R.lat. dorsi	F	13.15 (4.4)	11.51 (5.1)	9.77 (5.1)	8.45 (4.9)	7.34 (4.4)	5.39 (3.0)	3.44 (1.8)	1.45 (0.6)			
	M	21.68 (4.3)	19.53 (4.4)	16.61 (5.0)	14.10 (4.2)	12.03 (3.7)	8.96 (2.5)	6.22 (2.0)	2.71 (1.4)			
L.lat. dorsi	F	12.01 (4.7)	10.56 (4.9)	9.04 (4.9)	8.12 (4.8)	6.88 (4.3)	5.46 (3.0)	3.51 (2.4)	1.63 (0.7)			
	M	19.36 (5.2)	17.76 (4.4)	15.08 (4.9)	13.63 (4.6)	11.07 (4.0)	8.62 (2.8)	5.93 (2.3)	2.74 (1.5)			
R. er. spinae	F	7.63 (1.7)	8.38 (1.7)	9.56 (1.9)	10.92 (2.5)	11.69 (2.5)	13.67 (3.3)	15.68 (3.6)	15.43 (3.6)	12.37 (2.5)	2.81 (1.1)	
	M	12.96 (2.1)	13.91 (2.5)	15.38 (2.9)	17.28 (2.8)	19.65 (3.0)	22.49 (3.7)	25.60 (4.2)	25.03 (3.7)	20.08 (2.3)	4.95 (1.8)	
L. er. spinae	F	7.87 (1.6)	8.42 (1.9)	9.69 (2.3)	10.95 (2.5)	11.94 (2.7)	13.84 (3.0)	15.64 (3.5)	15.58 (3.2)	12.74 (2.4)	2.80 (1.1)	
	M	13.09 (2.2)	13.97 (2.4)	15.94 (3.1)	17.92 (3.5)	19.84 (3.5)	22.53 (3.7)	25.41 (4.2)	25.21 (4.1)	20.15 (2.7)	5.17 (1.7)	
R rect. abd	F					4.25 (0.7)	4.85 (1.0)	4.23 (1.2)	4.44 (1.3)	4.88 (1.8)	5.33 (1.5)	6.01 (2.2)
	M					5.80 (1.9)	6.39 (1.7)	6.02 (1.2)	7.32 (2.9)	7.05 (2.2)	8.53 (2.2)	8.86 (2.3)
L. rect. abd	F					4.54 (0.9)	4.89 (1.1)	4.43 (1.3)	4.51 (1.3)	5.04 (2.3)	5.41 (1.3)	6.14 (2.4)
	M					6.13 (1.9)	6.67 (2.1)	6.22 (1.4)	7.77 (2.7)	6.92 (2.4)	8.69 (2.4)	8.88 (2.4)
R. ext oblique	F					5.0 (1.1)	5.68 (1.2)	6.45 (1.3)	6.15 (0.9)	6.60 (1.0)		
	M					6.54 (1.5)	8.63 (1.9)	9.33 (1.9)	8.97 (1.8)	10.21 (2.0)		
L. ext. oblique	F					4.58 (0.7)	5.46 (1.1)	6.47 (1.3)	5.94 (1.1)	6.31 (1.0)		
	M					6.35 (1.6)	8.17 (1.8)	9.31 (2.1)	9.16 (2.1)	10.36 (2.0)		
R. int. oblique	F							3.51 (1.6)	3.73 (1.4)	6.17 (1.4)		
	M							3.79 (1.6)	6.38 (2.4)	9.96 (2.4)		
L. int. oblique	F							3.31 (1.8)	3.54 (1.4)	6.41 (1.1)		
	M							4.28 (1.8)	6.37 (2.3)	10.25 (2.5)		
R. psoas major	F						2.17 (1.2)	3.30 (0.9)	6.69 (1.8)	9.65 (1.7)	10.13 (1.7)	
	M						2.58 (–)	6.88 (2.3)	13.32 (3.1)	18.32 (3.6)	18.90 (3.8)	
L. psoas major	F						2.24 (0.4)	3.56 (0.9)	6.79 (1.7)	9.93 (1.8)	10.75 (1.8)	
	M						3.23 (1.4)	7.81 (2.5)	13.68 (2.7)	18.68 (3.1)	19.00 (2.9)	
R. quad. lumb.	F						1.71 (0.6)	1.88 (0.5)	2.11 (0.5)	1.97 (0.3)		
	M						2.50 (–)	3.04 (1.2)	5.20 (1.7)	3.56 (1.1)		
L. quad. lumb	F						1.71 (0.4)	1.91 (0.5)	2.39 (0.7)	2.28 (0.4)		
	M						2.71 (1.3)	3.03 (1.1)	5.38 (1.9)	3.59 (1.0)		
Vertebral body	F	7.28 (1.1)	7.80 (0.9)	8.43 (0.8)	8.93 (1.0)	9.37 (1.2)	9.49 (1.0)	10.11 (1.2)	10.89 (1.1)	11.25 (1.2)	11.80 (2.2)	12.75 (2.5)
	M	9.83 (1.8)	10.41 (2.1)	10.87 (1.7)	12.25 (1.8)	12.87 (1.9)	12.49 (2.1)	13.11 (2.4)	14.13 (2.0)	14.78 (2.4)	14.66 (2.2)	17.42 (2.6)
Trunk	F	482.30 (65.7)	466.05 (63.3)	444.05 (61.2)	430.92 (59.9)	425.51 (60.0)	415.98 (61.6)	399.13 (61.4)	377.56 (57.9)	388.82 (71.7)	471.66 (77.7)	533.20 (79.6)
	M	733.38 (110.8)	688.31 (90.2)	645.59 (82.6)	616.48 (85.5)	594.41 (84.6)	574.78 (79.3)	544.35 (81.1)	525.43 (87.7)	514.32 (101.8)	524.81 (88.2)	565.47 (77.0)

All male ACSAs are significantly larger than female ACSAs except where indicated in bold-italicized type (10).

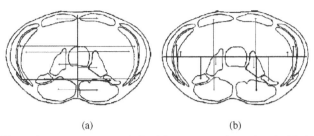

(a)   (b)

Figure 9.1 Moment arms derived from MRI and associated with the various trunk loading muscles at L3 assessed in the (**a**) coronal plane, and (**b**) sagittal planes of the body.

during this condition, indicating that the resulting loads were a consequence of factors other than body size differences.

When the lifting tasks involved whole-body free dynamic kinematics, loading differences between the genders occurred as a result of kinematic compensations. In terms of lift style, females flexed their hips about 6° more and had about 8° per second more hip motion during the lifts than the males. The greater reliance on the pelvis for the females may be reflective of the limited strength capacity in lumbar region. In this study, females exhibited 30% less extension strength than males during the maximum exertions.

Muscle coactivity patterns also played a significant role in the spine loading differences between males and females. Females exhibited significantly greater activity in the latissimus dorsi (about 12% of maximum) and right external oblique (about 3% of maximum) muscles than males (Fig. 9.3). Females needed to recruit muscles other than the primary agonist muscles (erector spinae) to complete the lifts, most likely due to the inferior mechanical advantage supplied by the erector spinae muscles compared to their male counterparts. The recruitment of additional secondary agonist muscles, such as the latissimus dorsi muscles, would increase stability but would also increase coactivity.

The level and nature of the spine loads would also be affected by differences in the muscle anatomy (as discussed earlier) between genders (e.g., muscle area, lines of actions, and moment arms of the muscles). Recruiting more oblique-oriented muscles in addition to the erector spinae muscles results in more complex loads—shear and compression. Since external oblique muscles are antagonists, they serve as trunk stabilizers and do not actually contribute to extensor moment generation. This also increases the coactivity, which may have occurred as a result of the limited strength capability of the females, causing the trunk to activate additional muscles to increase stability.

Females also have lower spine tolerances (15,16) and, thus, may be at greater risk of a low back injury. When spine loading is considered relative to the percentage of gender-specific compression tolerance, females' compression loads were about 47% of their tolerance as compared to males whose compression values represented about 38% of the tolerance value. On the basis of these tolerance values, females would be expected to be at a substantially higher level of risk than males when performing identical lifting tasks. Similar relative risk findings have been observed in more complex lifting situations. Specifically, when females lift heavier loads from either low vertical height origins or when lifting from asymmetric lift origins, spinal loads increase (17).

Epidemiological research supports this finding since females were found to report more low back pain compared to males when performing similar heavy physical jobs (18–20).

TABLE 9.2 Mean (SD) Coronal Plane Moment Arms (cm) for Each Muscle and Gender at Each Vertebral Level from T_8 to S_1 (From Reference 13)

Muscle	Gender	T_8	T_9	T_{10}	T_{11}	T_{12}	L_1	L_2	L_3	L_4	L_5	S_1
R. lat. dorsi	F	13.2 (1.0)	12.4 (0.9)	11.4 (0.9)	10.9 (0.9)	10.4 (0.9)	9.9 (0.9)	9.3 (1.0)	9.0 (1.1)			
	M	15.3 (1.0)	14.5 (0.9)	13.5 (1.0)	12.8 (0.9)	12.2 (0.8)	11.6 (0.6)	10.9 (0.7)	10.3 (0.8)			
L. lat. dorsi	F	13.1 (0.9)	12.2 (0.9)	11.4 (1.0)	10.8 (1.0)	10.4 (0.9)	10.1 (0.9)	9.4 (1.1)	9.2 (1.1)			
	M	15.0 (0.7)	14.0 (0.8)	13.2 (0.9)	12.6 (0.9)	12.1 (0.9)	11.6 (0.9)	11.0 (0.7)	10.5 (0.8)			
R. er. spinae	F	2.6 (0.3)	2.8 (0.3)	2.9 (0.3)	3.1 (0.3)	3.2 (0.3)	3.4 (0.3)	3.5 (0.3)	3.4 (0.3)	3.4 (0.3)	2.6 (0.6)	1.9 (0.3)
	M	3.1 (0.2)	3.2 (0.3)	3.4 (0.3)	3.6 (0.3)	3.6 (0.3)	4.0 (0.4)	4.1 (0.3)	3.8 (0.3)	3.6 (0.3)	3.0 (0.7)	1.9 (0.3)
L. er. spinae	F	2.7 (0.4)	2.8 (0.3)	3.1 (0.2)	3.2 (0.3)	3.4 (0.4)	3.5 (0.3)	3.5 (0.3)	3.3 (0.3)	3.5 (0.3)	2.7 (0.5)	1.9 (0.2)
	M	3.3 (0.4)	3.4 (0.4)	3.6 (0.3)	3.8 (0.3)	3.8 (0.3)	4.2 (0.3)	4.3 (0.4)	4.0 (0.2)	3.8 (0.3)	3.2 (0.5)	2.2 (0.2)
R rect. abd.	F					2.9 (0.8)	3.4 (0.9)	3.6 (0.8)	3.9 (0.8)	4.0 (0.8)	3.8 (0.9)	3.3 (0.7)
	M					3.9 (0.6)	4.6 (1.1)	4.9 (1.1)	4.7 (0.7)	4.6 (0.5)	4.1 (0.5)	3.8 (0.5)
L. rect. abd.	F					3.5 (0.5)	3.7 (0.7)	3.4 (0.8)	3.3 (0.9)	3.5 (0.8)	3.2 (0.8)	3.3 (0.6)
	M					3.5 (0.7)	4.1 (0.8)	3.9 (0.8)	4.0 (0.7)	3.6 (0.8)	3.3 (0.8)	2.9 (0.5)
R. ext. oblique	F					10.8 (0.8)	10.9 (0.8)	10.9 (0.8)	10.8 (0.7)	11.2 (0.8)	11.6 (0.3)	
	M					12.9 (1.0)	13.0 (1.2)	13.2 (1.0)	12.8 (0.7)	12.8 (0.7)	12.6 (0.6)	
L. ext. oblique	F					11.2 (1.0)	11.0 (1.0)	10.8 (1.0)	10.6 (0.9)	10.8 (0.9)	11.3 (1.1)	
	M					12.4 (0.9)	12.6 (0.9)	12.4 (1.1)	12.4 (1.0)	12.2 (0.9)	12.5 (1.1)	
R. int. oblique	F							9.9 (1.4)	9.7 (1.1)	10.1 (0.8)	10.4 (0.3)	
	M							11.4 (1.6)	11.5 (0.8)	11.4 (0.6)	10.9 (0.3)	
L. int. oblique	F							10.2 (1.5)	9.4 (1.4)	9.8 (0.8)	10.3 (1.0)	
	M							10.7 (1.3)	11.1 (1.4)	10.7 (0.8)	10.6 (0.9)	
R. psoas major	F						2.3 (0.2)	2.7 (0.2)	3.3 (0.2)	4.0 (0.3)	4.7 (0.4)	5.0 (0.4)
	M						2.6 (–)	3.3 (0.3)	3.9 (0.3)	4.7 (0.3)	5.3 (0.3)	5.6 (0.4)
L. psoas major	F						2.3 (0.1)	2.7 (0.1)	3.2 (0.2)	3.8 (0.3)	4.5 (0.3)	5.1 (0.3)
	M						2.8 (0.2)	3.3 (0.3)	3.9 (0.3)	4.4 (0.4)	5.0 (0.5)	5.4 (0.5)
R. quad. lumb.	F						3.8 (0.6)	4.1 (0.4)	5.5 (0.7)	6.8 (0.5)		
	M						3.8 (–)	5.0 (0.6)	6.4 (0.6)	7.5 (0.5)		
L. quad. lumb	F						3.7 (0.3)	4.2 (0.3)	1.5 (0.7)	6.8 (0.7)		
	M						4.4 (0.4)	4.7 (1.0)	6.5 (0.7)	7.3 (0.6)		

Italicized cells represent statistically significantly larger male than female moment arms ($P \leq 0.05$).

TABLE 9.3 Mean (SD) Sagittal Plane Moment Arms (cm) for Each Muscle and Gender at Each Vertebral Level from T_8 to S_1 (From Reference 13)

Muscle	Gender	T_8	T_9	T_{10}	T_{11}	T_{12}	L_1	L_2	L_3	L_4	L_5	S_1
R.lat. dorsi	F	−1.6 (10.2)	−1.9 (1.1)	−2.3 (0.9)	−2.6 (0.8)	−2.9 (0.8)	−3.2 (1.0)	−3.4 (1.1)	−3.1 (1.2)			
	M	−1.8 (0.9)	−2.2 (1.0)	−2.4 (0.9)	−2.7 (0.8)	−2.9 (0.7)	−3.8 (0.9)	−4.1 (0.7)	−4.2 (0.8)			
L.lal. dorsi	F	−0.7 (1.0)	−1.1 (0.9)	−1.6 (0.9)	−2.0 (0.8)	−2.6 (0.8)	−3.1 (1.0)	−3.9 (1.1)	−4.0 (1.2)			
	M	−0.7 (1.1)	−0.9 (1.1)	−1.3 (1.1)	−1.6 (1.0)	−2.2 (1.0)	−3.0 (1.2)	−4.0 (1.1)	−3.9 (1.1)			
R. er. spinae	F	−4.4 (0.3)	−4.5 (0.4)	−4.4 (0.4)	−4.4 (0.4)	−4.4 (0.4)	−4.7 (0.5)	−4.8 (0.4)	−5.0 (0.5)	−4.9 (0.4)	−5.4 (0.5)	−5.4 (0.5)
	M	−5.2 (0.4)	−5.3 (0.4)	−5.2 (0.4)	−5.1 (0.4)	−5.0 (0.4)	−5.2 (0.5)	−5.4 (0.7)	−5.7 (0.7)	−5.6 (0.6)	−6.1 (0.7)	−6.2 (0.7)
L. er. spinae	F	−4.2 (0.3)	−4.3 (0.3)	−4.2 (0.3)	−4.2 (0.4)	−4.3 (0.4)	−4.7 (0.5)	−5.1 (0.6)	−5.3 (0.6)	−5.3 (0.5)	−5.7 (0.6)	−5.6 (0.5)
	M	−4.9 (0.5)	−4.9 (0.6)	−4.8 (0.5)	−4.7 (0.5)	−4.8 (0.5)	−5.0 (0.6)	−5.4 (0.6)	−5.6 (0.6)	−5.7 (0.5)	−6.1 (0.7)	−6.3 (0.8)
R rect. abd	F					10.4 (0.9)	9.6 (1.0)	8.5 (0.9)	7.0 (0.9)	6.1 (0.9)	−6.5 (1.0)	7.5 (1.3)
	M					13.5 (1.7)	12.4 (1.2)	10.7 (1.2)	8.9 (1.3)	7.7 (1.5)	7.6 (1.4)	8.4 (1.2)
L. retc. abd	F					10.5 (1.0)	9.7 (1.1)	8.5 (1.1)	6.9 (0.9)	6.0 (0.9)	6.1 (1.0)	7.3 (1.2)
	M					13.7 (1.7)	12.7 (1.1)	10.8 (1.3)	9.2 (1.3)	7.8 (1.4)	7.6 (1.5)	8.2 (1.2)
R. ext. oblique	F					6.8 (0.7)	5.6 (1.2)	4.0 (1.1)	2.4 (1.2)	2.2 (1.2)	3.2 (2.0)	
	M					8.5 (1.2)	6.7 (1.0)	4.6 (0.6)	2.2 (1.0)	2.1 (0.8)	3.9 (1.2)	
L. ext. oblique	F					6.6 (1.2)	5.7 (1.3)	3.7 (1.2)	1.5 (1.3)	1.2 (1.3)	2.5 (0.9)	
	M					9.2 (1.4)	7.4 (1.3)	5.0 (1.4)	2.7 (1.4)	2.0 (1.1)	3.5 (1.2)	
R. int. oblique	F							5.5 (1.5)	3.3 (1.2)	2.1 (1.1)	3.6 (1.5)	
	M							5.2 (1.5)	3.4 (1.3)	2.5 (1.1)	4.5 (1.0)	
L. ini. oblique	F							7.2 (1.7)	3.0 (1.5)	1.6 (1.0)	3.0 (1.5)	
	M							7.7 (1.6)	4.3 (1.5)	2.7 (1.0)	4.5 (1.3)	
R. psoas major	F						−0.7 (0.9)	−0.9 (0.3)	−0.8 (0.4)	−0.4 (0.5)	0.7 (0.7)	2.3 (1.0)
	M						−0.5 (−)	−0.7 (0.5)	−0.4 (0.4)	−0.1 (0.3)	0.8 (0.5)	2.4 (0.7)
L. psoas major	F						−0.2 (0.7)	−1.0 (0.4)	−1.0 (0.5)	−0.7 (0.5)	0.2 (0.6)	2.0 (0.8)
	M						−0.9 (0.5)	−0.6 (0.5)	−0.3 (0.4)	−0.02 (0.5)	0.8 (0.6)	2.4 (0.7)
R. quad. lumb.	F						−2.9 (0.4)	−3.0 (0.4)	−3.1 (0.7)	−2.6 (0.8)		
	M						−27 (−)	−3.1 (0.6)	−3.1 (0.7)	−3.0 (0.6)		
L. quad. lumb	F						−26 (0.3)	−3.2 (0.6)	−3.6 (1.0)	−3.2 (1.0)		
	M						−3.0 (0.4)	−3.1 (0.6)	−3.1 (0.7)	−3.1 (0.6)		

Italicized cells represent statistically significantly larger male than female moment arms (P ≤ 0.05). Positive and negative moment arms correspond to anterior and posterior to vertebral body, respectively.

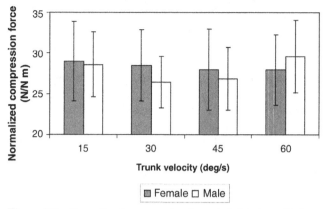

Figure 9.2 Normalized compression force (relative to sagittal moment) for males and females as a function of trunk velocity during the sagittally symmetric free-dynamic lifting. (From reference 14).

9.2.1 Personality

Recently, a limited number of studies have demonstrated that personality can play a role in the motor recruitment pattern of muscles (1,21,22) and the coactivity associated with increases in spine loading (1,21). Field observations have indicated that when employees' personalities were better matched with the nature of their work environment, they generally reported less anxiety and physical discomfort and more job satisfaction and social support than those employees whose personalities were mismatched with the work (23).

Biomechanically, it appears that certain personality characteristics are associated with increased coactivation of antagonistic muscles surrounding a joint when the worker is exposed to a work environment that is not compatible with his or her personality type. This has been observed in both the elbow joint (22) and the muscles surrounding the lumbar spine (1,21). However, it is important to understand that all of the studies that have been able to identify spine loading differences associated with load have done so only when personality traits are considered *in combination* or in terms of their interaction with other types of psychological or psychosocial stress.

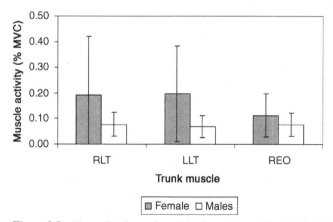

Figure 9.3 Normalized muscle activity for males and females for the left latissimus dorsi (LLT), right latissimus dorsi (RLT), and right external oblique (REO). (From reference 14).

One study (21) that tested a sufficiently large distribution of personality characteristics associated with spine loading while performing a lifting task under different levels of mental stress found that both gender and many of the Myers–Briggs personality indicators (24) affected spinal loads through the biomechanical responses of the body. When the spine loading, kinematic, kinetic, and muscle activity data were tested for response to personality traits alone, no meaningful statistically significant differences were found. However, the interactions of many personality traits with stress were significant, indicating that people with different personality traits *responded* to mental stress in different ways.

Table 9.4 summarizes the statistically significant trends associated with the reaction of the various personality traits to mental stress. This table indicates that most personality traits were associated with some sort of increase (either absolute or relative to moment supported) in spine compression when psychosocial stress was introduced. Spine shear loadings were also associated with personality traits. Extrovert, sensor, and feeler preferences were associated with large increases in lateral shear. Extroverts increased shear by increasing trunk acceleration and increasing the activity of the antagonist (external oblique) muscles, whereas sensors increased their lateral trunk motion. Mild A–P shear increases were associated with the extrovert and sensor traits. The horizontal vector component of the oblique muscles most likely resulted in an increases in spine shear. This table also indicates the degree of changes in spine loading that can be expected as a function of mental stress. As can be seen, lateral shear changes are the greatest with increases of up to 17%, followed by compression with changes of up to nearly 8%. A/P shear differences were much lower as a function of personality. The biomechanical responses associated with these changes in spine load indicate that the internal muscle responses are affected by personality traits and these responses result in changes in hip and trunk motion that interact with the muscle forces to ultimately change the nature of spine loading.

The other study to address changes in spine loading associated with personalities also used the Myers–Briggs classification of personality traits. This study found that when psychosocial stress associated with interpersonal confrontation was assessed, different personality traits correlated with increased spine loading (1). Figure 9.4 shows an example of the magnitude of the differences in three-dimensional loading associated with this type of stress. As can be seen, the increases are subtle yet significant enough to contribute to cumulative loading of the spine during work tasks.

A recent study also examined the role of personality while subjects lifted cases continuously over an 8-h workday (25). Since many of the personality traits relate to conditions that energize workers or frustrate them, one would expect that when an individual works under frustrating conditions (given the worker's personality type compared to the nature of the work environment), trunk muscle cocontraction would be expected to increase and would result in disproportionate increases in spine loading between personality types. Figure 9.5 demonstrates the difference in spine compression associated with the perceiver or judger personality traits. This figure indicates that perceivers not only have greater spine loading due to cocontraction, but also the subsequent spine loading increases more rapidly for perceivers as the load moment to which the worker is exposed increases.

One of the hallmarks of personality differences according to the Myers–Briggs personality inventory is related to the manner in which individuals respond to temporal aspects of activities. As indicated previously, the differences in personality appear to influence the manner in which people respond to situations in terms of the muscle coactivation, which in turn influences the loads imposed on the spine. Figure 9.6 shows how those workers who score high on the intuitor personality trait typically experience greater spine A/P shear (due to trunk muscle coactivation) than do their counterparts who score high on the sensor personality trait (25). Of particular interest is the fact that the

TABLE 9.4 Relative Percent Differences Between Simple and Complex Simultaneous Mental Processing as a Function of Personality Traits for the Spine Loads, Trunk and Hip Kinematics, Trunk Kinetics, Agonistic Muscle Activity, and Antagonistic Muscle Activity (numbers represent the additional percent change of the first characteristic relative to the second characteristic) (From Reference 21)

Individual characteristic	Spine loads			Biomechanical responses				
	Compression	Lateral shear	A–P shear	Trunk kinematics	Hip kinematics	Trunk moments	Agonistic muscle activity	Antagonistic muscle activity
Extroverts to introverts	7.8	12.0	2.4	0.8–2.0	10.0	1.0	3.1–9.8	9.0–20.4
Sensors to intuitors		15.2	2.7		−2.1 to −6.4		0.8–6.3	
Feelers to thinkers	6.1	17.3		4.1–9.7	−2.2	−2.5 to −3.3	−3.2–2.0	7.9–9.3
Judgers to perceivers	3.4			2.5		3.6–4.5	6.8	−8.1

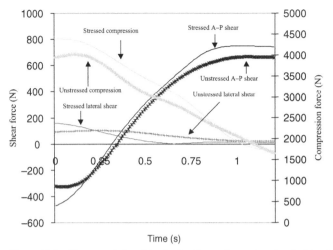

Figure 9.4 Representative data for the three-dimensional spinal loads for an unstressed and stressed lift. (From reference 1).

differences in spine loading between the sensors and intuitors is not evident until the workers were exposed to at least 2 h of repetitive lifting. These differences in spine loading remain significantly different through out the remainder of the 8-h workday.

9.3 EXPERIENCE

The literature also indicates significant interactions between personality and work experience in defining the biomechanical response of the back to physical work conditions over the course of an 8-h workday (25). In this study, workers were observed lifting for entire 8-h shifts while lifting at different lift frequencies during each workday. An interaction of experience and personality on spine compression was noted. This was an interesting interaction in that it has been observed only among experienced subjects where those

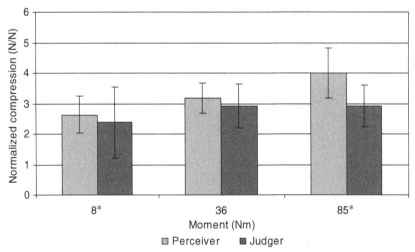

Figure 9.5 Interaction of moment and personality on compression (* indicates significant difference between perceivers and judgers) (N/N represents normalized to body weight). (From reference 25).

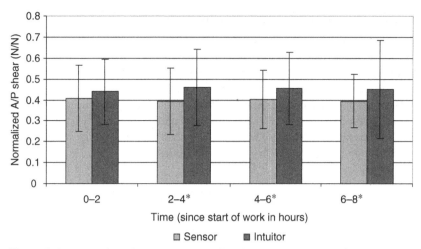

Figure 9.6 Interaction of time and personality SN on A P shear as a function of lifting duration exposure (* indicates significant difference between sensors and intuitors) (N/N represents normalized to body weight). (From reference 25).

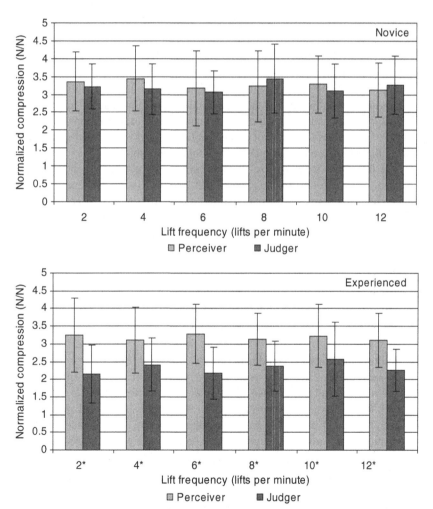

Figure 9.7 Interactive effect of frequency and personality perceiver/judger personality trait on novice (top) and experienced (bottom) workers' compression (* indicates significant difference between perceivers and judgers) (N/N represents normalized to body weight). (From reference 25).

workers with the perceiver personality trait displayed 27% higher compressive loading than did judgers. As shown in Fig. 9.7, experienced perceivers behaved similarly to all novice workers in terms of compressive loading on the spine. However, experienced workers with the judger personality trait experienced far less muscle cocontraction and spine compression compared to the experienced workers with the perceiver personality trait. Thus, as workers became more experienced, those who had the judger personality trait would be expected to suffer less cumulative trauma throughout the workday.

9.4   CONCLUSIONS

Individual factors have been suspected of influencing risk of low back pain for some time. However, until recently, few studies have been able to describe how individual factors influence the biomechanical functioning of the back and how the individual factors can activate the causal pathways discussed earlier. As this chapter indicates, the role of individual factors such as gender and personality is to mediate the response of the muscle recruitment pattern and subsequent biomechanical loading to workplace factors. It is likely that other individual factors (e.g., age) exist that may influence spine loading patterns when combined with work requirements; however, no studies exist that have explored the spine loading consequences of these factors in a quantitative manner.

It is also suspected that genetic polymorphisms may also be an individual characteristic that regulates the tolerance of the individual to spine loading, especially in response to cytokine upregulation that would initiate the muscle function disruption pathway to low back pain. However, the literature has not yet been able to describe the contribution of this effect in a manner that would be useful in defining a tolerance limit.

It is important to recognize that individual factors exert their influence through interactions. We are just beginning to understand the functioning of these interactions from a biomechanical standpoint. It appears that the interactions that exacerbate the pathways to back pain involve the individual factors such as gender, personality, experience, and most likely many other factors.

KEY POINTS

- Several individual differences between workers have been identified that can result in differences in spine tissue loading and may activate the various low back pain pathways.
- Studies have shown a significant difference in spine loading as a function of gender. Females' trunk muscle cross-sectional area and lines of action are different from those of males. Males and females also have demonstrated different muscle recruitment patterns even when exertions are normalized for differences in external spine load exposure. These different muscle recruitment patterns result in differences in spine loading characteristics, with females generally experiencing greater relative loading of the spine.
- Several studies have indicated that worker personality may also lead to different spine loadings. Personality appears to influence muscle recruitment and the resultant spine loading characteristics. However, personality interacts strongly with the psychosocial risk factor to influence trunk muscle recruitment patterns and the subsequent spine loading. Certain personality types are associated with greater levels of trunk muscle coactivation which increases the load imposed on the spine during task performance

when exposed to psychosocially stressful situations. The opposite personality type shows no increase in trunk muscle coactivation or spine loading in response to psychosocially stressful situations.

- Worker experience is another individual factor that can influence spine loading. Experienced workers use less trunk muscle coactivity and results in less overall spine loading when performing a work task.

REFERENCES

1. MARRAS WS, et al. The influence of psychosocial stress, gender, and personality on mechanical loading of the lumbar spine. Spine 2000;25(23):3045–3054.
2. ALLREAD WG. The effects of personality on musculoskeletal disorder risk, In Industrial and Systems Engineering. Columbus (OH): The Ohio State University; 2000.
3. KROEMER KHE. Engineering anthropometry, In KARWOWSKI W, MARRAS W, editors. The Occupational Ergonomcis Handbook.Boca Raton (FL); CRC Press; 1999. p. 139–165.
4. KUMAR S, DUFRESNE RM, Van SCHOOR T. Human trunk strength profile in flexion and extension. Spine 1995; 20(2):160–168.
5. KUMAR S, DUFRESNE RM, Van SCHOOR T. Human trunk strength profile in lateral flexion and axial rotation. Spine 1995;20(2):169–177.
6. KUMAR S. Axial rotation strength in seated neutral and prerotated postures of young adults. Spine 1997; 22(19):2213–2221.
7. KELLER TS, ROY AL. Posture-dependent isometric trunk extension and flexion strength in normal male and female subjects. J Spinal Disord Tech 2002;15(4): 312–318.
8. MIKA A, UNNITHAN VB, MIKA P. Differences in thoracic kyphosis and in back muscle strength in women with bone loss due to osteoporosis. Spine 2005;30(2):241–246.
9. CHAFFIN DB. Human strength capability and low-back pain. J Occup Med 1974;16(4):248–254.
10. MARRAS WS, et al. Female and male trunk geometry: size and prediction of the spine loading trunk muscles derived from MRI. Clin Biomech (Bristol, Avon) 2001;16(1):38–46.
11. McGILL SM, JUKER D, AXLER C. Correcting trunk muscle geometry obtained from MRI and CT scans of supine postures for use in standing postures. J Biomech 1996;29(5):643–646.
12. CHAFFIN D, et al. Lumbar muscle size and location from CT scans of 96 women age 40 to 63 years. Clin Biomech (Bristol, Avon) 1990;5:9–16.
13. JORGENSEN MJ, et al. MRI-derived moment-arms of the female and male spine loading muscles. Clin Biomech (Bristol, Avon) 2001;16(3):182–193.
14. MARRAS WS, DAVIS KG, JORGENSEN M. Spine loading as a function of gender. Spine 2002;27(22): 2514–2520.
15. JAGER M, LUTTMANN A. Compressive strength of lumbar spine elements related to age, gender, and other influences. J Electromyogr Kinesiol 1991;1: 291–294.
16. JAGER M, LUTTMANN A, LAURIG W. Lumbar load during one-hand bricklaying. Int J Ind Ergon 1991; 8:261–277.
17. MARRAS WS, DAVIS KG, JORGENSEN M. Gender influences on spine loads during complex lifting. Spine J 2003;3(2):93–99.
18. ANDERSSON GB. The epidemiology of spinal disorders, InFRYMOYER JW,editor. The Adult Spine: Principles and Practice. Philadelphia: Lippincott-Raven Publishers; 1997. p. 93–141.
19. BIGOS SJ, et al. Back injuries in industry: a retrospective study. III. Employee-related factors. Spine 1986;11(3):252–256.
20. MAGORA A. Investigation of the relation between low back pain and occupation. IMS Ind Med Surg 1970; 39(12):504–510.
21. DAVIS KG, et al. The impact of mental processing and pacing on spine loading: 2002 Volvo Award in biomechanics. Spine 2002;27(23):2645–2653.
22. GLASSCOCK NF, et al. The effect of personality type on muscle coactivation during elbow flexion. Human Factors 1999;41(1):51–60.
23. ALLREAD WG, MARRAS WS. Does personality affect the risk of developing musculoskeletal discomfort? Theor Issues Ergon Sci 2006;7(2):149–167.
24. MYERS P, MYERS K. Myers–Briggs Type Indicator. Consulting Psychologists Press :Palo Alto (CA);1998.
25. CHANY AM, et al. Changes in spine loading patterns throughout the workday as a function of experience, lift frequency, and personality. Spine J 2006;6(3): 296–305.

CHAPTER 10

PHYSICAL, INDIVIDUAL, AND PSYCHOSOCIAL/ORGANIZATIONAL RISK FACTOR INTERACTIONS

*T*HIS CHAPTER *reviews the influence of physical, psychosocial/organizational, and individual risk factors on the biomechanical functioning of the spine in a collective manner. A large biomechanical study is reviewed that has attempted to partition the influence of these various risk categories in their relationship to spine loading. The role of risk factor interactions is discussed. The chapter also discusses the need to better understand the contribution of risk factor influences through more well-designed studies.*

10.1   WHEN RISK FACTORS COLLIDE

We have seen that physical work environment factors, unique characteristics of the individual worker, and psychosocial/organizational work environment factors are each capable of influencing the loading of the spine's tissues, and this loading is sufficient to initiate pain pathways within the back. It should also be apparent from the previous discussion that all of these causal risk factors operate by way of a similar mechanism. The presence of these risk factors at sufficient levels can influence the recruitment patterns of the trunk's muscles and typically results in increased coactivation of these muscles. This coactivation, therefore, impose loads of greater magnitude and also in different directions of application on the spine's tissues and supporting structures.

Since all these risk factors share the same musculoskeletal control system, there are numerous opportunities for these risk factors to interact. It is this interaction that may account for individual variations and can explain why one worker develops a low back problem and another exposed to the same level of physical work does not.

In keeping with the biomechanical logic discussed earlier, variation can occur in either the tissue tolerance or the loading experienced by the tissue. *Tissue tolerance* can be influenced by anthropometry, tolerance due to conditioning, genetic differences in tissue strength, the probability that tissue load will lead to inflammation and result in pain (cytokine upregulation), the individuals techniques used during work, and the interaction of these components. For example, anthropometry can require a tall worker to bend more during the performance of a task and thus load the spine in a position where tissue strength is minimized. Similarly, Wolf's law suggests that tissues that have been *properly* conditioned and properly nourished are capable of withstanding more load than tissues that have been deprived of nutrients. A decrease in nutrient delivery may be a result of poor circulation, smoking, or an inability to adapt to a load. Maladaption occurs when the (load bearing) bony structures have not been able to remodel themselves as would be the case if increased loads were introduced in a gradual manner so that the structures become more resilient. Finally, genetic factors may influence the bone strength and work technique and experience might dissipate the external load among several structures so that stability is increased and tolerance is increased.

These same factors can influence tissue loading. The previous three chapters have demonstrated that physical work factors, psychosocial/organization work factors, and individual factors can all change the *loading profiles* of the spine structures. However, loading of the spine under these conditions is governed by the recruitment sequence of the trunk muscles. As previous chapters have demonstrated, trunk muscle recruitment patterns and the resultant spine tissue loading are influenced by many of the same factors that influence differences in tissue tolerance. The difference, however, is spine loading has a common feature in that trunk muscle recruitment patterns are the common link among physical work risk factors, the individual risk factors, and the psychosocial/organizational risk factors. In all cases, the causal pathway for each category of risk factor was an increase in unnecessary trunk muscle cocontraction thereby increasing the loads experienced by the spinal tissue. It is the unique combination or interaction of influences from each of these risk factors that define the spinal load experienced by the worker.

We have already seen some examples of how the various risk factors can interact to define muscle tension and spine structure loadings in the previous two chapters. We have observed that different personality factors interact with psychosocial factors and mental load and this interaction can result in a good deal of cocontraction in the trunk when exposed to workplace physical factors. Figure 8.2 documents the differences in spine loadings between extroverts and introverts when exposed to psychosocially stressful interactions, and Fig. 8.3 shows how these same psychosocially stressful situations affected people with the sensor or intuitor personality trait differently. Figure 9.6 domostrates how the perceiver versus judger personality traits defined differences in spine compression when workers were asked to lift loads of different weights. A strong interaction between these traits and work experience are also documented in Fig. 9.7. Finally, Figs. 8.3 and 9.4 indicate some complex interactions between gender and lifting motions in terms of both spine compressive force and muscle recruitment patterns.

10.2 THE MAGNITUDE OF INFLUENCE OF THE THREE RISK FACTOR CATEGORIES

These studies have demonstrated that the pathways to back pain, whether they are initiated by muscle tension or structure loading, involve a complex interaction of physical workstation exposure, psychosocial/organizational factor exposure, and the individual traits and characteristics that the worker brings to the work situation. However, although we know these factors interact, a significant issue involves the degree to which these various factors contribute to overall muscle tension and spine structure loading.

Some recent researchers have addressed this issue in a quantitative manner. In this study, a relatively large sample of subjects (60) were exposed to a series of moderately complex and taxing load lifting conditions (1). Even though this is a large sample size for a biomechanical study, the reader should also be cautioned that this is the only study that has attempted to assess these complex interactions. Thus, while this study is suggestive, more studies are needed to further delineate these findings.

The experimental conditions required people to lift two different weights (6.8 and 11.4 kg) and place them in one of two asymmetric destinations (90° clockwise, 90° counterclockwise). The task also involved different levels of mental concentration (none and number identification), different load precision placement requirements (general and specific), two different lift rates or pacings (two and eight lifts/min), and two different psychosocial environments (good and poor). Three-dimensional spine loading and muscle cocontractions were evaluated by an EMG-assisted biomechanical model so that specific reactions of the subjects were interpretable. The goal of this study was to observe the relative amount of variance that was explained by the various factors under these conditions.

Figure 10.1 shows that the relative contribution of the different risk factor components involved in the development of spine loads was dependent on the direction of the load (e.g., compression versus shear). This partitioning indicates that, for this particular combination of conditions, the combination of workplace physical job demands (load weight, task asymmetry, precision of load placement, and lift frequency) made the largest contribution to spine compression (explained 80.3% of the variance). However, this figure also indicates that the contribution of the physical work factors varies as a function of spine load direction. For example, the physical workplace factors were responsible for 65.1% of lateral shear loading but only 21.6% of anterior–posterior shear. Among these different dimensions of spine loading, the various factor components within each risk factor category contributed

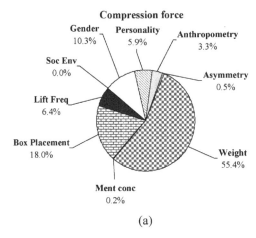

(a)

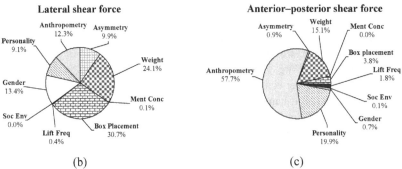

(b)   (c)

Figure 10.1 Spine compression force (**a**), lateral shear force (**b**), and anterior–posterior shear force (**c**) variance explained by the various risk physical work factors, psychosocial/organizational factors, and individual factors investigated in this experiment. (From reference 1).

differently to the different dimensions. For instance, the placement of the load (box placement) explained between 4% and 30% of the spine loading and the weight of the box lifted was responsible for between 15% and 55% of the spine loading in the various dimensions of spine loading.

Under these conditions, the psychosocial factors of mental concentration and social environment had a relatively small impact on the spinal loads (up to 0.2%). However, as we noted earlier, many of these risk factors would be expected to interact with individual risk factors or cause exacerbation of the risk.

Of the individual risk factors, personality contributed significantly to the variability in the spinal loads (about 6–19.9% of the explained variability) with the largest contribution occurring in anterior-posterior shear. Anthropometry played a large role in the shears (about 12–58%) but relatively minor role in the compressive forces (about 3%). Gender had a limited influence on the spinal loads (0.7–13.4%) under these conditions.

Figure 10.2 indicates the contribution of the workplace physical factors, psychosocial/ organizational factors, and individual factors on the agonistic (extensor) and antagonistic (flexor) muscle activities. By comparing the flexor and extensor activities, we can gain an appreciation for the relative coactivities or cocontraction potential of the different risk factors. Ideally, if spine tissue loads were minimal, only the extensor muscles would be active during a lift. However, when cocontraction occurs, the flexor activity increases. This flexor activity increases muscle tension as well as spine loading. In both cases, the weight of the box lifted (14–17%), anthropometry (17–20%), and gender (40–43%) had the largest

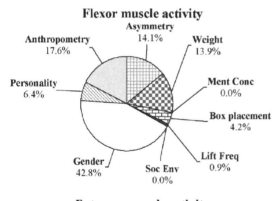

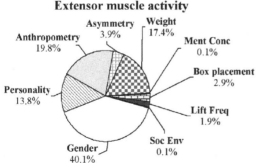

Figure 10.2 Amount of relative variance in *extensor* (latissimus dorsi, erector spinae, and internal obliques averaged) and *flexor* (rectus abdominus and external obliques averaged) *muscle activity* explained by the workplace job demands and modifiers (as predicted by the partial *r*-squares). (From reference 1).

impact on the muscle activity. Box placement (precision) also explained 3–4% of the relative variability, while task asymmetry explained about 4% of the extensor and 14% of the flexor activity variability.

Our previous investigations into factors that influence spine loadings have demonstrated that external load moment exposure, trunk velocity, and trunk posture all can contribute to spine loading and risk of low back pain. Figure 10.3 indicates the amount of variability in these measures that are associated with the various components of risk factors investigated in this study.

Individual factors (e.g., anthropometry, gender, and personality) played a large role in the trunk kinematic characteristics, accounting for more than 79% of the explained variability. Box weight, task asymmetry, and box placement (about 6–7%) were the job demands that had the greatest influence on the trunk postures, while lift rate had the highest impact on trunk velocity (4.5%). This analysis indicates that body dimensions of the individual had, by far, the greatest influence on the trunk postures and motions during the lifting tasks.

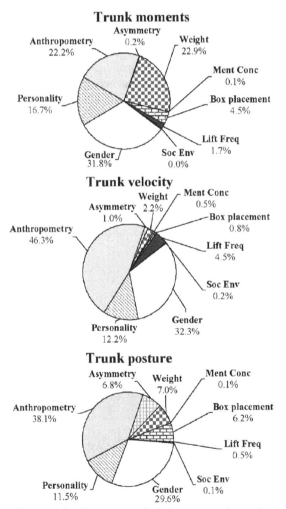

Figure 10.3   The amount of relative variance in *trunk moments* (sagittal, lateral, and twist averaged) and *trunk posture*, and *trunk velocity* (sagittal, lateral, and twist averaged) explained by the workplace job demands and modifiers (as predicted by the partial *r*-squares). (From reference 1).

The amount of variability explained by trunk moment exposure was relatively similar for gender, anthropometry, personality, and box weight (15–30%). However, the precision of box (load) placement was found to mildly influence the trunk moments during the lifting (4.5%). The explained variability was predominantly accounted for by both individual factors (e.g., anthropometry, gender, and personality) and load (box) weight lifted.

To understand the implications of these findings in perspective, one must understand several key issues relating to the study. One must be cautioned, once again, about the generalizability of the results. These results apply to *this* particular experiment and its specific conditions involving moderately taxing physical conditions, moderately taxing psychosocial conditions, and the individual characteristics represented by the 60 subjects in this particular study. A study with different experimental conditions may have different relative contributions of the specific factors with respect to the biomechanical responses (e.g., trunk kinetics and kinematics, muscle activity) and spine loads. Therefore, even though risk factors appear not to contribute to overall tissue loading via Figs. 10.1–10.3, a different set of experimental conditions may yield very different results. The point to be gained from these analyses is that many factors can contribute to spine loading and can impact the pain pathways described previously.

This work has demonstrated how different factors might impact different types of loading and the biomechanical responses that lead to them. This investigation provides an initial picture of the relative contribution of biomechanical and psychosocial workplace job demands as well as individual factors in the development of spine loading. As one would expect, load (box) weight lifted contributed significantly to compression force (more than 55% of the explained variability); however, box weight had a lesser role in the resulting shear forces (15–25%). Thus, controls that are driven solely by weight restriction limits are considering only a small portion of the big picture involved in low back pain causality.

It is also apparent from this work that individual factors such as personality, anthropometry, and gender play a larger role in the shear loads but have a relatively limited influence on compression. The potentially large contribution of anthropometry in the shear loading regression models suggests the importance of prescribing a workplace design specifically for an individual worker. Intervention controls in the form of adjustable equipment may normalize the negative impact of anthropometry. For example, by adjusting the workplace to the worker, the more extreme postures may have been reduced, and, thus, reducing the effect of taller standing heights or lessen the impact of heavier upper torso. Thus, workplace interventions that account for body dimensions and reduce the weight lifted are two of the few "controllable" workplace factors and they also have the greatest potential to impact the loads on the spine.

Psychosocial factors (mental concentration and social environment) have minimal contribution to the loads relative to the other factors. One explanation for this lack of impact for psychosocial factors (mental concentration and social environment) may be the relatively large contribution of personality. The variation explained by personality may account for similar variance due to the psychosocial factors. In other words, psychosocial reactions may be directly related to the personality of the individual. Another explanation is that psychosocial factors may have a relatively small impact on the spine loads and may act more as modifiers. In other words, psychosocial factors may contribute more interactively, actually magnifying the effect of the biomechanical factors. Next, it is extremely difficult to control psychosocial risk factors in a laboratory environment. Thus, psychosocial risk might be over represented or underrepresented in a laboratory study. A final explanation may be that the psychosocial manipulations used in this study were overridden by the physical demands of the tasks. As indicated in Fig. 2.7 it is suspected that psychosocial factors play more of a role under low physical load conditions.

The precision of load placement in lifting tasks can play a substantial role in accounting for load variance. This factor is a unique stressor, in that it has both biomechanical and psychosocial components. During precision controlled placement tasks, workers are required to hold the box at extended distances (biomechanical load) and concentrate on maintaining its position (a form of psychosocial demand) as the load is placed into position. Hence, mental processing occurs simultaneously with the biomechanical lifting of the load, potentially taxing multiple components of the musculoskeletal system and this interaction can lead to significant increases in trunk muscle cocontraction. The sizeable influence of box placement indicates the importance of considering nontraditional and more complex workplace factors when trying to reduce spine loading and control the development of low back disorders. This may be particularly important in lieu of the complexity of the workplace due to technological advances and modern work (i.e., lean manufacturing).

Hence, biomechanical workplace factors, individual characteristics, and psychosocial factors contribute to three-dimensional spine loading. On the basis of this study, load weight lifted was the major contributor to compression while individual characteristics accounted for the majority of A–P shear variability. Biomechanical workplace factors, individual characteristics, and load placement (combination of psychosocial and biomechanical aspects) contribute equally to the lateral shear forces. The results stress the importance of ergonomic controls, particularly, fitting the individual to the workplace. More importantly, this study points to the importance of considering a multitude of factors when attempting to control the load placed on the spine.

10.3 CAN RISK FACTOR INTERACTIONS BE PREDICTED?

Knowledge of the motor recruitment pattern can be a valuable tool in assessing the loads to which a worker is expected to be exposed under many condition. This reasoning suggests that unless an assessment tool is capable of assessing the specific recruitment patterns of the trunk muscles, the tool will probably not be able to accurately assess the loading and subsequent risk associated with work conditions. Furthermore, implicit in this argument is the fact that it is extremely difficult to assess muscular recruitment patterns and the subsequent spine loading that occurs in the workplace. As we will see in the following chapters, most workplace assessment tools that attempt to evaluate the biomechanical loading of the spine as a result of the workplace layout are able to only provide a crude assessment of spine loading. Because simplifying assumptions must be made in terms of which muscles are recruited to perform a task, most of these workplace assessments performed at the job site are incapable of assessing the coactivity of the trunk musculature necessary to realistically evaluate the loads that are imposed on the spine during the performance of the task. Most biomechanical models used to evaluate the spine under these conditions predict what muscle reactions would be expected if no cocontraction occurred. However, as we have seen, large cocontractions do not only control the load that must be moved but also respond to the worker's psychosocial response to the work situation and depend on individual characteristics of the worker.

Thus, it is of great significance to assess trunk muscle recruitment patterns if one is to accurately understand spinal loading. A great number of studies have attempted to assess recruitment patterns of trunk muscles (2–13). However, assessing recruitment patterns of trunk muscles experimentally is extremely tedious and costly. A number of investigators have attempted to develop means of predicting recruitment patterns using optimization theory. Early attempts to predict muscle activities attempted to predict muscle activities based on the minimization of spine loads (14–16) or minimization of the force required within a muscle (17–19). However, except under extremely artificial experimental conditions, the predicted activities of the trunk muscles seldom matched the observed muscle activities.

More sophisticated modeling techniques have been employed that involve fuzzy-logic estimates of muscle force based on the experimental conditions and these efforts have achieved some level of success but only when trunk external loads were of sufficient magnitude to minimize the influence of individual or psychosocial factors (20).

So the question is "what dictates the unique muscle recruitment patterns of an individual worker?" The answer to this question is probably a mixture or interaction of innate factors, training, experience, age, anthropometry, stress, personality, work conditions, and so on. One researcher has suggested that people employ their muscles according to a *satisfaction* principle (21). This theory suggests that over a lifetime, people establish a mental model of what muscles must be recruited to accomplish a specific activity. This mental model establishes an expectation of what muscles should be recruited given the situation that the musculoskeletal system must fulfill. Hence, if the expectation is satisfied, the body's control loop is closed and the system is satisfied and the mental model is reinforced. However, if the activity is accomplished unsuccessfully, the mental model is updated and the prediction system may become more unstable and erratic. This is often seen in sporting events, for example, when a basketball player misses an easy shot, the player may "over think" the shot and miss the next several shots because he is no longer relying on the natural recruitment patterns that have been established over time. Instead the athlete readjusts the muscle recruitment pattern and cocontracts to a greater extent and ends up in a cold streak until the natural pattern of muscle recruitment is reestablished. Similar changes in recruitment patterns occur when a worker experiences back pain. Under these conditions, the worker cocontracts the muscles to guard against pain; however, in reality, this cocontraction results in more loading of the spine. As will be discussed further in Chapter 14, this often results in a permanent reestablishment of the mental model (muscle recruitment pattern) and leads to long-term cocontraction and increases in cumulative loading of the spine.

Hence, when the numerous interactions between tissue tolerance and spine loading are considered, it is apparent that numerous unique interactions occur within an individual. As stated numerous times throughout this book, it is the mixture of risk factors that create the "perfect storm" for a given individual for work-related low back pain. This line of reasoning suggests that individual factors interact with the work-related factors of the physical environment and the psychosocial/organization environment to "tip the balance" of the load–tolerance relationship within the spine tissue and can result in exceeding the threshold limit for either damaging spine tissue, stimulating a nociceptor, or upregulating cytokines within the tissue so that pain is more easily experienced.

10.4 CONCLUSIONS

This brief review of the literature shows that there is a paucity of studies that have explored the interaction and contributions of the various risk factors on spine loading. While the study discussed here is certainly suggestive of an influence from many different types of potential risk factors on spine loading, it is just one piece of the puzzle. This one study does not provide definitive evidence of the nature of these relationships. The scarcity of studies should indicate that many more study efforts are needed to truly appreciate the contributions of the combinations of risk factors. The message from this chapter should be that there are many factors that may combine to influence spine loading.

KEY POINTS

- The mechanism resulting in increases in tissue loading is similar between the three categories of risk factors (physical, psychosocial/organizational, and individual). This mechanism involves increases in muscle cocontraction and a resulting increase in tissue load.

- Studies have documented how the various categories of risk factors contribute to overall variability in compression or shear loading of spine tissues. All categories of risk factors contribute to some extent to spine loads. However, the extent of the contribution to loading depends on the study conditions.

- Interactions between the risk factors also influence spine loading. Many of these interactions have been demonstrated previously (e.g., interactive influence of personality and psychosocial stress on spine load).

- Our ability to predict muscle cocontractions in response to the risk factors is poor and, thus, biologically assisted models provide the only means to accurately assess the impact of risk factors for a given work condition.

REFERENCES

1. DAVIS KG, MARRAS WS. Partitioning the contributing role of biomechanical, psychosocial, and individual risk factors in the development of spine loads. Spine Journal 2003;3(5):331–338.
2. NUSSBAUM MA, MARTIN BJ, CHAFFIN DB. A neural network model for simulation of torso muscle coordination. J Biomech 1997;30(3):251–258.
3. GRANATA KP, WILSON SE. Trunk posture and spinal stability. Clin Biomech (Bristol, Avon) 2001;16(8):650–659.
4. GRANATA KP, ORISHIMO KF, SANFORD AH. Trunk muscle coactivation in preparation for sudden load. J Electromyogr Kinesiol 2001;11(4):247–254.
5. NG JK, et al. EMG activity of trunk muscles and torque output during isometric axial rotation exertion: a comparison between back pain patients and matched controls. J Orthop Res 2002;20(1):112–121.
6. PEREZ MA, NUSSBAUM MA. Lower torso muscle activation patterns for high-magnitude static exertions: gender differences and the effects of twisting. Spine 2002;27(12):1326–1335.
7. HATZE H. The inverse dynamics problem of neuromuscular control. Biol Cybernet 2000;82(2):133–141.
8. DANNEELS LA, et al. Differences in electromyographic activity in the multifidus muscle and the iliocostalis lumborum between healthy subjects and patients with sub-acute and chronic low back pain. Eur Spine J 2002;11(1):13–19.

9. VAN DIEEN JH, CHOLEWICKI J, RADEBOLD A. Trunk muscle recruitment patterns in patients with low back pain enhance the stability of the lumbar spine. Spine 2003; 28(8):834–841.
10. MCGILL SM, et al. Coordination of muscle activity to assure stability of the lumbar spine. J Electromyogr Kinesiol 2003;13(4):353–359.
11. SILFIES SP, et al. Trunk muscle recruitment patterns in specific chronic low back pain populations. Clin Biomech (Bristol, Avon) 2005;20(5):465–473.
12. HODGES P, et al. Intervertebral stiffness of the spine is increased by evoked contraction of transversus abdominis and the diaphragm: in vivo porcine studies. Spine 2003;28(23):2594–2601.
13. HODGES PW, RICHARDSON CA. Inefficient muscular stabilization of the lumbar spine associated with low back pain. A motor control evaluation of transversus abdominis. Spine 1996;21(22):2640–2650.
14. SCHULTZ A. et al. Loads on the lumbar spine. Validation of a biomechanical analysis by measurements of intradiscal pressures and myoelectric signals. J Bone Joint Surg [Am] 1982;64(5):713–720.
15. SCHULTZ A, et al. Use of lumbar trunk muscles in isometric performance of mechanically complex standing tasks. J Orthop Res 1983;1(1):77–91.
16. SCHULTZ AB, ANDERSSON GB. Analysis of loads on the lumbar spine. Spine 1981;6(1):76–82.

17. HUGHES RE, BEAN JC, CHAFFIN DB. Evaluating the effect of co-contraction in optimization models. J Biomech 1995;28(7):875–878.

18. HUGHES RE, et al. Evaluation of muscle force prediction models of the lumbar trunk using surface electromyography. J Orthop Res 1994;12(5):689–698.

19. BEAN JC, CHAFFIN DB, SCHULTZ AB. Biomechanical model calculation of muscle contraction forces: a double linear programming method. J Biomech 1988;21(1):59–66.

20. LEE W, et al. A neuro-fuzzy model for estimating electromyographical activity of trunk muscles due to manual lifting. Ergonomics 2003;46(1–3):285–309.

21. ERLANDSON RF, FLEMING DG. Uncertainty sets associated with saccadic eye movements-basis of satisfaction control. Vision Res 1974;14(7):481–486.

CHAPTER 11

ENGINEERING CONTROLS TO MEDIATE BACK PAIN AT WORK: TOOLS FOR THE ASSESSMENT OF PHYSICAL FACTOR IMPACT ON SPINE LOADS AND INTERVENTION EFFECTIVENESS

THE ROLES of engineering controls-based interventions intended to mediate the influence of physical risk factors are discussed. Common risk assessment techniques that are relevant to the spine tissue loading discussions of previous chapters are reviewed. Studies demonstrating engineering control effectiveness in mediating low back pain reporting are presented.

11.1 INTRODUCTION

Chapter 6 has introduced biomechanical logic that underpins the accurate assessment of spine loading and is fundamental to the interpretation of low back pain loading due to risk factor exposure. We have seen how sophisticated biomechanical assessment techniques (such as EMG-assisted biomechanical models) can be employed in laboratory studies to evaluate the potential risks associated with exposure to physical workplace characteristics (Chapter 7) that are common to many workplaces. These studies have resulted in a rich body of literature that can be used as a guide for worker exposure to many generic work conditions. However, given the large variety of workplace situations present in industrial settings, there is often a need to evaluate specific work conditions that may not have been explored in these laboratory studies. This is especially true for the exploration of interactions among risk factors that may be unique to a given work environment.

The more robust methods for assessing spine loads that are used in laboratory studies (e.g., EMG-assisted models) are often impractical for the assessment of risk *at* the work site since they require extensive instrumentation. However, there are several techniques that have been developed to provide rough estimates of biomechanically based risk associated with work situations that do not require a high level of biomechanical expertise and are available to those wishing to perform assessments at the worksite. This section reviews the commonly used methods and tools available for these worksite assessments and reviews the literature that supports their usage.

11.2 STATIC STRENGTH PREDICTION PROGRAMS

The two-dimensional static strength prediction program logic has been described previously. The same single equivalent muscle vector logic has been used to expand this tool to a three-dimensional static strength prediction program (3DSSPP). The program considers the load–tolerance relationship from two aspects. First, an estimate of spine compression is generated and compared to the generally accepted tolerance limits of 3400 N. Second, the load imposed by the task on each of six joints is compared to a static strength database of the population strength that considers the strength capacity of workers relative to these six joints.

As shown in Fig. 11.1, the model presents a stick figure in three-dimensional space. This figure must be oriented to mimic a static component of the task (one frozen posture) performed by the worker. The model logic assumes that the internal loads can be assessed by working backwards from knowledge about the external loads to which a worker is exposed under static conditions. The model calculates the torque generated about each of the six joints that make up the stick figure and sums the net resulting force imposed on the low back. The load imposed about low back (L5/S1) is considered to be supported by a single equivalent back muscle so that the external load is counterbalanced and equilibrium is maintained in the model.

The relationship between the torque imposed at a joint and the available strength of the joint has been defined as a lifting strength rating (LSR) and was used to prospectively assess low back injuries in an industrial environment (1).

The LSR is defined as the weight of the maximum load lifted on the job divided by the lifting strength measured in the same lifting posture for a large, strong man. One study concluded that "the incidence rate of low back pain (was) correlated (monotonically) with higher lifting strength requirements as determined by assessment of both the location and

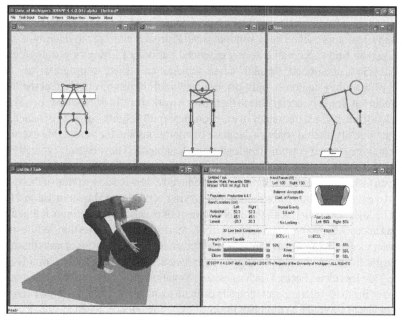

Figure 11.1 Example of 3D static strength prediction program (SSPP). (Courtesy of D. Chaffin).

magnitude of the load lifted." This was one of the first quantitative studies to conclude that not only was the magnitude of the load lifted potentially hazardous, but it was also important to consider the load location when assessing risk. Thus, strength is highly dependent on body posture. The study also suggested that exposure to moderate lifting frequencies appeared to be protective, whereas high or low rates of lifting were common in jobs with greater reports of back injury.

An industrial study using both the LSR and estimates of back compression forces (predicted by this program) observed jobs over 3 years in five large industrial plants where 2934 material handling tasks were evaluated (2). The results suggested a positive correlation between the lifting strength ratio and back incidence rates. The study also reported that musculoskeletal injuries were twice as likely for predicted spine compression forces that exceeded 6800 N. However, this trend was not evident for back-specific musculoskeletal incidents specifically. The study also suggested that prediction of risk was best associated with the most stressful tasks (as opposed to indices that represent risk aggregation). However, more recent studies in an automobile assembly plant found an increase in low back pain reporting in workers exposed to prolonged static postures, but did not find an associated increase in low back forces when they were evaluated using this method (3). This may indicate a different pathway or mechanism of low back pain for these low- to moderate-load jobs.

The advantage of this model is that it is relatively straightforward and easy to use. Thus, it can be used routinely to assess both structure-based load and muscle load on a large scale in a plant. The model is often used as a "first pass" type of assessment to determine whether a task requires more sophisticated analyses. The limitations of the model are its moderate costs and that it cannot assess the effects of motion. In addition, it does not account for trunk muscle coactivations that can uniquely define tissue loads and are important contributors to both structure-based and muscle-based low back pain risk. Thus, this model appears to be best suited to the assessment of jobs that require sustained static postures and involve large external forces.

11.3 PSYCHOPHYSICAL TOLERANCE LIMITS

Another approach attempting to identify safe exertion limits for the back has been the psychophysical approach. The psychophysical approach attempts to determine how much force a person finds acceptable during extended periods of lifting or pushing/pulling. The psychophysical documents strength when subjects are asked to progressively adjust the amount of load they can push, pull, lift, or carry until they subjectively feel the load is of a magnitude that would be acceptable to them over a work shift. Task variables such as lift origin, height, load dimensions, frequency of exertion, push/pull heights, carrying distance, and so on are systematically altered so that a database of conditions and the acceptable exertion ranges can be cataloged for a spectrum of male and female subjects. These data are typically presented in tables that indicate the percentage of subjects who would find a particular load acceptable for a given task. Snook and colleagues have produced extensive description of these tolerances (4–9). An example of this information for carrying activities is shown in Table 11.1.

The logic associated with the establishment of psychophysical limits it that this assessment can account for motion and fatigue over extended periods of exertion. While mechanical tissue tolerance limits appear to be reasonable thresholds for the analysis of tasks that may lead to an acute trauma event, their application to repetitive tasks (that may lead to cumulative trauma disorder) are less clear. Factors such as tissue adaptation may play a role, making quantitative analyses of the load–tolerance relationship difficult to quantify. Thus, some have resorted to the psychophysical approach to establish limits of exposure. Hence, when mechanical tolerances are not available, some have adopted psychophysical limits as the tolerance.

TABLE 11.1 Psychophysical Assessment of Maximum Acceptable Weight of Carry as a Function of Frequency and Height of Carry (From Reference 9)

Height[a]	Percent[b]	2.1 m carry — One carry every							4.3 m carry — One carry every							8.5 m carry — One carry every						
		6 s	12 s	1 min	2 min	5 min	30 min	8 h	10 s	16 s	1 min	2 min	5 min	30 min	8 h	18 s	24 s	1 min	2 min	5 min	30 min	8 h
Males																						
111	90	10	14	17	17	19	21	25	9	11	15	15	17	19	22	10	11	13	13	15	17	20
	75	14	19	23	23	26	29	34	13	16	21	21	23	26	30	13	15	18	18	20	23	27
	50	19	25	30	30	33	38	44	17	20	27	27	30	34	39	17	19	23	24	26	29	35
	25	23	30	37	37	41	46	54	20	25	33	33	37	41	48	21	24	29	29	32	36	43
	10	27	35	43	43	48	54	63	24	29	38	39	43	48	57	24	28	34	34	38	42	50
79	90	13	17	21	21	23	26	31	11	14	18	19	21	23	27	13	15	17	18	20	22	26
	75	18	23	28	29	32	36	42	16	19	25	25	28	32	37	17	20	24	24	27	30	35
	50	23	30	37	37	41	46	54	20	25	32	33	36	41	48	22	26	31	31	35	39	46
	25	28	37	45	46	51	57	67	25	30	40	40	45	50	59	27	32	38	38	42	48	56
	10	33	43	53	53	59	66	78	29	35	47	47	52	59	69	32	38	44	45	50	56	65
Females																						
105	90	11	12	13	13	13	13	18	9	10	13	13	13	13	18	10	11	12	12	12	12	16
	75	13	14	15	15	16	16	21	11	12	15	15	16	16	21	12	13	14	14	14	14	19
	50	15	16	18	18	18	18	25	12	13	18	18	18	18	24	14	15	16	16	16	16	22
	25	17	18	20	20	21	21	28	14	15	20	20	21	21	28	15	17	18	18	19	19	25
	10	19	20	22	22	23	23	31	16	17	22	22	23	23	31	17	19	20	20	21	21	28
72	90	13	14	16	16	16	16	22	10	11	14	14	14	14	20	12	12	14	14	14	14	19
	75	15	17	18	18	19	19	25	11	13	16	16	17	17	23	14	15	16	16	17	17	23
	50	17	19	21	21	22	22	29	13	15	19	19	20	20	26	16	17	19	19	20	20	26
	25	20	22	24	24	25	25	33	15	17	22	22	22	22	30	18	19	21	22	22	22	30
	10	22	24	27	27	28	28	37	17	19	24	24	25	25	33	20	21	24	24	25	25	33

Italicized values exceed 8 h physiological criteria (see text).

[a] Vertical distance from floor to hands (cm).

[b] Percentage of industrial population.

Few investigations have formally validated whether the design of work tasks through psychophysical tolerance limits is protective and minimizes low back pain at work. However, Snook (5) has observed that low back related injury claims were three times more prevalent in jobs exceeding the psychophysically determined strength tolerance of 75% of men compared with jobs demanding less strength.

The advantage of this approach is that it is quick and easy to apply and simply requires one to assess the task conditions and match these conditions to psychophysical tables. In addition, the application of the approach requires virtually no expense. The disadvantage of the approach is that people do not necessarily know their appropriate tolerance limit. Given our knowledge of pain perception and the back (Chapter 5), it is unlikely that people could perceive when microfractures occur in the vertebral end plate or when proinflammatory cytokines are about to be released. Hence, it is questionable as to whether this approach is accurately identifying pain or damage thresholds.

11.4 JOB DEMAND INDEX

Yet another approach that combines concept similar to the LSR along with psychophysically determined strength was reported in the literature (10) in terms of a job severity index or JSI. This index considers the ratio of the job demands relative to the lifting capacities of the worker. Job demands include factors such as the weight of the object lifted, the frequency of lifting, exposure time, and lifting task origins and destinations. A comprehensive task analysis is required to assess job demands. The worker capacity includes the strength and body size of the worker. Strength is determined via psychophysical testing. A prospective study using the JSI was reported in the literature (11). Although this approach does not assess structure loading, it is of value in assessing potential trunk muscle over exertions and may have some relevance to the muscle dysfunction pathway described earlier. Results suggested a threshold of a job demand relative to worker strength above which the risk of low back injury increased.

The authors suggest that this method could identify the more costly injuries. The JSI is not a biomechanical assessment of the lift, so it is not able to quantify loads imposed on spine tissues that might activate a low back pain pathway. In addition, a low level of task quantification reduces the specificity of the technique. However, it may reflect a psychophysical component of work in that it can help define situations that are subjectively more or less acceptable to the worker. No literature has assessed the validation of this approach.

11.5 NIOSH LIFTING GUIDE AND REVISED EQUATION

11.5.1 The 1981 Lifting Guide

The National Institute for Occupational Safety and Health (NIOSH) has developed two assessment tools or guides to help determine the risk associated with manual materials handling tasks. These guides are the tools typically used by federal agencies (i.e., OSHA) to assess risk associated with a particular work situation. The lifting guide was originally developed in 1981 (12) and applies to lifting situations where the lifts are performed in the sagittal plane and to motions that are slow and smooth. Two benchmarks or limits were defined by this guide. The first limit is called the *action limit* (AL) and represents a magnitude of weight in a given lifting situation that would impose a spine load corresponding to the beginning point of low back disorder risk along a risk continuum. The AL was associated with the point at which people under 40 years of age just begin to experience a risk of vertebral end plate microfracture (3400 N of compressive load). Microfractures are one method by which disk degeneration is believed to occur (see Chapter 5). The guide estimates the force imposed on the spine of a worker as a result of lifting a weight and compares the spine load to the AL. If the weight of the object results in a spine load that is below the AL, the job is considered safe. If the weight lifted by the worker is larger than the AL, there is some level of risk associated with the task. The general form of the AL formula is defined according to Equation 11.1.

$$AL = k(HF)(VF)(DF)(FF) \tag{11.1}$$

where

$\quad$ AL = the action limit in kg or pounds and

$\quad\quad k$ = load constant (40 kg or 90 lb), which is the greatest weight a subject could lift if all lifting conditions are optimal.

$\quad$ HF = horizontal factor defined as the horizontal distance from a point bisecting the ankles to the center of gravity of the load at the lift origin. Defined algebraically as $15/H$ (cm) or $6/H$ (in.).

$\quad$ VF = vertical factor or height of the load at lift origin. Defined algebraically as $(0.004)|V-75|$ (cm) or $1 - (0.01)|V - 30|$ (in.).

$\quad$ DF = distance factor or the vertical travel distance of the load. Defined algebraically as $0.7 + 7.5/D$ (cm) or $0.7 + 3/D$ (in.).

$\quad$ FF = frequency factor or lifting rate defined algebraically as $1 - F/F_{max}$.

$\quad F$ = average frequency of lift and F_{max} is between 12 and 18 lifts per minute.

$\quad\quad$ This equation assumes that if the lifting conditions are ideal, a worker could safely hold (and implicitly lift) the load of the load constant (k) magnitude (40 kg or 90 lbs). However, if the lifting conditions are not ideal, the allowable weight is "discounted" according to the four factors HF, VF, DF, and FF. These four discounting factors are shown in Fig. 11.2. According to the relationships indicated in these figures, the HF, which is associated with external moment exposure, has the most dramatic effect on acceptable lifting conditions (Fig. 11.2a). Both a vertical height modulator (VF) (indicating the original lift height of a load) and a vertical distance modulator (DF) (indicating the distance traveled during the lift) are associated with the back muscle's length–strength relationship (Fig. 11.2b and c). Finally, FF attempts to account for the cumulative effects of repetitive lifting (Fig. 11.2d).

$\quad\quad$ The second benchmark associated with the 1981 lifting guide is the *maximum permissible limit* or MPL. The MPL represents the point at which significant risk, defined in part as a significant risk of vertebral end plate microfracture, occurs. The MPL is associated with a compressive load on the spine of 6400 N, which corresponds to the point at which 50% of the people would be expected to suffer a vertebral end plate microfracture. The MPL is a function of the AL and is defined as follows in Equation 11.2:

$$MPL = 3(AL) \tag{11.2}$$

The weight that the worker is expected to lift in a work situation is compared to the weight limits prescribed by the AL and MPL. If the magnitude of weight falls below the AL, the work is considered safe and no work adjustments are necessary. If the magnitude of the weight falls above the MPL, then the work is considered to represent a significant risk and engineering changes involving the adjustment of HF, VF, and/or DF are required to reduce the AL and MPL. If the weight falls between the AL and MPL, then either engineering changes or administrative changes, defined as selecting workers who are less likely to be injured or rotating workers, would be appropriate.

$\quad\quad$ The AL and MPL were also indexed relative to nonbiomechanical benchmarks. NIOSH (1981) states that these limits also correspond to strength, energy expenditure, and psychophysical acceptance points. Weights below the AL are expected to represent tasks

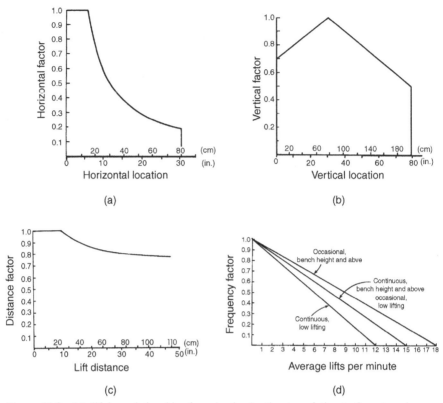

Figure 11.2   Modifying relationships for spine load estimates relating to the external moment (**a**), length–strength relationship of the muscle (**b** and **c**), and the temporal components of the work (**d**) (from reference 12).

within the static strength capability of 75% for females and 99% for males. Hence, matching tasks relative to this limit may be protective from a muscle dysfunction risk standpoint (Chapter 5). However, it is not known how dynamic strength (involved in much of modern work) compares to this criterion.

The guide was designed to be used for primarily sagittally symmetric lifts that were slow and smooth. Only one evaluation of the guide's effectiveness could be found in the literature (13). Comparing the predictions with historical data of back injury reporting in industry, this evaluation indicated an odds ratio of 3.5 with good specificity but low sensitivity. Thus, while this equation did a reasonable job of identifying jobs that were not particularly risky, it did not identify problematic jobs well.

Overall, the benefit of this guide is that it is straightforward to use and free. In addition, given the specificity, if a task is identified as problematic, it probably is worth an intervention. The disadvantages of the guide include a lack of sensitivity to nonsymmetric lifts and dynamic movement. In addition, the sensitivity is such that it will most likely not identify jobs that may be problematic.

11.5.2   The 1993 Revised Equation

The 1993 NIOSH revised lifting equation was introduced to address those lifting jobs that violate the sagittally symmetric lifting assumption of the original 1981 lifting guide (14). While NIOSH recommends the use of this revised equation, some prefer to use the original

1981 Lifting Guide. The concepts of AL and MPL were replaced with a concept of a *lifting index* or LI, intended for ease of use. The LI is defined in Equation 11.3 as:

$$LI = \frac{L}{RWL} \tag{11.3}$$

where L = load weight or the weight of the object to be lifted. RWL = recommended weight limit for the particular lifting situation. LI = lifting index used to estimate relative magnitude of physical stress for a particular job.

If the LI is greater than 1.0, an increased risk of suffering a lifting-related low back disorder exists. The RWL is similar in concept to the 1981 Lifting Guide AL equation (Eq. 11.1) in that it contains factors that discount the allowable load according to the horizontal distance, vertical location of the load, vertical travel distance, and frequency of lift. However, there were also a couple of adjustments made to the equation. The load constant was reduced from 40 kg (90 lb) to 23 kg (51 lb), thereby reducing the maximum allowable lift weight. In addition, the form of these discounting factors was adjusted to account for the lower load constant. Also, two additional discounting factors have been included. These additional factors include a lift asymmetry factor that accounts for asymmetric lifting conditions and a coupling factor that accounts for whether or not the load lifted has handles. The RWL is represented in Equations 11.4 (metric units) and 11.5 (US units).

$$RWL(kg) = 23(25/H)(1-(0.003|V-75|))(0.82 + 4.5/D))(FM)(1-(0.0032A))(CM) \tag{11.4}$$

$$RWL(lb) = 51(10/H)(1-(0.0075|V-30|))(0.82 + 1.8/D))(FM)(1-(0.0032A))(CM) \tag{11.5}$$

where H = horizontal location forward of the midpoint between the ankles at the origin of the lift. If significant control is required at the destination, then H should be measured both at the origin and destination of the lift (in centimeters or inches). V = vertical location at the origin of the lift (in centimeters or inches). D = vertical travel distance between origin and destination of the lift (in centimeters or inches). FM = frequency multiplier shown in Table 11.2. A = angle between the midpoint of the ankles and the midpoint between the hands at the origin of the lift (degrees). CM = coupling multiplier ranked as either good, fair, or poor and described in Table 11.3.

Two assessments of the revised equation, comparing its estimates to injury reporting, have been performed. One assessment compared the ability of the tool to identify high and low risk jobs based on a historical database (13). This assessment yielded an odds ratio of 3.1. Further analyses indicated higher sensitivity than the 1981 guide but lower specificity. Thus, the 1993 revised equation yields a more conservative (protective) prediction of work-related low back disorder risk. This version of the model tended to identify problematic jobs well (from a low back risk perspective), but unfortunately, also often identified nonrisky jobs as problematic.

A second analysis using a different data set compared risk odds ratios to the predicted LI for various jobs (16). For LIs between 1 and 3, the odds ratios ranged from 1.54 to 2.45 indicating an increasing odds ratio with increasing low back pain reporting. However, the odds ratio for LIs over 3 was lower (odds ratio of 1.63) indicating a nonmonotonic relationship between the LI and risk.

The advantages of this tool are that it is relatively simple to use and cost free. However, it appears to be unnecessarily protective and may require the changing of jobs that do not necessarily place workers at risk. In addition, the tool is also unable to consider the effects of dynamic movements upon risk.

TABLE 11.2   Frequency Multiplier Table (FM)

| Frequency lifts/min $(F)^a$ | Work Duration | | | | | |
| | ≤ 1 h | | >1 but ≤ 2 h | | >2 but ≤ 8 h | |
	$V < 30$	$V \geq 30$	$V < 30$	$V \geq 30$	$V < 30$	$V \geq 30$
≥ 0.2	1.00	1.00	0.95	0.95	0.85	0.85
0.5	0.97	0.97	0.92	0.92	0.81	0.81
1	0.94	0.94	0.88	0.88	0.75	0.75
2	0.91	0.91	0.84	0.84	0.65	0.65
3	0.88	0.88	0.79	0.79	0.55	0.55
4	0.84	0.84	0.72	0.72	0.45	0.45
5	0.80	0.80	0.60	0.60	0.35	0.35
6	0.75	0.75	0.50	0.50	0.27	0.27
7	0.70	0.70	0.42	0.42	0.22	0.22
8	0.60	0.60	0.35	0.35	0.18	0.18
9	0.52	0.52	0.30	0.30	0.00	0.15
10	0.45	0.45	0.26	0.26	0.00	0.13
11	0.41	0.41	0.00	0.23	0.00	0.00
12	0.37	0.37	0.00	0.21	0.00	0.00
13	0.00	0.34	0.00	0.00	0.00	0.00
14	0.00	0.31	0.00	0.00	0.00	0.00
15	0.00	0.28	0.00	0.00	0.00	0.00
>15	0.00	0.00	0.00	0.00	0.00	0.00

Reprinted from NIOSH, Applications Manual for the Revised NIOSH Lifting Equation (from reference 15).
^{a}For lifting less frequently than once per 5 min, set $F = 0.2$ lifts/min.
^{b}Values of V are in inches.

TABLE 11.3   Coupling Multiplier

Coupling type	$V < 30$ in. (75 cm)	$V \geq 30$ in. (75 cm)
Good	1.00	1.00
Fair	0.95	1.00
Poor	0.90	0.90

Reprinted from NIOSH, *Application Manual for Revised NIOSH Equation, 1994* (from reference 15).

11.6   VIDEO-BASED BIOMECHANICAL MODELS

A Canadian group of researchers (17) used a quasi-dynamic 2D biomechanical model to assess cumulative biomechanical loading of the spine in 234 automotive assembly workers. This study identified four independent risk factors for low back disorder reporting consisting of integrated load moment (over a work shift), hand forces, peak shear force on the spine, and peak trunk velocity. They concluded that workers in the top 25% of loading exposure on all risk factors were at about six times the risk of reporting back pain than those in the bottom 25% of loading.

While this model has helped identify dynamic risk factors, it also requires significant effort as well as the expense of software to perform the assessments.

11.7   LUMBAR MOTION MONITOR RISK ASSESSMENT

In an attempt to consider the contribution of trunk dynamics as well as the traditional biomechanical factors in workplace assessment of risk, a study (18,19) biomechanically evaluated over 400 industrial jobs (with documented low back disorder risk history) by observing 114 workplace and worker-related variables. The study compared primarily physical workplace characteristics (including dynamic motions to which the workers were exposed) in those workers performing lifts in high risk jobs (average of 26 low back pain reports per 100 workers) to low risk lifting jobs (0 low back pain reports per 100 workers).

Of the variables explored, exposure to load moment (load magnitude × distance of load from spine) was found to be the single most powerful predictor of low back disorder reporting. This study also identified 16 trunk kinematic variables that resulted in statistically significant odds ratios associated with risk of low back disorder reporting in the workplace. None of the single kinematic variables were as strong a predictor as load moment; however, when load moment was combined with three kinematic variables (relating to the three dimensions of trunk motion) along with an exposure frequency measure (indicating the temporal aspects of loading), a strong multiple logistic regression model resulted that described reporting of back disorder well (OR = 10.7). The analysis indicated that risk was multivariate in nature and that exposure to the *combination* of the five variables described reporting well.

This information was incorporated into a tool that included this predictive functional risk model (Fig. 11.3) and is capable of accounting for trade-offs between risk variables. For example, a job task that exposes a worker to low magnitude of load-moment can represent a high risk situation if the other four variables in the model were of sufficient magnitude. Hence, the model recognizes the trade-offs among the interactive risk factors.

To aid in interpretation of risk, the model has color coded the probability of high risk group membership into a green (safe), yellow (moderate risk), and red (high risk) groups (Fig. 11.3). The model has been validated in a prospective workplace intervention study (20).

However, to perform this assessment, one must assess the three-dimensional dynamic motions to which the worker is exposed during repetitions of the job task. To provide this information to the model, a lumbar motion monitor (LMM) is worn by the worker when the

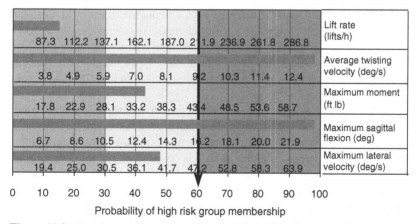

Figure 11.3   Lumbar motion monitor (LMM) risk model. The probability risk of high risk (of low back pain) group membership is quantitatively indicated for a particular task for each of five risk factors indicating how much exposure is too much exposure for a particular risk factor. The vertical arrow indicates the overall probability of high risk group membership due to the combination of risk factors. The risk "zone" is also color coded to help in interpretation.

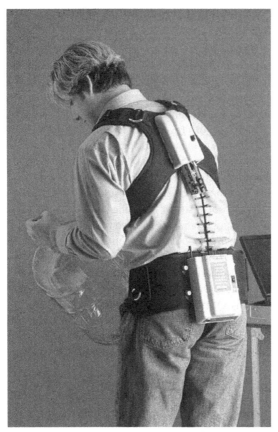

Figure 11.4   A lumbar motion monitor (LMM) worn by a worker can document worker exposure to dynamic work conditions. This information is used as part of the input to the risk model described in Fig. 11.3.

job is performed (Fig. 11.4). This lightweight device offers little resistance to worker motion and simply moves along with the worker's back without interfering with the job tasks. The LMM measurements are linked via a radio telemetry system to the risk model described above via a computer program to document trunk motion exposure on the job. Load moment is input to the model by simply measuring the distance of the lifted object from the worker's spine multiplied by the object weight. Temporal aspects of the job (lift rate) are also input to the program by the analyst.

The advantage of this assessment is that it can account for the dynamic components of task demands as well as the external loads to which the worker is exposed. Another advantage is that, since the analyses are computerized, the results are available immediately after data collection has been completed. This makes it possible to get immediate feedback and intervention feasibility can be easily achieved via a "trial and error approach." The disadvantage of this approach is the cost of the equipment and program needed to perform the assessment. However, given costs of low back disorders to industry, the device can more than pay for itself by eliminating one work-related low back problem.

When the findings from these studies are considered in conjunction with previous epidemiologic evidence at the workplace (3), it is clear that work associated with activity performed in nonneutral postures increases the risk to the back. Collectively, these studies indicate that as trunk posture becomes more extreme or the trunk motion becomes more rapid, reporting of back disorders is greater. While this model is not a direct assessment of spinal loads associated with the task, it represents the only means to indirectly consider the interaction among risk factors by assessing loading and risk due to dynamic motion exposure in the workplace.

Each of the risk factor scales shown in Fig. 11.3 has also been assessed from a biomechanical standpoint. Biologically assisted models of spine loading have been used to assess the range of lift frequency (21,22), trunk twisting (23), load moment (24–26), sagittal flexion (26), and the trunk's lateral bending velocity (27). These studies have demonstrated why the lower values on each risk factor scale relate to lower spine loading compared to greater scale values. Thus, this assessment tool enjoys the benefit of a biomechanical validation.

A database of 126 jobs including LMM information was evaluated (28) to precisely quantify and assess the complex trunk motions of groups with varying degrees of low back disorder reporting. They determined that groups with greater reporting rates exhibited complex trunk motion patterns involving high magnitudes of combined trunk velocities, especially at extreme sagittal flexion, whereas the low risk groups did not exhibit these patterns. This study suggested that elevated levels of complex simultaneous velocity patterns along with key workplace factors (load moment and frequency) were unique to those with increased low back disorder risk.

A validation study of this technique (described in Chapter 7) was also used to assess which interventions were effective in reducing low back pain reporting in this assessment (20). This same study observed the interventions that were chosen to control low back pain on the job. As shown in Fig. 11.5, under these circumstances, only lift tables and lift aids (such as hoists and cranes) had any appreciable effect on incident rates. In general, interventions such as redesign and equipment changes were no more effective than no interventions at all (control) over the observation period. It is worth noting that the effectiveness (or lack of effectiveness) of these interventions (as measured by incidence rates) were predictable by the LMM risk model. Thus, if appropriate measurements techniques are employed, that are capable of identifying the nature of the risk (e.g., dynamic loading), it is possible to identify both risky work conditions and appropriate interventions.

The advantages of the LMM risk model include the consideration of dynamic movement during the task, a strong prediction capability, a historical and biomechanical underpinning, and a prospective validation. Disadvantages of the system are associated with the cost of the device and the need to instrument the worker to perform an assessment.

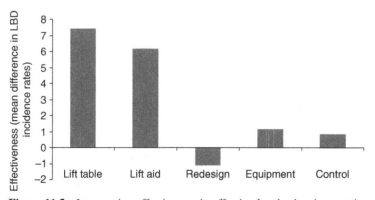

Figure 11.5 Intervention effectiveness in affecting low back pain reporting at the job classified according to four different intervention categories and a control group (no intervention over the observation period). (From reference 20).

11.8   LIFTING THRESHOLD LIMIT VALUES (TLVs)

The lifting threshold limit values or TLVs represent the most recent lifting assessment tool to be used in the workplace. The TLV was developed by considering predictions from biomechanical loading from an EMG-assisted model (29), a database of historical risk associated with different lifting conditions (19), as well as the 3DSSPP and NIOSH lift guide predictions when estimating risk associated with lifts from different lifting "zones." The TLVs identify workplace lifting conditions under which it is believed that nearly all workers may be repeatedly exposed, day after day, without developing workrelated low back disorders associated with repetitive lifting tasks (30). Appropriate control measures should be implemented any time the lifting TLVs are exceeded or lifting-related musculoskeletal disorders are detected.

The TLVs consists of three charts: the chart used to determine the TLVs is a function of the lifting duration and lifting frequency. Then, based on one of four categories for height of the lift (floor to mid-shin height, mid-shin to knuckle height, knuckle height to below shoulder, and below shoulder to 30 cm above shoulder) and one of three categories of horizontal lift distance (close, intermediate, and extended), TLVs for weight are given. Thus, this approach considers both horizontal moment and origin of lift height to define lift "zones" in one measure. In some cases, the tables indicate that there is no known safe limit for repetitive lifting under those conditions.

The TLV is limited to two-handed mono-lifting tasks performed within 30° of the sagittal plane, so tasks requiring a large amount of trunk twisting should not be analyzed with this tool.

If any of the conditions listed below are present, then professional judgment should be used to reduce weight limits below those recommended in the TLVs:

- Lifting at a frequency higher than 360 lifts per hour.
- Extended work shifts: lifting performed for longer than 8 h per day.
- High asymmetry: lifting more than 30° away from the sagittal plane.
- One-handed lifting.
- Lifting while seated or kneeling.
- High heat and humidity.
- Lifting unstable objects (e.g., liquids with shifting center of mass).
- Poor hand coupling: lack of handles, cut-outs, or other grasping points.
- Unstable footing (e.g., inability to support the body with both feet while standing).

The lifting TLV does incorporate relatively complex data into a format that is quick, easy to use, and easy to interpret; hence, it is a very useful tool to quickly assess many lifting tasks. The results can also direct the user to job redesign strategies. For example, if the lifting conditions exceed the TLV, the user can then find cells in the table that would not exceed the TLV, and then redesign the job accordingly. Since the results are presented in a straightforward, intuitive format, the TLV also can be useful when requesting support from management for resources to institute ergonomic interventions.

The following represent step-by-step instructions for determining the lifting TLV:

1. Understand the limitations and basis of the TLVs.
2. Determine if the task duration is less than or equal to 2 h per day or greater than 2 h per day.
3. Determine the lifting frequency as the number of lifts a worker performs per hour.
4. Use the TLV table that corresponds to the duration and lifting frequency of the task. (Table 11.4 can be used to determine the appropriate TLV table given the frequency and the duration.)

TABLE 11.4   TLV Table Corresponding to Specified Levels of Lifting Frequency and Lifting Duration (From Reference 30)

	Duration of Task Per Day	
Lifts per Hour	≤2 h	>2 h
≤60	Table 11.5	
≤12		Table 11.5
>12 and ≤30		Table 11.6
>60 and ≤360	Table 11.6	
>30 and ≤360		Table 11.7

5. Determine the lifting zone height based on the location of the hands at the beginning of the lift. (Fig. 11.6).

6. Determine the horizontal location of the lift by measuring the horizontal distance from the midpoint between the inner ankle bones to the midpoint between the hands at the beginning of the lift.

7. Determine the TLV for the lifting task, as displayed in the table cell that corresponds to the lifting zone and horizontal distance in the appropriate table, based on frequency and duration (Tables 11.5–11.7).

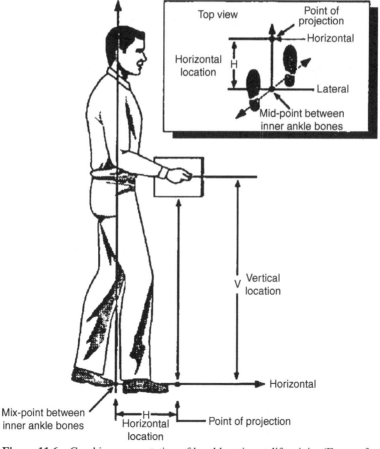

Figure 11.6   Graphic representation of hand location at lift origin. (From reference 15).

TABLE 11.5 TLVs for Lifting Tasks ≤2 h per Day with ≤60 Lifts per h or >2 h per Day with ≤12 Lifts per h (From Reference 30)

Lifting height zone	Horizontal location of lift	Close lifts: origin <30 cm from midpoint between inner ankle bones	Intermediate lifts: origin 30–60 cm from midpoint between inner ankle bones	Extended lifts: origin >60–80 cm from midpoint between inner ankle bones[a]
Reach limit[b] from 30 cm above to 8 cm below shoulder height		16 kg	7 kg	No known safe limit for repetitive lifting[c]
Knuckle height[d] to below shoulder		32 kg	16 kg	9 kg
Middle shin height to knuckle height[d]		18 kg	14 kg	7 kg
Floor to middle shin height		14 kg	No known safe limit for repetitive lifting[c]	No known safe limit for repetitive lifting[c]

[a]Lifting tasks should not be started at a horizontal reach distance more than 80 cm from the midpoint between the inner ankle bones (Fig. 11.2).
[b]Routine lifting tasks should not be conducted from starting heights greater than 30 cm above the shoulder or more than 180 cm above floor level (Fig. 11.2).
[c]Routine lifting tasks should not be performed for shaded table entries marked "no known safe limit for repetitive lifting." While the available evidence does not permit identification of safe weight limits in the shaded regions, professional judgment may be used to determine if infrequent lifts of light weights may be safe.
[d]Anatomical landmark for knuckle height assumes the worker is standing erect with arms hanging at the side.

TABLE 11.6 TLVs for Lifting Tasks >2 h per Day with >12 and ≤30 Lifts per h or ≤2 h per Day with >60 and ≤360 Lifts per h (From Reference 30)

Lifting height zone	Horizontal location of lift	Close lifts: origin <30 cm from midpoint between inner ankle bones	Intermediate lifts: origin 30–60 cm from midpoint between inner ankle bones	Extended lifts: origin >60 to 80 cm from midpoint between inner ankle bones[a]
Reach limit[b] from 30 cm above to 8 cm below shoulder height		14 kg	5 kg	No known safe limit for repetitive lifting[c]
Knuckle height[d] to below shoulder		27 kg	14 kg	7 kg
Middle shin height to knuckle height[d]		16 kg	11 kg	5 kg
Floor to middle shin height		9 kg	No known safe limit for repetitive lifting[c]	No known safe limit for repetitive lifting[c]

[a]Lifting tasks should not be started at a horizontal reach distance more than 80 cm from the midpoint between the inner ankle bones (Fig. 11.2).
[b]Routine lifting tasks should not be conducted from starting heights greater than 30 cm above the shoulder or more than 180 cm above floor level (Fig. 11.2).
[c]Routine lifting tasks should not be performed for shaded table entries marked "No known safe limit for repetitive lifting." While the available evidence does not permit identification of safe weight limits in the shaded regions, professional judgment may be used to determine if infrequent lifts of light weights may be safe.
[d]Anatomical landmark for knuckle height assumes the worker is standing erect with arms hanging at the side.

TABLE 11.7   TLVs for Lifting Tasks >2 h per Day with >30 and ≤360 Lifts per Hour (From Reference 30)

Lifting height zone	Horizontal location of lift	Close lifts: origin < 30 cm from midpoint between inner ankle bones	Intermediate lifts: origin 30–60 cm from midpoint between inner ankle bones	Extended lifts: origin >60–80 cm from midpoint between inner ankle bones[a]
Reach limit[b] from 30 cm above to 8 cm below shoulder height		11 kg	No known safe limit for repetitive lifting[c]	No known safe limit for repetitive lifting[c]
Knuckle height[d] to below shoulder		14 kg	9 kg	5 kg
Middle shin height to knuckle height[d]		9 kg	7 kg	2 kg
Floor to middle shin height		No known safe limit for repetitive lifting[c]	No known safe limit for repetitive lifting[c]	No known safe limit for repetitive lifting[c]

[a]Lifting tasks should not be started at a horizontal reach distance more than 80 cm from the midpoint between the inner ankle bones (Fig. 11.2).
[b]Routine lifting tasks should not be conducted from starting heights greater than 30 cm above the shoulder or more than 180 cm above floor level (Fig. 11.2).
[c]Routine lifting tasks should not be performed for shaded table entries marked "no known safe limit for repetitive lifting." While the available evidence does not permit identification of safe weight limits in the shaded regions, professional judgment may be used to determine if infrequent lifts of light weights may be safe.
[d]Anatomical landmark for knuckle height assumes the worker is standing erect with arms hanging at the side.

If the weight being lifted in the task exceeds the TLV, then changes must be made to the task to ensure that the weight is within the limit. Factors such as the characteristics of the task, type of industry, and economics will dictate the appropriate task redesign strategy. The following hierarchy of controls is suggested when redesigning manual material handling tasks:

1. *Eliminate unnecessary lifting:* Whenever possible, eliminate manual materials handling by combining operations or shortening the distances that material must be moved. Look at material flow through the facility and eliminate any unnecessary lifts. By doing so, you eliminate worker exposure to the musculoskeletal disorder risk factors. In addition, the overall efficiency of a facility is generally improved as time previously required to manually handle materials can be used for other productive tasks.

2. *Automate or mechanize lifting:* If it is not possible to eliminate the lift, consider automating the lifting task or using a mechanical lifting device. Devices such as hoists, cranes, and manipulators can eliminate the forces on the spine associated with manual materials handling. Therefore, the likelihood of back injuries is also reduced.

3. *Modify the job to fit within worker capabilities:* If material must still be handled manually (or until one of the above approaches can be implemented), design the task to reduce the stress on the body as much as possible, with emphasis on ensuring that the weight lifted is below the lifting TLV. Some strategies for job design include the following:

   • Allow for lifting loads as close to the body as possible. Some techniques to reduce reaching distances are (a) eliminate any barriers such as the sides of bins or boxes, (b) use a turn table for loads on pallets, and (c) use a tilt table to allow for better access into bins.

- Place the load as close to waist height as possible. This may be accomplished by using adjustable lift tables or inclined conveyors to locate the object to be handled at waist height.

- Reduce the need to twist the trunk by reorienting the lifting origins and destinations.

- Reduce the weight of the load being lifted so that the weights are within the lifting TLV.

There are several advantages of the TLV. It incorporates the benefits of several biomechanical assessment tools into an "easy to use" assessment method. In addition, biomechanical loads as well as dynamic risk factors are imbedded in the analyses. Finally, the logic has been tied to historical observations of risk. The disadvantage is, as with several of the other measures, the specific information about the task (precision of load placement, specific trunk motion requirements, etc.) is not considered. However, overall, this is the single "easy to use" tool that considers several different types of information in one assessment tool.

11.9   WORKPLACE ASSESSMENT COMPARISONS

The findings of recent quantitative field studies used to assess workplace low back pain risk using available workplace risk factor measures are summarized in Table 11.8. The studies are consistent in that even though these studies have not evaluated spinal loading directly, the exposure measures included were indirect indicators of spinal load and suggest that as these risk factors increase in magnitude the risk increases. Load location or strength ratings both appear to be indicators of the magnitude of the load imposed on the spine. The exposure metrics (load location, kinematics, and three-dimensional analyses) are important from a biomechanical standpoint because they mediate the ability of the trunk's internal structures to support the external load. As these metrics change, they can change the nature of the loading on the backs internal structures.

Table 11.9 shows how the various available assessment tools discussed in this section compare relative to identified risk factors affecting loading of the spine and potentially influencing the low back pain pathways discussed earlier. As shown in this table, most of the assessment tools are sensitive to various components of the physical risk factors discussed in Chapter 7. Several findings are apparent from this table. First, few of the assessment tools are sensitive to all of the physical risk factors. Thus, one must consider the nature of the physical risk and then choose the appropriate risk assessment tool if one is to understand the impact of physical factors on spine loading due to the physical work environment. Second, all of the estimates of spine loadings used in these assessments are based on crude estimates of loading. Since none are direct results of biologically assisted models, the loadings are all simply approximations and not particularly sensitive. Third, none of the assessment techniques is able to comprehensively evaluate the influence of psychosocial/organizational or individual risk factors. Thus, the influence of interactions between these risk factors is typically not evaluated through the use of these tools. Given these constraints, all assessments should be used in conjunction with the realization that the dimensions of the risk factors not evaluated by the assessment tool may play a role in spine loading and resulting risk of low back pain.

Collectively, these studies demonstrate that when meaningful biomechanical assessments are performed at the workplace, associations between biomechanical factors and risk

TABLE 11.8 Comparisons of Field Risk Assessment Studies as a Function of the Specificity of Risk Factors Identified

References	# Jobs	Capacity/demand ratio	Load location	Load moment	Frequency	Kinematics	2D	3D	Multiple factors	Odds ratio
					Risk factors identified					
3	95 case 124 refferant					×		×	×	Max flex 5.7 (1.6–20.4) Twist/lat 5.9 (1.6–21.4)
18,19	403		×	×	×	×		×	×	5 var = 10.7 (4.9–23.6)
17	104 cases 130 refferant			×		×	×		×	4 var = 5.7 (1–31.2)
16	36	×	×	×	×			×	×	Max OR = 2.45 (1.29–4.85)

[a]Note tht the greater the level of risk factor quantification, the better the ability to properly identify risk (odds ratio).

TABLE 11.9 Sensitivity of the Commonly Used Physical Environment Assessment Tools to Physical Risk Factors, Psychosocial/Organizational Risk Factors, and Individual Risk Factors

Risk factor	3DSSPP	NIOSH WPG	NIOSH Revised Equation	Psychophysical tables	LMM risk model	ACGIH TLV
Physical factors						
3D load						
• Compression	×	×	×		×	×
• Shear	×				×	×
• Torsion					×	×
Moment sensitive	×	×	×	×	×	×
Posture sensitive	×				×	
Motion sensitive					×	
Asymmetry	×		×		×	
Temporal factors		×	×	×	×	×
Psychosocial organizational factors						
• Environment						
• Mental stress						
• Pacing		×	×		×	×
Individual factors						
• Gender	×			×		
• Personality						
• Experience						
• Strength	×			×		

of low back disorder reporting are stronger. Several common components of biomechanical risk assessment can be derived from these studies. First, increased low back pain reporting is associated with work primarily when the specific load location relative to the body (load moment or load location) is quantified in some way. Most studies have shown that these factors are closely associated with increased low back pain reports. Second, many studies have shown that increased reporting of low back pain can be well characterized when the three-dimensional kinematic demands of the work are described. Finally, nearly all of these assessments have demonstrated that risk is multidimensional in that there is a synergy among risk factors that is often associated with increased reporting of low back pain. Several studies have also suggested that some of these relationships are nonmonotonic.

In summary, these efforts have suggested that the better the lifting dimensions can be characterized in terms of biomechanical demand, the better the association with risk. This review also suggests that there are several assessment techniques that are available, many of which are based on different risk factors or a combination of risk factors. The most appropriate assessment tool depends on the nature of the risk associated with the job (static versus dynamic activities, large force versus low level force, etc.)

11.10 CONCLUSIONS

This review has shown that low back disorders are common in the workplace and are associated with occupational tasks when the risk factors of manual materials handling, bending, and twisting are present. The load–tolerance relationship represents a sound biomechanically plausible avenue to support the epidemiologic findings. Sophisticated biologically assisted biomechanical models have been developed that have been used to quantitatively assess many situations (in the laboratory) that are common to workplaces. There are also a host of quantitative workplace assessment tools available to assess risk directly at the worksite. Some of these workplace tools have incorporated the findings of these sensitive laboratory tools. These tools appear to be most sensitive if they are multifactorial in nature, assess the load moment exposure, and torso kinematic responses to work situations in three-dimensional space and employ assessment techniques that are well matched with the nature of the risk on a particular job (e.g., static versus dynamic risk). The more precisely these job requirements are documented, the better the association with risk.

This review has also shown that all tools have their strength and weaknesses. Additionally, the strengths and weaknesses vary between tools. For example, some tools are more sensitive to static loading risk (e.g., the 3DSSPP), whereas other tools are sensitive to dynamic movement loading risk (e.g., the LMM risk model). Therefore, it is important for the tool user to determine which risk factor is present in the work situation and then select an appropriate tool that is sensitive to the nature of the risk. Hence, different tools will be appropriate for different situations. Likewise, certain tools will be inappropriate for a given situations. Remember, these are simply tools that should be used in conjunction with the knowledge and judgments of the person performing the assessment. No tool will represent the "final word" on LBP risk for all work situations.

KEY POINTS

- Engineering control assessment tools are intended to assess the aspect of work that have the potential to influence risk and are able to be changed. Thus, assessment tools typically assess the physical components of work.

- Different assessment tools are based on different assumptions about risk and, therefore, are sensitive to different components of risk.

- It is important to match the assessment tool to the nature of the risk (e.g., static, dynamic, etc.) expected at work for the tool to be sensitive in identifying risk.

- Assessment tools that are easy to use are generally insensitive to the specific nature of the risk factors. Those tools that are more sensitive to risk generally require more instrumentation and are more expensive.

- While engineering control assessment tools assess different aspects of physical exposure risk, few are able to account for interactive effects due to the psychosocial/organizational environment or the influence of individual worker.

REFERENCES

1. CHAFFIN DB, PARK KS. A longitudinal study of low-back pain as associated with occupational weight lifting factors. Am Ind Hygiene Assoc J 1973;34(12): 513–525.
2. HERRIN GD, JARAIEDI M, ANDERSON CK. Prediction of overexertion injuries using biomechanical and psychophysical models. Am Ind Hygiene Assoc J 1986; 47(6):322–330.
3. PUNNETT L, et al. Back disorders and nonneutral trunk postures of automobile assembly workers. Scand J Work Environ Health 1991;17(5):337–346.
4. CIRIELLO VM, et al. The effects of task duration on psychophysically-determined maximum acceptable weights and forces. Ergonomics 1990;33(2):187–200.
5. SNOOK SH. The design of manual handling tasks. Ergonomics 1978;21(12):963–985.
6. SNOOK SH. Psychophysical considerations in permissible loads. Ergonomics 1985;28(1):327–330.
7. SNOOK SH. Psychophysical acceptability as a constraint in manual working capacity. Ergonomics 1985;28(1): 331–335.
8. SNOOK SH. Approaches to preplacement testing and selection of workers. Ergonomics 1987;30(2):241–247.
9. SNOOK SH, CIRIELLO VM. The design of manual handling tasks: revised tables of maximum acceptable weights and forces. Ergonomics 1991;34(9):1197–1213.
10. AYOUB MM, et al. Determination and Modeling of Lifting Capacity. Lubbock (TX): Texas Tech University; 1978.
11. LILES DH, et al. A job severity index for the evaluation and control of lifting injury. Human Factors 1984;26(6): 683–693.
12. (NIOSH). Work practices guide for manual lifting. Cincinnati (OH): Department of Health and Human Services (DHHS), National Institute for Occupational Safety and Health (NIOSH); 1981.
13. MARRAS WS, et al. The effectiveness of commonly used lifting assessment methods to identify industrial jobs associated with elevated risk of low-back disorders. Ergonomics 1999;42(1):229–245.
14. WATERS TR, et al. Revised NIOSH equation for the design and evaluation of manual lifting tasks. Ergonomics 1993;36(7):749–776.
15. NIOSH. Application Manual for the Revised NIOSH Lifting Equation. U.S. Department of Health and Human Services. NIOSH; 1994.
16. WATERS TR, et al. Evaluation of the revised NIOSH lifting equation. A cross-sectional epidemiologic study. Spine 1999;24(4):386–394; discussion 395.
17. NORMAN R, et al. A comparison of peak vs cumulative physical work exposure risk factors for the reporting of low back pain in the automotive industry. Clin Biomech (Bristol, Avon) 1998;13(8):561–573.
18. MARRAS WS, et al. The role of dynamic three-dimensional trunk motion in occupationally-related low back disorders. The effects of workplace factors, trunk position, and trunk motion characteristics on risk of injury. Spine 1993;18(5):617–628.
19. MARRAS WS, et al. Biomechanical risk factors for occupationally related low back disorders. Ergonomics 1995;38(2):377–410.
20. MARRAS WS, et al. Prospective validation of a low-back disorder risk model and assessment of ergonomic interventions associated with manual materials handling tasks. Ergonomics 2000;43(11):1866–1886.
21. MARRAS WS, GRANATA KP. Changes in trunk dynamics and spine loading during repeated trunk exertions. Spine 1997;22(21):2564–2570.
22. MARRAS WS, et al. Spine loading as a function of lift frequency, exposure duration, and work experience. Clin Biomech (Bristol, Avon) 2006;21(4):345–352.
23. MARRAS WS, GRANATA KP. A biomechanical assessment and model of axial twisting in the thoracolumbar spine. Spine 1995;20(13):1440–1451.
24. GRANATA KP, MARRAS WS. An EMG-assisted model of loads on the lumbar spine during asymmetric trunk extensions. J Biomech 1993;26(12):1429–1438.

25. MARRAS WS. Toward an understanding of dynamic variables in ergonomics. *Occup Med* 1992;7(4):655–677.

26. MARRAS WS, SOMMERICH CM. A three-dimensional motion model of loads on the lumbar spine. II. Model validation. *Hum Factors* 1991;33(2):139–149.

27. MARRAS WS, GRANATA KP. Spine loading during trunk lateral bending motions. *J Biomech* 1997;30(7):697–703.

28. FATHALLAH FA, MARRAS WS, PARNIANPOUR M. The role of complex, simultaneous trunk motions in the risk of occupation-related low back disorders. *Spine* 1998; 23(9):1035–1042.

29. MARRAS WS, GRANATA KP. The development of an EMG-assisted model to assess spine loading during whole-body free-dynamic lifting. *J Electromyogr Kinesiol* 1997;7(4):259–268.

30. American Conference of Governmental Industrial Hygienists; 2005 TLVs and VEIs Book; 2005.

31. American Conference of Governmental Industrial Hygienists; 2004 TLVs and VEIs Book; 2004.

CHAPTER 12

ADMINISTRATIVE CONTROLS FOR THE WORKPLACE: PSYCHOSOCIAL AND ORGANIZATIONAL INTERVENTIONS

*T*HIS CHAPTER *discusses the ability of administrative controls to influence risk of low back pain reports in the workplace. The process of psychosocial and organization change and the thinking behind influencing the low back pain pathways is discussed. Administrative practices such as ergonomics processes, lift training, and back belts are considered.*

12.1 IMPLEMENTING PSYCHOSOCIAL AND ORGANIZATIONAL CHANGE

Recent findings have shown that there are substantial links and interactions between trunk muscle cocontraction levels caused by psychosocial factors and the subsequent biomechanical loading of the spine (1,2). This increase in biomechanical loading of the spine may be significant enough to initiate one of the low back pain pathways discussed earlier. Hence, to effectively impact low back pain risk in the workplace as well as to maximize the effectiveness of the physical workplace interventions, it is necessary to consider the psychosocial and organizational environment surrounding the intervention.

Psychosocial factors can be related to the worker acceptance of physical workplace interventions. Thus, psychosocial factors should be considered in conjunction with physical adjustments to the workplace. One can develop the world's best engineering solution to minimize back stress at work. However, if the workers do not accept the change and use the intervention, the intervention becomes useless. In addition, the worker may become resentful of the situation and this may lead to a poorer psychosocial environment. There are numerous reasons why a worker might not accept a physical change to the workplace. It is typical to hear workers proclaim that they like the way the job is designed and they have not had any problems yet, so they are not going to use the intervention. From the worker's perspective, change can be uncomfortable. The first reaction is usually to reject the intervention. Most interventions take some getting used to and workers rarely give the new solution a chance by using it for more than a few cycles of the job. Besides, workers take ownership of their workplace and if you are going to change it, their first reaction is to feel violated. In addition, few workers are familiar with how back pain occurs in terms of the delayed effects of nutrition disruption to the disc or the cumulative nature of spine loading. Therefore, if they are not feeling pain, there is little incentive for the worker to accept change.

The key to helping the worker accept the change or intervention without risking negative attitudes is to pay attention to the psychosocial and organizational situation surrounding the workplace. Two key components of intervention acceptance involve training and worker involvement in the intervention solution. Training should involve a discussion regarding the progressive nature of back pain. Basic anatomy of the spine, the fundamentals of biomechanics, and the process of disc degeneration should be covered at a minimum. However, this training should be performed in a functional manner and should be presented by someone with credibility in the worker health field.

Worker involvement in the solution should make the worker realize they are part of the design and the key to the solution. It is often the case that one understands exactly which physical interventions are necessary to correct a low back risk situation. However, if one spends some time talking to the workers performing the operation and ask them for their insight, they may arrive at a similar conclusion as your intervention. The key is to help the worker take ownership of the idea. If the worker realizes that it is his or her intervention that is being implemented and that you are simply helping them fulfill their ideas, there is a good chance they will use the intervention. This is one of the main advantages of a psychosocially acceptable intervention.

A review of workplace systems interventions (3) has shown that such interventions can reduce workers' compensation costs if they are implemented correctly. Thus, it is incumbent upon management to provide well thought through interventions that can interface well with the work situation. However, experience has also shown that unless the workers are accepting of workplace redesign, the interventions will not be effective.

A proven method to maximize the effectiveness of workplace interventions is to implement an ergonomics process. These processes are designed to address occupational health issues in a timely manner and create an environment that makes the workers accepting of engineering interventions. Ergonomics processes grew out of efforts to control musculo-skeletal disorders in meat-packing facilities (4). The logic behind this approach is to develop a system or process to identify and correct musculoskeletal problems associated with work. The process deals with systems changes in the organization. The goal is to develop an organization where the workers feel empowered and take ownership for their own health. Labor and management are involved collectively in the design and control of work so that everyone has a stake in the success of the process. An important aspect of this practice is that it is considered an ongoing process instead of a program since it is intended to become an ongoing surveillance and correction component of the business operation instead of a one-time effort.

The process is intended to encourage management and labor to communicate and work as a team to accomplish a common goal of worker health. To address the psychosocial issues in the workplace, a key component of an ergonomics process is worker empowerment. Workers are encouraged to take an active role in the process and take control and ownership of work design suggestions and changes. Thus, the process encourages a participatory approach. Benefits of such an approach include increased worker motivation, job satisfaction, and greater acceptance of change. The goal is to create an environment where the success of the operation is the objective as opposed to the interests of any given individual. Thus, changing the attitude of the organizational unit is expected to minimize the trunk muscle cocontractions responses associated with certain personality types and, thereby, minimize the prolonged muscle tensions and subsequent spine loading patterns that can lead to low back pain.

12.2   ELEMENTS OF THE PROCESS

There are several functions of a successful organizational intervention process. These functions include management leadership and commitment, employee participation, job analysis leading to injury prevention and control, training, medical management, program evaluation, and documentation. A successful process begins with the creation of an occupational health committee (often called an ergonomics committee). The committee composition should be balanced between management and labor to encourage a balanced effort to work toward the common goal. A balance is needed so that the committee is not controlled by either management or labor. All members should have an equal vote on the committee and members must not feel intimidated or unwilling to communicate substantive issues regarding worker health concerns and potential solutions.

Committee members should include those involved with the design of work layout as well as those empowered to dictate scheduling. In addition, labor representatives to the committee should include those employees who have broad experience with many of the jobs in the facility as well as those employees who can communicate well with the majority of the work force. This committee then becomes the center of all intervention-related activities within the facility.

This process consists of a *system* of components where the different components of the system interact to produce the desired effect. The interactions within this system are shown in Fig. 12.1. This figure indicates that a steering committee is at the heart of the interactions with all the components of the process. The process begins with management involvement. Ergonomic processes must be driven from top down. Thus, management must initiate the process and visibly demonstrate commitment to the process. In addition, management must provide resources to the committee. These resources should include financial resources so that physical interventions can be implemented as well as the access to information such as injury records, production schedules, and so on.

As indicated in Fig. 12.1, the fundamental responsibilities of the steering committee are threefold. First, the committee must monitor the workplace to determine where clusters of

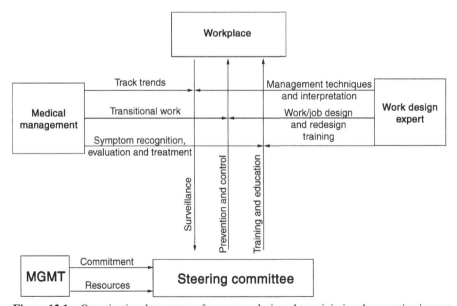

Figure 12.1   Organizational structure of a process designed to minimize the negative impact of psychosocial problems and help implement effective physical workplace interventions.

work-related low back disorders are located. Techniques for surveillance include monitoring OSHA recordable injury reports and medical reports as well as surveying workers for low back pain symptoms. The objective of this surveillance effort is to identify which job processes or organizational units may be associated with an increased risk of low back pain. For the intervention efforts to become preventive rather than reactive, it is important to solicit the cooperation of the labor workforce in this effort. Medical personnel can help facilitate this effort by helping the committee interpret the trends in an objective fashion.

The second responsibility of the committee is the prevention and control of occupationally related musculoskeletal disorders and in particular low back pain. For the purposes of low back pain, the techniques discussed earlier can be employed to help isolate the nature of any potential problems associated with the design of work. The issue of interest here is often "how much exposure to risk factors is too much exposure?" Thus, quantitative methods can be used to help determine which changes are needed and their likely impact. As indicated in the figure, work design experts can be useful in assisting the committee in performing these assessments.

The third responsibility of the committee is the training and education of the workforce. Several levels of training are typically necessary. All workers should receive short-duration awareness training to inform them that an occupational health process is in place, familiarize them with risk factors, and explain to them how to interact with the process. In addition, workers should receive training about the types of symptoms that need to be reported to the committee for prevention to be successful. This training should also include a brief review of the spine's structure and organization and a review of basic back health information including basic biomechanics. This information will provide a basic understanding of low back pain causality for the worker and provide the worker with the knowledge necessary to motivate them to use an intervention.

Higher level training should also be provided to engineers and supervisors. In general, training should be of sufficient detail so that management understands the functioning of the process and they do not become an impediment to the process success. Both medical professionals and ergonomic specialists can facilitate these activities. It is also imperative to set management expectations for the process. Once the work force is educated about the types of symptoms that should be reported, it is not unusual for incident reporting to increase dramatically. This is because early symptom reporting is being encouraged. Therefore, traditional injury reports (that would have occurred without encouragement) are occurring along with early symptom reports. This combination increases overall reporting. However, management should not panic since the early symptom reports typically do not incur lost time. Therefore, lost time drops and soon after incident rates also drop since the problems are addressed before lost time events occur.

Medical management and the workplace experts serve as resources to the committee for the process responsibilities. The goal of a process is not to make the ergonomics committee into ergonomics experts, but to encourage them to actively involve experts to accomplish the goals of the process. These experts can be valuable in terms of advising the committee as to how and when to perform surveillance activities as well as suggesting appropriate interventions for a given situation.

It is imperative that the program be evaluated regularly to justify its continuation. Issues such as the achievement of program goals, reductions of musculoskeletal disorders, hazard reduction, and employee feedback should be considered. Corrective actions should be taken in response to the evaluation. Finally, documentation is an important part of a successful program. Records should be kept that document the changes made to the workplace and can serve as justification of expenditures. These records can also be used to transfer knowledge to new team members.

Such a process can have a significant impact on musculoskeletal risk, but only if the process is performed correctly and maintained. Keys to process maintenance include strong direction, realistic goals, establishment of a system to address employee concerns, early intervention success, and publicity for the intervention. Although there are few well-planned studies that explore the success of these processes from an epidemiological perspective, numerous anecdotal reports of process successes have been reported in the literature (5).

12.3   TRADITIONAL ADMINISTRATIVE CONTROLS

12.3.1   Worker Selection

Administrative controls and interventions constitute a means to control risk when it is difficult or impossible to change the physical exposure to risk in the workplace. Administrative controls basically involve two approaches: (1) identifying workers who are least likely to suffer a low back disorder when exposed to the work and (2) controlling the length of exposure time to the risk. Some of the literature has indicated that worker conditioning is an important factor in determining risk of low back pain in physically demanding jobs (6,7). A few organizations have based worker selection criteria on conditioning and strength criteria. However, these practices are not supported by the literature at this time. In addition, some have noted that employing such criteria for worker selection reduces the potential work pool to a very small number and creates staffing problems.

Genetics is believed to play a role in the development of low back pain. However, it is unclear to what extent genetics plays a role in causality relative to physical risk factors. Several researchers claim that genetic factors account for the majority of risk (8–12), whereas other studies have attributed low back disorder risk to physical activities (13–17). As stated earlier, it is highly likely that both categories of factors interact to set the stage for the occurrence of low back disorders at the workplace.

From a practical standpoint, there are several problems with attempting to employ administrative controls based on genetic predisposition to back pain. This approach sets up a situation for worker selection based on genetics. Until the literature becomes much clearer with regard to the percent of low back pain variance explained by genetics independent of work exposure, the legality of worker selection will represent a problematic issue for employers.

12.3.2   Worker Rotation

Probably the most common administrative control involves worker rotation. Rotation attempts to control cumulative exposure risk by spreading the risky exposure over a larger population of workers so that no worker is exposed to the risk for a long period of time. The problem with worker rotation is that our understanding of time-dependent risk exposure is poor. Many of the physical exposure interventions are able to assess whether work conditions are risky for the low back or safe. However, when risk is present, difficulties arise when one attempts to assess how much exposure to a risk is too much exposure to a risk. Most rotation schemes are arbitrary and are not grounded in the scientific literature. Thus, one rotation scheme may happen to converge on correct risk exposure limits for a group of workers, whereas another may not. While many believe that job rotation results in a reduction of low back pain risk, several studies have shown that risk can actually increase with job rotation (18,19). These studies have observed that increases in low back pain reporting typically occur in the group that was previously not exposed to the low back risk factor. The increase in risk to this previously unexposed group typically does not offset the reduction in risk to the high exposure group. Thus, most studies that have attempted to control low back pain risk have had difficulty determining a safe level of temporal exposure to the risk factor. These findings are consistent with surveillance risk models that have found the exposure to extremes of risk was more indicative of risk than the length of time exposed to the risk factor (20,21).

12.3.3 Training

Traditionally, workers have been led to believe that there are correct or incorrect ways to lift an object. It is a common occurrence to hear one suggest that one "lifts with the legs not the back" or use a squat lift instead of a stoop lift. While it is appealing to think that one can control low back risk through technique training, the literature does not support this notion. Early biomechanical assessments of liftstyle revealed that the liftstyle that minimizes spine load is highly dependent on the worker's size and shape (anthropometry) and the conventional thinking that minimal spine load occurred while lifting with the legs was not born out by the biomechanical analyses (22,23). Later studies using more robust biomechanical assessment techniques have confirmed that spine loads are not necessarily lower during squat lifts compared to stoop lifts (24). In addition, since squat lifting requires more energy, workers tend to gravitate to stoop lift styles as they become more fatigued (25). Thus, even if squat lifts were an effective means of controlling spine loads, workers would tend to use more stoop lifting as the workday progressed. In addition, one needs to consider how training might affect risk to the other parts of the body. For example, more squat lifts might increase risk to the lower extremities.

From a biomechanical standpoint, the only way that training could be effective is if one was able to train workers to minimize the distance at which the load is lifted relative to the spine, thereby reducing the spine's load moment exposure. One technique has used sophisticated instrumentation to train distribution center workers how to lift while minimizing this loading. Recently, the effectiveness of the training was evaluated in a prospective study where nearly 2000 employees were trained and followed over the course of a year (26). Overall, no difference in low back reporting was noted between the group receiving training and the control group. However, those workers who were observed to impose lower twisting moments on the initial training were less likely to report low back pain. These findings are consistent with the notion that lifting muscle recruitment patterns are developed over long periods of time during one's development and cannot be easily altered. However, the study results also point to the fact that load exposure does indeed relate to risk of work-related low back pain reporting.

12.3.4 Stretching Programs

Some companies have adopted stretching programs prior to work to minimize the risk of low back pain. While these programs have been popular for a number of years, the research does not support the use of stretching to reduce musculoskeletal injury risk. On the contrary, the literature is much stronger in demonstrating that there is no reduction in muscle soreness symptoms after stretching (27–29), and no statistically significant reduction in musculo- skeletal injury rates after stretching programs are initiated (30,31).

In addition, they may introduce additional risks in terms of microfiber muscle tears, increased tolerance, and analgesia that can increase the risk of damage (32). Hence, extensive literature reviews of stretching have concluded that the benefits of stretching programs do not outweigh the potential problems (27,32,33). Therefore, ergonomic practitioners do not often recommend such programs to minimize the risk of low back pain in industrial environments (32).

12.3.5 Back Belts

Several studies have explored the use of orthoses, back belts, or lifting belts and their relationship to low back disorder risk. Several comprehensive reviews have appeared in the literature (34–39), and few preventive benefits of belt wearing have been reported. Studies have explored the ability and willingness of workers to lift loads when wearing back belts. One study indicated that subjects were capable of lifting about 19% more weight while wearing belts (40). However, it is not clear if any more tolerance is afforded to the spine while wearing back belts. Some studies have indicated physiological costs to belt wearing including increased blood pressure (41,42). Others have investigated biomechanical correlates such as range of motion (42,43), muscle recruitment patterns (44), and intra-abdominal pressures (45).

Only recently have the effects of back belts on spinal loading been investigated (35). One of the first studies to examine spine loading while wearing belts explored the three-dimensional spinal loads associated with lifting loads of two magnitudes from sagittally symmetric and asymmetric lift origins to an upright posture with the feet fixed on a force plate. Three types of lifting belts (leather weight lifting belt, elastic belt, and orthotic belts) were compared to lifting without a lifting belt. This study confirmed previous findings that lifting belts reduced peak trunk angles, velocities, and accelerations in the sagittal, lateral, and transverse planes. Only the elastic belt reduced trunk motions in all three dimensions. The orthotic belt increased the load moment associated with a given weight. Minor redistributions in muscle recruitment patterns were noted with belts with slightly less antagonistic coactivity of the trunk musculature. Reductions in antagonistic muscle activations were also reported by others under similar conditions (46). When spinal loads were assessed, only the elastic belt resulted in a reduction in compression and A/P shear spinal load at L5/S1 (Fig. 12.2). Further analyses indicated that the reduction in load was associated strongly with the asymmetric lifts and was a function of the design of the elastic

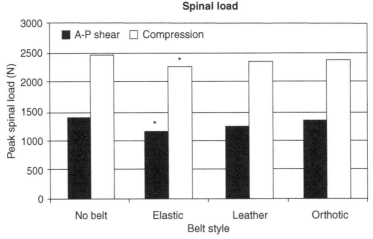

Figure 12.2 Spine loading associated with lifting using three different types of belts compared to a no-belt condition (from reference 35) (*indicates level in significantly P < 0.01 different than no-belt condition).

belt. Only the elastic belt was large enough (vertically) to connect the thorax with the pelvis. This connection served to force the torso to act as a unit, thereby reducing the required antagonistic coactivity typically needed to stabilize the trunk. The other belts were not tall enough to connect the thorax with the pelvis and demonstrated no difference in spine loading compared to the no-belt condition. Since few occupational conditions require workers to lift asymmetrically without allowing them to move their feet (as were the asymmetric lifting conditions in this study), the study was replicated except that the participants were permitted to move their feet during the asymmetric lifting conditions (47). When participants were allowed to move their feet, as would be expected under occupational conditions, no statistically significant differences in spine loading were observed between the belt and no-belt conditions.

Some belt manufacturers have claimed that belts are only effective if they are tensioned properly. One study explored the effect of belt tension on the electromyographic activity of the 10 power-producing (and spine loading) trunk muscles (48). When three different belt tension levels were compared with a no-belt condition under a range of trunk extension moment exertions, no statistically significant differences were noted.

Collectively, these studies have indicated that there are no significant biomechanical benefits of back belt usage in terms of protecting the back from excessive loads under occupational conditions for healthy workers. In addition, a potential problem lies in the fact that workers are willing to expose themselves to larger loads when wearing belts (40). Moreover, some studies have noted some negative health effects of belt usage (34,41,49,50,51). There is some evidence of positive benefits of belt usage, but only for those who have already suffered back problems and then only for intermittent use (52).

12.4 SUMMARY

The goal of administrative controls to manage low back pain risk is to impact the potential biomechanical spine loading that can occur as a result of poor psychosocial or organizational environments. This brief review has indicated that many administrative controls, by themselves, are not effective at controlling low back pain risk. Many traditional administrative controls such as worker selection, conditioning programs, worker rotation scheduling, stretching programs, and supplying workers with back belts have not proven effective in prospective investigations in reducing injury reporting or in reducing the exposure to the low back pain pathways discussed earlier. For the most part, these programs lack any biomechanical foundation or the proper implementation of the intervention has not been achieved and documented.

The only administrative control that has been shown to be effective consists of process controls or ergonomics processes. When such a process is correctly and systematically employed in a work environment, it provides a means to increase communication among the organization and lessens the probability that workers will respond to the organizational and psychosocial environment by impacting biomechanical loading of the spine. Perhaps the greatest benefit of this process is that it is a means to gain acceptance for the engineering controls. Engineering controls are preferable to administrative controls because of their potential to mediate biomechanical loads imposed on the spine. However, they are only effective if they are used by the workers. Administrative controls can help ensure acceptance and use of these improvements to the workplace.

KEY POINTS

- Administrative controls can impact psychosocial and organizational risk in the workplace. When deployed properly, they can influence back risk by reducing the degree of muscle coactivation and reducing the subsequent loading of the spine.

- Traditional administrative controls techniques such as worker selection, conditioning programs, stretching, rotation, and back belts, by themselves, have not been proven effective at reducing low back pain. Although rotation schedules do have the potential to control risk if implemented properly.

- To be effective, administrative controls should be part of a broader, multidimensional ergonomics process.

- An ergonomics process is one proven way to organize and control the acceptance of job interventions and gain worker acceptance. An ergonomics process can also influence productivity, quality control, and injury/illness reporting and costs.

- Ergonomics processes are most effective when they are integrated and employed along with engineering controls.

REFERENCES

1. DAVIS KG, et al. The impact of mental processing and pacing on spine loading: 2002 Volvo Award in biomechanics. Spine 2002;27(23):2645–2653.
2. MARRAS WS, et al. The influence of psychosocial stress, gender, and personality on mechanical loading of the lumbar spine. Spine 2000;25(23):3045–3054.
3. GAO, Worker Protection: Private Sector Ergonomics Programs Yield Positive Results, Government Accounting Office; 1997.
4. OSHA Ergonomics Program Management Guidelines for Meatpacking Plants. Occupational Safety and Health Administration,Washington (DC): U.S. Department of Labor; 1993.
5. NRC, Musculoskeletal disorders and the workplace: low back and upper extremity. Panel on Musculoskeletal Disorders at the Workplace, editor.Washington (DC): National Academy of Sciences, National Research Council, National Academy Press; 2001. p. 492.
6. CADY LD, et al. Strength and fitness and subsequent back injuries in firefighters. J Occup Med, 1979;21(4): 269–272.
7. CADY LD, Jr, THOMAS PC, KARWASKY RJ. Program for increasing health and physical fitness of fire fighters. J Occup Med, 1985;27(2):110–114.
8. BATTIE MC, et al. Similarities in degenerative findings on magnetic resonance images of the lumbar spines of identical twins. J Bone Joint Surg [Am] 1995; 77(11):1662–1670.
9. BATTIE MC, et al. 1995 Volvo Award in clinical sciences. Determinants of lumbar disc degeneration. A study relating lifetime exposures and magnetic resonance imaging findings in identical twins. Spine 1995;20(24):2601–2612.
10. BATTIE MC, VIDEMAN T, PARENT E. Lumbar disc degeneration: epidemiology and genetic influences. Spine 2004;29(23):2679–2690.
11. LEBOEUF-YDE C. Back pain — individual and genetic factors. J Electromyogr Kinesiol 2004;14(1):129–133.
12. VIDEMAN T, et al. Intragenic polymorphisms of the vitamin D receptor gene associated with intervertebral disc degeneration. Spine 1998;23(23):2477–2485.
13. VIDEMAN T, et al. The long-term effects of physical loading and exercise lifestyles on back-related symptoms, disability, and spinal pathology among men. Spine 1995;20(6):699–709.
14. BURDORF A, van der BEEK AJ. In musculoskeletal epidemiology are we asking the unanswerable in questionnaires on physical load?Scand J Work Environ Health 1999;25(2):81–83.
15. HOOGENDOORN WE, et al. Flexion and rotation of the trunk and lifting at work are risk factors for low back pain: results of a prospective cohort study. Spine 2000;25(23):3087–3092.
16. HOOGENDOORN WE, et al. Physical load during work and leisure time as risk factors for back pain [see comments]. Scand J Work, Environ Health 1999; 25(5):387–403.
17. NORMAN R, et al. A comparison of peak vs cumulative physical work exposure risk factors for the reporting of low back pain in the automotive industry. Clin Biomech (Bristol, Avon) 1998;13(8):561–573.

18. FRAZER MB, et al. The effects of job rotation on the risk of reporting low back pain. Ergonomics 2003;46(9): 904–919.

19. KUIJER PP, et al. Effect of job rotation on need for recovery, musculoskeletal complaints, and sick leave due to musculoskeletal complaints: a prospective study among refuse collectors. Am J Ind Med 2005;47(5): 394–402.

20. HERRIN GD, JARAIEDI M, ANDERSON CK. Prediction of overexertion injuries using biomechanical and psycho-physical models. Am Ind Hygiene Assoc J 1986;47(6): 322–330.

21. MARRAS WS, et al. The role of dynamic three-dimensional trunk motion in occupationally-related low back disorders. The effects of workplace factors, trunk position, and trunk motion characteristics on risk of injury. Spine 1993;18(5):617–628.

22. CHAFFIN DB, ANDERSSON GBJ, MARTIN BJ. Occupational Biomechanics, 3rd ed., John Wiley & Sons, Inc.; New York: 1999. p. 579.

23. FREIVALDS A, et al. A dynamic biomechanical evaluation of lifting maximum acceptable loads. J Biomech 1984;17(4):251–262.

24. van DIEEN JH, HOOZEMANS MJ, TOUSSAINT HM. Stoop or squat: a review of biomechanical studies on lifting technique. Clin Biomech (Bristol, Avon) 1999;14(10): 685–696.

25. TRAFIMOW JH, et al. The effects of quadriceps fatigue on the technique of lifting. Spine 1993;18(3):364–367.

26. LAVENDER SA, LORENZ EP, ANDERSSON GB. Can a new behaviorally oriented training process to improve lifting technique prevent occupationally related back injuries due to lifting? Spine 2007;32(4):487–494.

27. HERBERT RD, GABRIEL M. Effects of stretching before and after exercising on muscle soreness and risk of injury: systematic review. Br Med J 2002;325 (7362):468.

28. JOHANSSON PH, et al. The effects of preexercise stretching on muscular soreness, tenderness and force loss following heavy eccentric exercise. Scand J Med Sci Sports 1999;9(4):219–225.

29. POPE RP, et al. A randomized trial of preexercise stretching for prevention of lower-limb injury. Med Sci Sports Exerise 2000;32(2):271–277.

30. POPE R, HERBERT R, KIRWAN J. Effects of ankle dorsi-flexion range and pre-exercise calf muscle stretching on injury risk in Army recruits. Aust J Physiotherapy 1998;44(3):165–172.

31. SHRIER I. Stretching before exercise does not reduce the risk of local muscle injury: a critical review of the clinical and basic science literature. Clin J Sport Med 1999;9(4):221–227.

32. JOFFEE M.Exploring the myth behind stretching programs. In 7th Annual Applied Ergonomics Conference;2004.

33. SILVERSTEIN B, CLARK R. Interventions to reduce work-related musculoskeletal disorders. J Electromyogr Kinesiol 2004;14(1):135–152.

34. National Institute for Occupational Safety and Health (NIOSH),Workplace Use of Back Belts. Cincinnati (OH); 1994.

35. GRANATA KP, MARRAS WS, DAVIS KG. Biomechanical assessment of lifting dynamics, muscle activity and spinal loads while using three different styles of lifting belt. Clin Biomech (Bristol, Avon) 1997;12(2):107–115.

36. MCGILL SM. Abdominal belts in industry: a position paper on their assets, liabilities and use. Am Ind Hygiene Assoc J 1993;54(12):752–754.

37. van POPPEL MN, et al. Mechanisms of action of lumbar supports: a systematic review [in process citation]. Spine 2000;25(16):2103–2113.

38. van POPPEL MN, et al. A systematic review of controlled clinical trials on the prevention of back pain in industry. Occup Environ Med 1997;54(12):841–847.

39. Van TULDER MW, et al. Lumbar supports for prevention and treatment of low back pain. Cochrane Database System Rev 2000;(3):CD001823.

40. McCOY M, et al. The role of lifting belts in manual lifting. Int J Ind Ergono 1988;2:256–259.

41. HUNTER G, et al. The effect of weight training on blood pressure during exercise. J Appl Sport Sci Res 1989; 3(1):13–18.

42. MCGILL S, SEGUIN J, BENNETT G. Passive stiffness of the lumbar torso in flexion, extension, lateral bending, and axial rotation. Effect of belt wearing and breath holding. Spine 1994;19(6):696–704.

43. LAVENDER SA, et al. Effect of lifting belts, foot movement, and lift asymmetry on trunk motions. Hum Factors 1995;37(4):844–853.

44. LAVENDER SA, et al. Effects of a lifting belt on spine moments and muscle recruitments after unexpected sudden loading. Spine 2000;25(12):1569–1578.

45. LANDER JE, HUNDLEY JR, SIMONTON RL. The effectiveness of weight-belts during multiple repetitions of the squat exercise. Med Sci Sports and Exercise 1992; 24(5):603–609.

46. CHOLEWICKI J. The effects of lumbosacral orthoses on spine stability: what changes in EMG can be expected?J Orthop Res 2004;22(5):1150–1155.

47. MARRAS WS, JORGENSEN MJ, DAVIS KG. Effect of foot movement and an elastic lumbar back support on spinal loading during free-dynamic symmetric and asymmetric lifting exertions. Ergonomics 2000;43(5):653–668.

48. JORGENSEN MJ, MARRAS WS. The effect of lumbar back support tension on trunk muscle activity. Clin Biomech (Bristol, Avon) 2000;15(4):292–294.

49. BOBICK TG, et al. Physiological effects of back belt wearing during asymmetric lifting. Appl Ergono 2001;32(6):541–547.

50. REDDELL C, et al. An evaluation of weight-lifting belt and back injury prevention training class for airline baggage handlers. Appl Ergono 1992;22(5):319–329.

51. WALSH NE, SCHWARTZ RK. The influence of prophylactic orthoses on abdominal strength and low back injury in the workplace [see comments]. Am J Phys Med Rehabil 1990;69(5):245–250.

INTEGRATING RISK INTERVENTIONS INTO THE WORKPLACE

*E*XAMPLES OF *how biomechanical assessments can lead to effective reductions in low back pain reports through engineering and administrative intervention implementations are discussed. Examples from patient handling and distribution center intervention efforts are used to demonstrate the importance of integrating engineering and administrative controls.*

13.1 INTRODUCTION

We have seen that there are three main risk factor contributors to low back pain. These include physical exposure to physical risk factors, psychosocial and organizational risk factors, and individual-based risk factors. For the most part, it is not possible to alter individual risk factors. Individual factors such as genetics, metabolic processes, and pain response patterns are not modifiable. We have also seen (Chapters 8 and 9) that personality and its interaction with psychosocial factors play a major role in trunk muscle recruitment patterns and can influence the loading of the spine. Thus, there are few opportunities to modify risk by way of the individual risk factors since most of these are inherent qualities of the worker. Furthermore, we are in the early phases of understanding how these individual factors interact with other risk factors. Thus, worker selection and screening, while currently used, are more difficult to employ successfully since the science associated with worker selection is relatively weak.

13.2 SYSTEMS INTERVENTION

Physiological conditioning represents one of the few modifiable individual risk factors available to control low back pain risk. For optimum back health, it is the responsibility of the worker to keep in reasonable physical shape. Some of the low back pain pathways discussed in Chapter 5 are associated with disruption of blood flow and a resultant lack of tissue oxygenation, cardiovascular fitness, and strength has been shown to significantly reduce the risk of low back pain in jobs where few other risk factors can be modified (1,2). Factors that influence cardiovascular fitness such as smoking are also modifiable. However, from a practical standpoint, in most workplace environments, it is impractical if not impossible to demand that workers become and remain physically conditioned. While conditioning may improve over a short period, long-term success in maintenance of physical conditioning is difficult on a large scale.

Wellness programs have become popular over the last several years as a mechanism to improve overall worker health. These programs typically involve the promotion of healthy lifestyles, some of which may improve health and fitness factors that can influence low back pain risk. These include stress reduction, proper diet, and exercise. Wellness programs may also improve the attitudes of workers in that they may enhance the feeling of well being, which, in turn, may modify reaction to psychosocial stress factors.

Overall, an intervention strategy that only focuses on the individual risk factors of the worker can only be minimally effective, since many of the most potent risk factors work as interactions between categories of risk factors. Thus, the most effective efforts to minimize risk modify several risk factors and create a system of interventions that attempt to affect the interdependency and interaction throughout the entire human system (Fig. 1.2).

13.3 EXAMPLES OF INTERVENTION EFFECTIVENESS

Because of the difficulty in performing intervention research at the worksite, the body of literature demonstrating intervention effectiveness for any type of intervention is limited. As we have seen, risk is multidimensional, and most intervention effectiveness studies have only observed the influence of a single intervention on a small group of workers. Much of the intervention evidence is also anecdotal in nature, which makes it less valuable from a scientific perspective. Thus, in an attempt to demonstrate these interactions, some examples of the degree to which risk can be influenced by different categories of interventions for specific populations of workers are presented.

13.3.1 Patient Handling Interventions

A population at high risk for low back pain consists of those who are involved in patient handling (lifting). Nurses aides have the highest incidence of disabling back injuries in the United States (3). The low back pain incidence rate for nurse's aides is higher than the more traditional heavy physical occupations such as construction workers and garbage collectors. Both licensed practical nurses and registered nurses have low back pain incidence rates similar to that of construction workers and garbage collectors. Nurses' aides accounted for 3.6 worker compensation claims due to back injuries per 100 workers, which was higher than material handlers (3.4) and construction workers (2.8) (4). Furthermore, nurses' aides were more than three times as likely to suffer a low back pain compared to registered nurses (5). It has been estimated that the incidence rate of low back pain for patient handlers was 83 per 100 full-time nursing personnel in the United States (6).

An analysis of tasks associated with patient handling reveals that most of the patient handling involves transfer of patients between the bed, chairs, and commodes, as well as repositioning the patient in bed (7). Some have suggested that two-person patient handling would minimize the risk to a point where the lifts would be safe from a low back pain perspective. Using a static single-equivalent muscle model to assess spine compression and risk of low back pain, one study suggested that two-person handling of patients would be expected to control the risk of low back pain among patient handlers (8). However, a study employing both the LMM risk model and an EMG-assisted biomechanical model to assess the contribution of muscle coactivation during patient handling came to a very different conclusion (7). Figure 13.1 shows the LMM risk associated with the various one-person and

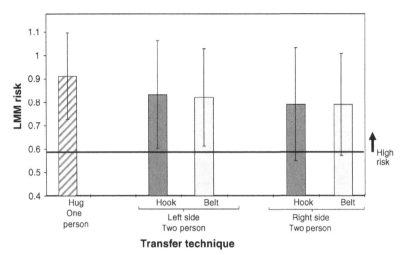

Figure 13.1   LMM risk associated with the various one-person and two-person lifting tasks involved in patient handling. (From reference 7).

two-person lifting tasks involved in patient handling. Figure 13.2 summarizes the spine compression loading associated with these same tasks. As indicated in these figures, neither the one-person nor the two-person lifting situations result in risk or spine loading conditions that would be considered safe from a risk or biomechanical perspective.

These studies indicated that, based on historical risk measures (LMM risk model) and the biomechanical assessments of loads imposed on the lumbar spine, the risk of low back problems was substantial during patient lifting. Furthermore, when the proposed intervention of two-person lifting was considered, the biomechanical trade-offs were such that the increase in risk associated with shear forces did not adequately offset the decrease in risk associated with a reduction in spine compression. The study evaluating the risk of one-person versus two-person patient handling concluded that the only means by which low back pain

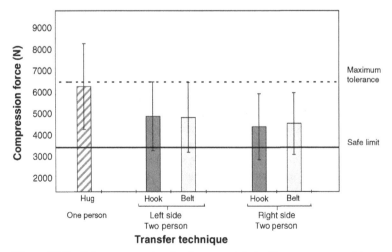

Figure 13.2   Spine compression loading associated with one-person and two-person lifting tasks involved in patient handling. (From reference 7).

TABLE 13.1 Musculoskeletal Disorder Rate Changes (#MSDs/employee-hours worked)*200,000) Between Baseline and Follow-Up for Interventions in Patient Handling (From Reference 9)

Type of intervention	n	Baseline median (range)	Follow-up median (range)	Rate Ratio (FU/BL MSD rate)
Reduce bending	16	9.89 (0.0–42.65)	6.65 (0.0–59.51)	0.66
Zero lift	44	15.38 (0.0–87.59)	9.25 (0.0–28.27)	0.54
Reduce carrying	8	6.47 (0.0–15.80)	0.33 (0.0–6.70)	0.15
Multiple interventions	38	11.97 (0.0–60.34)	7.78 (0.0–25.94)	0.56
All	100	12.32 (0.0–87.59)	6.64 (0.0–59.51)	0.52

would be expected to be reduced would be to incorporate mechanical patient lifting devices and eliminate lifting patients manually (7). Hence, this evaluation suggested that an intervention to minimize the impact of the biomechanical loading was necessary during patient handling.

To assess the effectiveness of such an intervention, a large-scale field intervention study was performed (9). This study explored the incidence rate of patient handlers before and after the introduction of patient-handling devices in 86 health care facilities. In this study, several interventions were investigated. These interventions consisted of (1) interventions that reduced bending such as adjustable beds, (2) interventions that eliminated lifting, such as patient hoists, (3) interventions that reduced carrying, such as sliding devices, and (4) multiple interventions that often included the introduction of not only physical alterations but also organizational and psychosocial changes (although this category was mixed with those interventions that involved only multiple physical alterations).

The study observed musculoskeletal disorders over a 1–2 year baseline period (averaging 445 days) and compared incidence rates to a follow-up period (averaging 629 days). Effectiveness was measured by comparing the follow-up normalized incidence rate to the baseline normalized incidence rate producing a rate ratio. This rate ratio indicates the percentage of musculoskeletal disorders observed during the follow-up period compared to those observed prior to the intervention. Thus, a rate of 0.75 indicates that only 75% of those incidences were observed after the intervention compared to before the intervention, or in other words, a 25% reduction. Table 13.1 shows the rate ratio for the various categories of interventions. These reductions in rates were statistically different for all types of interventions. There are several points of interest worth noting in this data. First, all interventions were effective. On average, the reduction in risk was about 48%. Second, interventions that eliminated the need to exert force (carrying and lifting) reduced the risk to a greater extent than those interventions that only addressed postural changes.

These data evaluated the impact of interventions on all musculoskeletal disorders associated with patient handling. However, the motivation for most of the interventions was the rate of low back disorders. The effects of interventions for low back pain alone are shown in Table 13.2. This table indicates similar or more dramatic improvements compared to all

TABLE 13.2 Change in MSD Rates for the Back versus Other Body Parts (baseline to follow-up) in 100 Patient Handling Units (From Reference 9)

Part of body	Number of units decreased or no change	Number of units increased	Median rate ratio
Back	79 (79%)	21 (21%)	0.43
Other Parts of Body*	73 (73%)	27 (27%)	0.51

*Other body parts include shoulder, upper extremity, lower extremity, head, neck, and multiple body parts (excluding back).

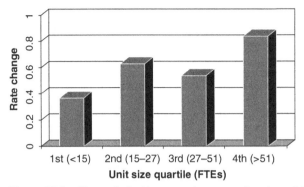

Figure 13.3 Change in incident rate shown as a function of the size of the unit observed (in quartiles) defined in terms of full-time equivalent workers or FTEs. Smaller units were impacted by a greater amount by the intervention than the larger units. (From reference 9).

musculoskeletal disorders. Notice in this table the fact that nearly 80% the units observed decreased their rates (or no change) of back pain and about one-fifth increased their rate of back pain. In addition, when changes were implemented to improve the risk of low back pain, other parts of the body enjoyed a reduction in risk also.

Thus, these data indicate that, overall, minimizing the physical risk alone reduces the low back risk by nearly 60%. However, one must also be cognizant of the fact that there may be other factors that may affect these outcomes. First, in a large study such as this, there is very little control over whether the interventions were actually being used. Figure 13.3 shows the effectiveness of the intervention based on the size of the unit observed. We can speculate that the compliance with the intervention was much better in the smaller facilities, thus these units enjoyed a greater reduction in risk. Second, this study was not able to determine whether preexisting back problems were reaggravated or whether new back problems were occurring during the follow-up. However, Fig. 13.4 does provide evidence that the longer the intervention, the greater the benefit from a low back pain standpoint. Hence, it appears to be the case that fewer new back pain reports were occurring as the follow-up period progressed.

13.3.2 Types of Physical Interventions

Another example of intervention effectiveness can be seen in a study that explored the ability of risk prediction indicators to identify changes in low back pain risk once interventions were

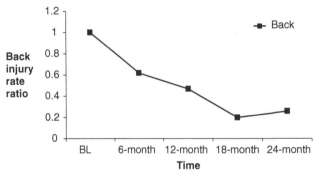

Figure 13.4 Two-year follow-up trends with back injuries. Rate ratio indicates follow-up rate compared to baseline (BL) rate at 6-month intervals following intervention. (From reference 9).

implemented (10). In this study, different categories of intervention were implemented in an industrial setting and the differences in low back pain incidence rates 3 years before and 3 years after an intervention implementation were observed. These differences in rates were used as a measure of intervention effectiveness. Of the four classes of interventions observed (as well as a control condition where no interventions were employed), only the lift table and lifting aid (e.g., overhead lift) interventions produced a positive benefit in injury rates (Fig. 11.5). Furthermore, the reduction in incidence rates due to these interventions was rather substantial. This study indicates that not all interventions are equally effective. In fact, Fig. 11.5 shows that some interventions were no more effective than no intervention at all. However, the figure also indicates that the intervention must be appropriate for the risk present. Implicit in this study was the fact that for interventions to be effective one must employ assessment tools that can effectively pinpoint the conditions that contribute to the physical risk and are capable of quantifying the extent of the benefit associated with a potential intervention. Hence, there is a dire need to quantitatively evaluate the nature of the risk to the low back by using accurate measurement tools if one is to optimize the probability that the problem will be corrected.

13.4 IMPLEMENTING BOTH PHYSICAL AND PSYCHOSOCIAL INTERVENTIONS

One of the more systematic studies of the effectiveness of implementing an ergonomics process to impact both the physical environment and the organizational/psychosocial environment was performed by the United States General Accounting Office in 1997 (11). In this evaluation, musculoskeletal injury rates were observed in five companies of varying size and with different physical risk factors. These rates were observed before and after the implementation of an ergonomics process similar to the one described in Chapter 12. Of the five companies observed, two (Navistar and Sisters of Charity) had significant rates of low back pain reporting. The interventions included not only physical interventions to minimize the physical exposures to factors that would be expected to increase low back loading but also organizational changes to encourage more employee involvement and worker empowerment. Figure 13.5 indicates the results of these observations. Substantial reductions in musculoskeletal injury rates were noted for all of these work environments. It is also interesting to note that the reductions reported here were generally much larger than those in patient-handling facilities (discussed previously) that only addressed physical problems in many instances (without the introduction of a process).

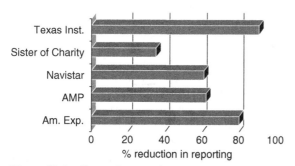

Figure 13.5 Change in musculoskeletal disorder reporting in five companies before versus after implementation of an ergonomics process (11). (Adapted from reference 11).

13.4.1 Distribution Center Interventions

One of the environments that has been associated with significantly high rates of low back pain involve distribution centers. These environments are becoming more prevalent in the United States as more products are being produced in other nations. This means that fewer products are made in the United States; however, more products are stored and distributed in the United States. Workers in these environments known as "pickers" are required to select a number of cases of a particular product and build an order on a pallet that is to be sent to a particular store. Thus, high frequencies of lifting occur in these facilities and these environments represent one of the highest risk occupations for low back disorders.

The Biodynamics Laboratory at The Ohio State University was involved with a case study of one of these environments. The study observed musculoskeletal incident rates in the facility (primarily low back complaints) before and after implementation of some interventions. The interventions consisted of a process to address psychosocial and organizational problems (as described in Chapter 12) as well as some physical interventions such as changing the lifting requirements (by elevating loads and bringing them closer to the worker) as well as altering the "picking order" so that the high intensity work was distributed throughout the workday. Figures 13.6 and 13.7 show the change in lost time and restricted time over the study, respectively. The interventions were introduced in 1996. It is interesting to note the "spike" in reporting at the time of process implementation (as noted in the last chapter). However, within 2 years of implementation, both lost time and restricted time were significantly reduced in this facility. However, implementation of such a process requires continual maintenance or the incidence rates will return to the original level.

13.5 SUMMARY

This chapter has reviewed several instances of implementing interventions to control low back pain in the workplace. While intervention examples are often difficult to interpret because of the potential confounding issues associated with field observations, these findings are consistent with the pattern of evidence that has been presented throughout this book. First, physical interventions, by themselves, can be effective in controlling low

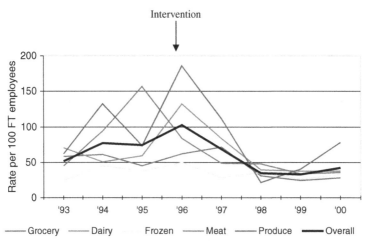

Figure 13.6 Changes in musculoskeletal reporting rates before and after implementation of a process to address psychosocial/organizational issues and the introduction of engineering controls (in 1996).

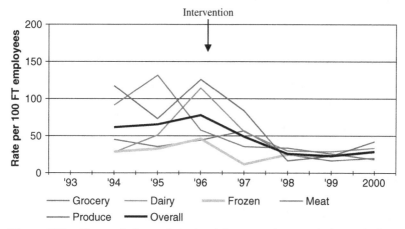

Figure 13.7 Changes in lost and restricted time reporting rates before and after implementation of a process to address psychosocial/organizational issues and the introduction of engineering controls (in 1996).

back pain reporting, but only if the correct intervention is selected for the situation at hand. It is clear from these case studies that quantitative measures of risk are necessary to ensure that the correct physical aspects of the job are being adequately addressed. Second, when multiple interventions are implemented, risk is further reduced. Finally, when engineering controls are combined with administrative controls (typically involving psychosocial and organizational interventions) risk can be most effectively reduced.

These findings lend indirect support to the notion that both physical and psychosocial/organizational pathways to low back pain can be mediated through a combination of changes to the physical exposures as well as adjustments to the social environment so that the torso muscle cocontraction pattern and subsequent spine loading pattern are optimized under the particular work situation. Hence, this information provides further evidence that we must address the human *system* in response to the work environment if we are to control the risk of low back pain.

KEY POINTS

- There is evidence that physical interventions can reduce incidence rates in musculo-skeletal disorders, particularly in the low back.
- Incidence rate reductions are dependent on the size of the facility (probably due to compliance), and low back incidence rates decline over time after intervention implementation.
- Other studies have shown that not all interventions are equally effective. In fact, a large difference in effectiveness among physical interventions was noted.
- Government studies have shown large reductions in incidence rates with the implementation of ergonomics processes in different industries.
- Implementation of engineering controls along with an ergonomics process has been observed to result in large decreases in incidence rates as well as decreases in lost time in distribution center environments.

REFERENCES

1. CADY LD, et al. Strength and fitness and subsequent back injuries in firefighters. J Occup Med 1979;21(4): 269–272.
2. CADY LD, Jr, THOMAS PC, KARWASKY RJ. Program for increasing health and physical fitness of fire fighters. J Occup Med 1985;27(2):110–114.
3. JENSEN RC. Disabling back injuries among nursing personnel: research needs and justification. Res Nurs Health 1987;10(1):29–38.
4. KLEIN BP, JENSEN RC, SANDERSON LM. Assessment of workers' compensation claims for back strains/sprains. J Occup Med 1984;26(6):443–448.
5. FUORTES LJ, et al. Epidemiology of back injury in university hospital nurses from review of workers' compensation records and a case-control survey. J Occup Med 1994;36(9):1022–1026.
6. GARG A, OWEN B. Reducing back stress to nursing personnel: an ergonomic intervention in a nursing home. Ergonomics 1992;35(11):1353–1375.

7. MARRAS WS, et al. A comprehensive analysis of low-back disorder risk and spinal loading during the transferring and repositioning of patients using different techniques. Ergonomics 1999;42(7):904–926.
8. GRAG A, OWEN B. Prevention of Back Injuries in Healthcare Workers. Int J Ind Ergon 1994;14: 315–331.
9. FUJISHIRO K, et al. The effect of ergonomic interventions in healthcare facilities on musculoskeletal disorders. Am J Ind Med 2005;48(5):338–347.
10. MARRAS WS, et al. Prospective validation of a low-back disorder risk model and assessment of ergonomic interventions associated with manual materials handling tasks [in Process citation]. Ergonomics 2000;43(11): 1866–1886.
11. GAO, Worker Protection: Private Sector Ergonomics Programs Yield Postive Results. Government Accounting Office; 1997.

CHAPTER 14

UNDERSTANDING RECURRENT LOW BACK PAIN AND IMPLICATIONS FOR RETURN TO WORK

*T*HIS CHAPTER *emphasizes the importance of considering how pain pathways behave once a low back pain event occurs. The biomechanical consequences of low back pain involve greater muscle coactivation and more tissue load. It is also reasonable to expect that recurrent back pain is accompanied by lower biochemical pain thresholds. These concepts are similar to previous LBP pathway discussions, however, the system becomes more complex because factors such as pain behavior, memory, societal pressures, and so on can exacerbate the response. To objectify impairment, a functional impairment measurement system is presented and its relationship to low back disorder status is established. Next, studies that have established the differences in trunk muscle recruitment patterns and spine loading between asymptomatic and patients with low back pain are reviewed. The relationship between functional impairment measures and predicted changes in spine loading is reviewed. Finally, field tests predictive of low back pain recurrence are reviewed showing that the biomechanically relevant measures are predictive of recurrence.*

14.1 INTRODUCTION

A continuing dilemma for those involved in the design of work for those returning to the workplace after a low back pain experience is the prevention of *recurrent* or *secondary* low back pain. A previous episode of low back pain, in and of itself, signals a greater risk of another low back pain event. It has been well documented that one of the strongest predictors of future low back pain is a previous history of low back pain (1,2).

Recurrent or secondary low back pain is more complex than the initial low back pain incident for several reasons. First, it is often difficult to determine whether a low back pain episode is a new low back problem or an exacerbation of a previous problem. Second, we expect that the low back pain pathways for recurrent low back pain is similar to the pathways described earlier; however, they are more complex. Since patients with low back pain are more cautious of pain, there is more guarding and more fear avoidance behavior. This can increase tissue loading. In addition, once pain pathways are initiated, we expect that the upregulation of proinflammatory cytokines would lower the threshold for pain. This process would further exacerbate the biomechanical guarding response and most likely initiate a viscous cycle of pain responses. Thus, theoretically, we expect that recurrent back pain initiates a complex sequence of events that can make the pathways described previously more responsive at lower levels of tissue loading.

A review of risk factors for low back pain found that 80% of the studies examined concluded that previous history of low back pain was associated with an increased risk of symptoms (3). Those with a history of previous low back pain have twice the rate of new low back episodes compared to those without a history of low back pain (4). It has also been reported that the more frequently back pain occurs, the greater the risk of new back pain. For example, the odds ratio for new episodes of low back pain in those material handlers reporting back pain more than twice in a year is 9.8 (2), which represents an extremely high odds ratio risk. However, it is unclear whether reports of "new episodes" in these studies were truly new or reoccurrences of previous episodes. One might speculate that patients who do not fully recover from a low back episode might be predisposed to further exacerbation of a low back pain event. Furthermore, given our knowledge of how pain sensing and perception behaves, these trends may indicate that central pain is involved and much more difficult to control.

Few studies have evaluated the costs associated with recurrent back pain. The limited literature that does exist suggests that recurrent low back costs are substantial. A descriptive study of recurrent low back trends reports that the median disability costs associated with recurrent back pain episodes were greater than those for nonrecurrent low back pain (5). Similarly, Washington State Workers' Compensation data indicated that "gradual onset" (chronic) back injuries represent two-thirds of the award claims and 60% of lost workdays attributed to back injuries (6). Likewise, a recent analysis performed on low back related workers' compensation claims in Ohio indicated that 16% of the back injuries accounted for 80% of back injury costs. Further evaluations suggested that "these high cost back injuries often result from re-injury of an existing condition" (7). Hence, recurrent low back injuries could represent a rather large and costly problem.

Unfortunately, we know little about what triggers recurrent low back pain. Although we know that the risk for back pain increases once a low back pain event has occurred, we do not know what factors put a worker at risk of recurrent back pain. We know little about how the biomechanical loads differ in the spine when a worker is retuning to work with low back pain compared to a worker who has never experienced back pain. Furthermore, few studies have addressed how exposure to physical and/or psychosocial/organizational risk factors activate the low back pain pathways discussed earlier. If one could understand, quantitatively, the characteristics of spine loading in those with LBP, then situations that might further exacerbate a low back disorder could be avoided when returning a worker to the workplace. However, the mechanisms by which a history of low back pain increases risk have been poorly understood.

Thus, the goal of this discussion will be to review the body of knowledge related to recurrent back pain and examine how it might relate to work factors from the same systematic pattern of evidence standpoint that was used to assess initial risk of low back pain in earlier chapters. This section will explore the results of biomechanical tissue loading studies designed to assess how the impaired spine responds to work demands. Finally, we will examine how low back impairment can be quantified and how quantification may help us predict the spine loads experienced by individuals with low back pain.

14.2 THE NATURAL HISTORY OF LOW BACK PAIN RECOVERY

While the history of low back pain can vary greatly between individuals, there are some typical responses that have been reported in the literature as a function of time (8). There are several issues associated with the interpretation of these trends via the literature. First, different studies report on different aspects of low back pain. Some studies discuss trends associated with incidents, while others discuss lost work time or pain symptom reporting. Different measures could find different trends in the history of low back pain. Second, work-related versus nonwork-related low back pain events can lead to different findings. Third, different outcome measures can lead to different results. Some studies use pain question-naires as a measure, while others use functional performance measures. Hence, one must pay close attention to which aspect of low back pain system one is documenting to make valid comparisons.

The typical time sequence for low back pain typically is initiated by an acute pain phase that lasts for up to 6 weeks followed by steady progress. For those patients in whom the pain lasts for more than 3 months, this is typically the point at which the low back pain is described as chronic. Chronic pain can often last for years.

One study has described the recovery pattern of a group of 32 subjects over time of up to 6 months (8). Different categories of low back pain recovery were tracked including, symptoms, activities of daily living, work status, and functional performance. The pain symptoms, activities of daily living, and functional performance all displayed increases in performance over the fist 3 months. After 3 months, the different measures vary more in terms of recovery over time, with pain reports decreasing more readily than the return of functional performance. Return to work appeared to be the least sensitive measure with very dissimilar responses to the other measures.

Nonetheless, it appears that the general trend for recovery involves first, a gradual increase in pain reporting, followed by increases in return to activities of daily living, followed by functional performance return. All these measures return monotonically over a 3 month period. Improvement in return to work lagged these other measures by a large amount. At the end of 3 weeks, half of the workers that missed work due to low back pain had returned to the workplace. However, relatively few workers (20%) missed work to begin with. Thus, return to work is only a measure of recovery for a small portion of those with low back pain.

14.3 HOW CAN ONE QUANTIFY THE EXTENT OF LOW BACK PAIN?

From a biomechanical perspective, if one is to understand how the experience of low back pain is influenced by work factors in a quantitative manner, it is necessary to objectively quantify the degree of back pain experienced by a worker. It is reasonable to assume that workers with severe back pain might have a dramatically different response to potential risk factors than workers with mild back pain. Therefore, attempts to understand the quantitative relationship between low back pain status and the extent of spine loading that could lead to low back pain must establish quantifiable measures. Only then can the demands of the workplace be matched to the capabilities of the worker returning to work from a low back pain event. Unfortunately, most descriptions of low back pain, used for medical diagnostic purposes, are rather subjective in nature and do not necessarily describe quantitatively the functional capability of the worker in biomechanically meaningful terms. In the medical profession, there is an abundance of subjective perception scales, as well as ability tests that ascertain the patient's current pain perception status. However, the ability of these scales and measures to compare the functional ability of the patient's spine on different days is poor since pain is a subjective experience. Hence, these evaluations do little to reveal much about the biomechanical capability of the worker in terms that can be useful in a quantitative biomechanical assessment.

One measure reflecting patient status, and potentially spine loading, could be trunk kinematics. Trunk kinematics has been shown to be related to occupational low back pain risk (9–11) as well as spine biomechanical loading (12–18) in asymptomatic subjects. Since trunk motion plays an important role in defining muscle coactivation and the subsequent spine loading in asymptomatic people, it is logical that trunk motion might also provide information about the condition of the muscle recruitment system in symptomatic individuals.

Over the past decade, there have been substantial efforts to understand the role of trunk kinematics in describing the extent of functional impairment associated with low back pain (19–22). Studies have been able to demonstrate that torso *kinematic compromise* can be a sensitive indicator of the degree of low back pain impairment. The torso kinematic profile is monitored as a function of patient-controlled free-dynamic flexion–extension task exertions (while the trunk is *not* exposed to external loads, e.g., not lifting) and is believed to reflect the torso's motor recruitment patterns adopted by the patient.

14.3.1 Impairment Assessment

Severity measures have been recognized as an essential element of medical assessment (23). Specifically, quantification of function has been regarded as a key to functional restoration (24). However, an accurate assessment can be problematic. Pathoanatomic (anatomy-based disorder) diagnosis is rare (25), and the assessment of a low back pain has been subjective at best.

Traditionally, functional assessments have involved attempts to assess the amount of weight that patients can handle in a particular position without experiencing pain or have focused on the range of motion (ROM) available to a patient. The problem with such assessments is that these outcome measures are influenced by patient motivation and are thus subjective. They generally do not account for symptom magnification and have little relationship to the loading experienced by the spine, since trunk moment exposure is rarely controlled.

Quantitative assessment of low back pain is important for several reasons. First, without a quantitative measure of low back status, identification of the extent of low back pain and the extent of the low back disorder is difficult. In the absence of a quantitative measure, it is difficult to separate normal variability in function from a true disorder. Second, without a quantitative measure of low back pain, treatment management becomes subjective. Patients have different pain thresholds and distinguishing different pain tolerances from different levels of impairment can become difficult. A review of the medical impairment criteria for low back pain have suggested that measures be developed that are far more quantitative (26). Third, a quantitative measure would provide insight into functional status that can be meaningfully compared at different points in time as one recovers from low back pain to assess progress. Currently, motivation and desire for secondary gain can influence assessments of low back pain. A quantitative measure would provide a more objective means to assess capabilities and would relate less to motivation. Finally, quantitative measures may provide a benchmark of when one is ready to return to a job without increasing the risk of exacerbating the disorder. This is important because exacerbation of the low back pain could also contribute to chronicity (increasing the probability that central pain is established), and ultimately, disability. Thus, society would benefit greatly from a quantitative measure of low back pain.

Quantifying the extent of a low back pain is necessary as a measure of physical impairment. Physical impairment should not be confused with other low back pain definitions. Physical impairment is an *objective* assessment of structural limitations and

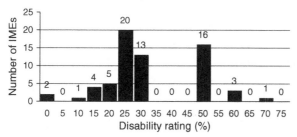

Figure 14.1   Range of disability rating of one patient as assessed by 65 independent medical examiners (IMEs). (From reference 30).

is solely a medical responsibility. It relates to a pathological or anatomical loss (abnormality of structure) or a physiological loss or limitation leading to loss of ability (functional impairment) (23). Disability, on the contrary, is assessed based on a patient's *subjective* report but relates to the ability to perform work tasks. The U.S. Bureau of Disability Insurance (27) specifies that loss or limitation evaluation be objective and "demonstrable by medically acceptable clinical and laboratory diagnostic techniques."

Quantification of low back impairment has traditionally been extremely difficult and elusive. Currently, impairment ratings of LBD vary by as much as 70% (28). As an example, Fig. 14.1 shows the disability ratings of the same patient by 65 independent medical examiners (IMEs). The figure shows that the range of disability varied from 0% to 70%. The problem with such subjective assessments that lack objective criteria is apparent from the lack of convergence of the assessments. It has been estimated that a precise diagnosis is unknown in 80–90% of disabling LBDs, emphasizing the need for more quantitative measures (29).

Traditionally, attempts to judge impairments have tried to identify anatomic sources of the low back pain. Imaging techniques such as CT scans, MRI, and myelograms are used to assist in the identification of the structure that has been compromised. However, over 85% of LBDs do not have a pathoanatomic diagnosis (25).

This finding is not surprising since few current imaging techniques are able to observe anatomic anomalies while subjects are positioned in a functionally painful posture. For example, most high quality imaging such as MRI is performed while the patient is lying supine on a table. When lying supine, the vertebrae experience minimal spine force and any damaged disc will not have enough force imposed on them to divulge a bulging disc on an image if it were present in more natural work postures (e.g., standing or bent over). Hence, most traditional imaging is of minimal benefit for identifying spine mechanical problems due to mismatch of spine loading with spine tolerance.

Given these difficulties, recent attempts to develop a measurement system for low back pain have centered on functional measures of impairment. Several approaches or methodologies have been identified in the literature. These include (1) the use of EMG to observe flexion–relaxation and/or temporal features of the torso muscles, (2) observation of muscle fatigue via EMG spectral analysis, (3) observation of EMG activity level, (4) trunk strength, and (5) documentation of trunk motion components. Table 14.1 summarizes the features of the more notable studies. Several limitations are associated with many of these studies (21). First, many of these previous studies suffer from small population samples that limit their applicability to the general population. Second, examination of the *sensitivity-specificity* column in Table 14.1 indicates that few of these previous studies have considered the issues of classification error. Furthermore, few of the previous investigations have been able to identify patients with low back pain from a sufficiently large (normally distributed)

TABLE 14.1 Summary of Low Back Pain Measurement Studies (Adapted From Reference 21)

Methodology	References	Number of subjects	Objective of study	Methods	Statistical methods and major findings	Sensitivity and specificity and error rate
Temporal aspects/ flexion–relaxation	31	6 controls and 7 low back pain	Evaluate paraspinal muscles in controls and LBP group	Surface EMG erector spinae temporal and amplitude	The time-normalized bilateral paraspinal envelope was significantly different	Not reported
	32	40 LBP patients and 40 controls	Examine EMG patterns in CLBP patients and controls	Activity levels of surface EMG measured	Multivariate discriminant function model of EMG activity	Sensitivity 84.6%, specificity 87.5%, error 14%
	33	41 LBP patients and 7 controls	Measure ROM, strength ratio of ext/flex, and flexion–relaxation phenomenon	Surface EMG measured on erector spinae and rectus abdominus.	Two-way ANOVA was used. Flexion–relaxation was absent in patients	Not reported
	34	10 normals and 10 LBP patients	Compare hip–spine motion in controls and patients	Performance measured using EMG and electrogoniometers	Relaxation index was significantly higher in patients than in controls.	Not reported
	35	20 controls 70 CLBP	Develop reliable flexion relaxation ratio	Surface EMG applied at L1/2, L4/5	Discriminant analysis. Flexion–relaxation ratio was significant between control and patients	Sensitivity 93%, specificity 75%
	36	24 controls 14 LBP	Compare temporal activation pattern in between controls and patients	Surface EMG measured on rectus abdominus, exerternal obliques, erector spinae, multifidus	Two factor (muscle and group) mixed model ANOVA was used. All muscle in controls had similar temporal patterns whereas patients had greater variation	Not reported
	37	20 controls and 20 CLBP	Analyze muscle activation pattern in LBP patient and controls	Surface EMG of erector spinae, rectus abdominus, gastrocnemius, anteriror tibialis	Chi-square test, logistic regression. Subjects with LBP were four times more likely to have asymmetric muscle activation than controls	Not reported

	Sample	Objective	Method	Analysis	Results
38	19 controls and 19 chronic LBP	Compare muscle function during sagittal flexion and exention	Surface EMG of paraspinal muscles, biceps femoris and gluteus maximus	t-tests. Gluteus maximum activity had a shorter duration in both flexion and extension for LBP patients compared to controls	Not reported
39	20 controls and 20 LBP	Compare patters of paraspinal and abdominal muscles in flexion/extension	Surface EMG of erector spinae L1/2 L4/5, abdominals	ANOVA, in flexion, there was a significant difference in EMG patterns between patients and controls	Not reported
40	14 controls and 14 chronic recurrent LBP	To evaluate changes in recruitment organization between controls and patients	Fine wire EMG of transverse abdominis internal and external obliques. Surface EMG anterior and middle detoid, rectus abdominus	ANOVA. In controls reaction time of the deltoid and rectus abdominis increased with task complexity, whereas reaction time in transverse abdominis was constant. In patients, transverse abdominis reaction time increased with all other muscles	Not reported
Fatigue analysis or frequency analysis					
41	18 normals and 21 LBP patients	Develop model to classify normal and patients	Surface EMG analysis included median frequency, slope	Logistic regression model of initial median frequency and slope from the dominant multifidus was found	*Test:* sensitivity = 100%, specificity = 75%
42	Training: 28 LBP, 42 controls; Test: 57 LBP, 6 controls	Distinguish muscle impairment between patients and controls	Surface EMG measuring initial median frequency and median frequency slope.	Discriminant analysis model of IMF and MF slope	*Training:* 85%, 86%, Error 14%; *Test:* Sensitivity 88%, specificity. 100%, error 6%
43	17 non-LBP rowers and 8 LBP rowers	Difference between athletes and LBP athletes	Surface EMG of low back musculature	Discriminant function model using percentage median frequency recovery	Sensitivity 66% specificity 71%, error rate 31%

continued

TABLE 14.1 (continued)

Methodology	References	Number of subjects	Objective of study	Methods	Statistical methods and major findings	Sensitivity and specificity and error rate
	44	11 healthy controls, 10 LBP patients	Spectral EMG differences in patients and controls	Surface EMG measuring spectral parameters	t-test showed significant differences on spectral slopes between controls and patients	Sensitivity 40%, no specificity reported
	45	22 normals and 27 patients (avoider 9 and confronter 15)	The objective was to systematically evaluate spectral parameters	Surface EMG of the iliocostalis muscle	Discriminant analysis model of spectral parameters identified 88.9% of avoiders, 67% of confronter, and 59% of controls	Sensitivity 78%, specificity 59%, error rate 31%
	46	20 controls and 20 patients	Develop reliable EMG indicator of back muscle impairment	Surface EMG of multifidus L5, iliocostalis lumborum L3 and longissimus L1, T10	Intraclass correlation coefficients (ICC). The ICCs for the medial back muscles range from 0.68 to 0.91. The EMG fatigue indices had an ICC of 0.74–0.79	Not reported
	47	20 controls, and 14 LBP patients	Test hypothesis that patients redistribute activation pattern which creates an imbalance in EMG	Surface EMG of longissimus L1, illiocostales L2 and multifidus L5	ANOVA. Median frequency imbalances were significantly greater in patients at segmental as well as across lumbar levels	Not reported
	48	15 controls and 20 CLBP	To compare muscle fatigability between controls and patients	Surface EMG of lumbar paraspinal muscles at L3/4, L5/S1, and gluteus maximus	MANOVA, t-test. Time to endurance and MVC were significantly lower in patients compared to controls	Not reported
EMG activity level	49	15 controls, 28 history of LBP, 83 with LBP symptoms	The objective was to distinguish among the groups	Measure surface EMG of paraspinal muscles in different postures	No significant difference between controls and history of symptom group. Current LBP subjects had EMG activity above controls.	Not reported

	50	28 normals and 20 patients	Examine paraspinal muscle function in controls and LBP	EMG on paraspinal muscles	EMG was significantly greater in patients compared to controls	Not reported
	51	40 normal and 40 LBP patients	Compare strength and EMG in controls and LBP patients	Measure trunk position with goniometer and EMG activity of erector spinae	Controls were significantly stronger than patients but did not have significantly higher EMG.	Not reported
	52	16 CLBP patients and 12 controls	Describe strength and EMG in controls and LBP	Surface EMG of paraspinal muscles	The groups showed significantly different IEMG fatigue slopes	Not reported
	53	19 CLBP patients, and 14 controls	Examine erector spinae muscle activity level at various walking speeds	Surface EMG of the erector spinae at T12, L2, and L4.	Principle component analysis, T-test. ES amplitude at L2 and L4 was significantly greater during the swing phase in LBP patients compared to controls	Not reported
	54	30 CLBP patients and 30 controls	Examine changes in RMS during submaximal trunk rotation	Surface EMG of latissimus dorsi, erector spinae, upper and lower gluteus maximus, hamstrings	Mixed models. There were significant differences between groups with the LBP group having greater EMG amplitude in several muscles	Not reported
	55	77 controls, 24 acute LBP, and 51 chronic LBP	Compare level of back muscle activity	Surface EMG of multifidus and iliocostalis lumborum pars throacis	Kruskall-Wallis test. Chronic LBP had significantly lower EMG level during exercise but no difference during stabilizing activities	Not reported
Strength testing	56	21 controls US postal workers and 59 LBP patients	Distinguish controls and LBP patients with functional performance measures	Evaluated ROM, strength and cardiovascular fitness	Isometric and isokinetic peak force and torque tests failed to show significant differences between low back pain and workers	Not reported

(continued)

TABLE 14.1 (continued)

Methodology	References	Number of subjects	Objective of study	Methods	Statistical methods and major findings	Sensitivity and specificity and error rate
	57	65 normals and 68 patients	Compare controls to chronic LBP patients	Isokinetic strength	Paired *t*-tests showed that patients lifted significantly less weight compared to controls	Not reported
	58	73 controls and 10 LBP	Develop database of controls	Flexion extension and lateral flexion strength	The patient isokinetic strength was 9–40% less than the reference controls group	Not reported
	59	12 control and 38 chronic LBP	Measure spinal ROM in controls and patients	Evaluated ROM using inclinometers and X-ray	Descriptives for two groups but not statistics to compare controls and patients	Not reported
	60	32 normals and 23 patients	Compare controls to LBP patients	Measure strength ROM, velocity, and oscillation angle	Average velocity was significantly different between controls and patients at $P<0.001$	Not reported
	61	36 normals, and 91 intermittent LBP, and 21 CLBP	Compare groups in strength, endurance, and body composition	Trunk strength measures at 30° per second, calipers measure body composition	Significant difference in isometric endurance between normals and intermittent LBP as well as between CLBP and intermittent LBP	Not reported
	62	70 controls and 120 CLBP	Standardize testing methods with controls and LBP group	Measure strength, ROM, fatigue, and endurance	ICCs on controls were above 0.80. Differences in sex but not age or body weight	Sensitivity 85–90%, specificity 77–80%, error 15–19%

63	37 controls and 61 LBD	Compare strength in trunk and knee between group	Measure isokinetic strength at 120° per second knee strength at 126° per second	*t*-tests showed that the LBP group had significantly lower strength in both the trunk and knee compared to the control group	Not reported
64	90 controls and 100 CLBP	Compare controls and CLBP group	Endurance was measured in time person could hold position	*t*-tests showed that the controls group had longer endurance time than CLBP patients	Not reported
65	191 chronic LBP compared to normative data	Evaluate isokinetic trunk strength before and after functional restoration	Trunk strength measured at 60 per second and 150 per second	Studentized t-test showed significant improvement. The percent control analysis indicated residual strength decrements	Not reported
66	53 controls and 53 LPB	Quantify performance differences during isodynamic lifting	Lifts performed on a work simulator	MANOVA, controls completed significantly more lifts and lifted more weight than patients	Not reported
67	15 controls and 16 LBD	Compare isometric force production	Time to peak force, time to peak force variability, peak force variability	Linear regression, LBD had two subgroup one similar to controls and second showed time to peak force much higher than control. Regression explained 84–97% of variance	Not reported

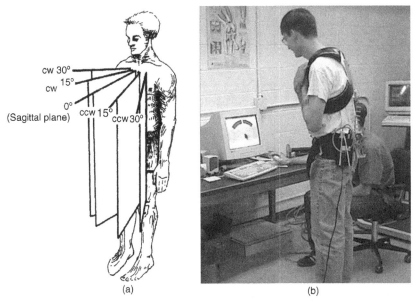

(a)   (b)

Figure 14.2 (a) Asymmetric planes used to solicit the range of musculoskeletal kinematic performance from patients. Patients interact with a computer and play a computer game with their back as they flex and extend as fast as they can in each plane of motion. (CW = clockwise, CCW = counterclockwise) (from reference 21) (**b**) Kinematic testing using the lumbar motion monitor to monitor spine motion while subject interacts with a computer to control motion.

population of asymptomatic and subjects with low back pain. Finally, few of these studies have attempted to validate their findings using multiple robust evaluation techniques.

An alternative approach to assessing the extent of low back pain has been suggested [19–22,71]. This approach documents the symmetric and asymmetric back *motion characteristics* of a patient and compares these motion characteristics to that of a normal, unimpaired subject population adjusted for age and gender. Patients are tested in different torso asymmetries so that different combinations of the trunk's muscles must be recruited to flex and extend the trunk (see Fig. 14.2). Patients are asked to flex and extend their trunk as fast as possible within these various planes of motion (Fig. 14.2a). To control their movement within each plane, they watch and respond to computer feedback that displays their twisting position. Thus, in effect, the patients are playing a computer game with their back under these testing conditions.

The motion profile observed during repeated flexion and extension of the torso at different trunk asymmetries is believed to be a reflection of the trunk's musculoskeletal central control program (mental model) often referred to as the "central set" (72). For asymptomatic subjects, this control program has been well developed over the person's lifetime. However, for a patient with low back pain, it is thought that this musculoskeletal control program must be adjusted to compensate for limitations due to muscle functions, structural restrictions, and guarding behavior.

Early studies (19) were able to show that the best discriminators between healthy people and patients with low back pain involved more dynamic trunk motion indicators (velocity). Later efforts described trunk velocity and acceleration characteristics as well as expected variability for a large normal population of subjects (71). This study indicated that age and gender as well as back disorders independently influence trunk motion characteristics and suggested that motion characteristics could be normalized for age and gender. The study showed that once age and gender was accounted for, the deficit in trunk motion was an accurate reflection of the degree of low back impairment.

Recent studies (20,21) compared the activities of asymptomatic subjects to patients with low back pain and concluded that (1) the trunk motion measures were extremely repeatable and (2) only dynamic motion characteristics (not ROM) varied as a function of low back pain. Hence, a common measure of disability, range of motion, showed no statistically significant difference between a low back pain group and an asymptomatic group of subjects. However, trunk velocity and acceleration were able to distinguish well between the two groups.

Measures of trunk instantaneous position, velocity, and acceleration were recorded and compared to a previously established normative database of trunk motions (71). Previous studies have indicated that trunk kinematics, once adjusted for age and gender, are indicative of the degree of low back impairment (20). In this study, kinematic compromise was operationally defined as the subject's deficit in low back motion characteristics (kinematics) relative to the expected trunk motions (defined by the normative database) and adjusted as a function of the subject's gender and age. The kinematic compromise summary measure, "probability of normal" or $p(n)$, was used to concisely indicate the degree of low back impairment of an individual compared to the normative database (20,21). This measure is composed of a combination of sagittal plane range of motion, velocity, and acceleration characteristics, frontal plane and transverse plane motion as well as the ability to complete the five conditions shown in Fig. 14.2a.

The $p(n)$ measure has been independently validated and reports good sensitivity (92%) and specificity (97%) (21) in its ability to distinguish between individuals with and without low back pain and is considered a quantifiable measure of the extent of a low back disorder impairment (19–22). This was accomplished by determining how well the quantification tool was able to distinguish between a large group of normal and participants with. Table 14.2 shows the ability of the kinematic-based assessments to distinguish between asymptomatic and patients with low back pain as a function of various statistical methods. As can be seen, by using some advanced statistical methods one is able to distinguish extremely well between low back pain and asymptomatic patients using just kinematic measures of performance. The 5% error

TABLE 14.2 Effectiveness of the Kinematic Measure to Distinguish Between Asymptomatic Patients and those Low Back Pain with Using Different Test Sets and Different Statistical Methods (CART = classification and regression trees; CUS = classification using splines; MCUS = modified classification using splines) (From Reference 21)

Data set		Statistical method			
		Disciminant function	CART	CUS	MCUS
Method 1	Sensitivity (%)	85	90	84	
Cross-validation	Specificity (%)	95	86	94	
	Error rate	0.1002	0.1213	0.1027	
Method II	Sensitivity (%)	83	88	85	86
Training set	Specificity (%)	93	87	96	95
	Error rate	0.1177	0.122S	0.0852	0.0877
Test set	Sensitivity (K)	90	91	90	92
	Specificity (%)	94	92	96	37
	Error rate	0.0792	0.0870	0.0710	0.0581

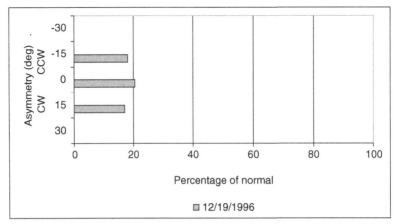

Figure 14.3 Trunk sagittal acceleration performance shown as function of the five test planes of motion. The horizontal axis shows the patient impairment relative to asymptomatic individuals of the same age and gender.

rate for the independent test set is a marked improvement over traditional methods of evaluating low back impairment that do not assess motion characteristics (Table 14.1).

Figure 14.3 shows how kinematic performance and impairment can be documented. This figure displays the performance of a given measure of kinematics (in this case, trunk acceleration in the sagittal plane) normalize relative to patient age and gender. The horizontal axis shows the percentile performance relative to the performance expected of someone who has not experienced low back pain. The vertical axis identifies the different asymmetric testing planes of motion (Fig. 14.2a). Thus, this evaluation indicated that the patient was only able to generate between 16% and 21% of the trunk acceleration that would be expected given her age and gender. As impairment decreases, the performance bars would move further to the right. To track performance at different point in time, different patterned bars document the change in performance (Fig. 14.4). As can be seen in this figure, the patient improved when moving in counterclockwise planes but not in clockwise planes. These differences were tracked to tension on the left nerve root when moving clockwise that indicated a disc bulge on that side of the back. In this manner, these kinematic analyses can be extended to all kinematic variables. Figure 14.5 shows the kinematic profiles for a patient in terms of ROM, flexion velocity,

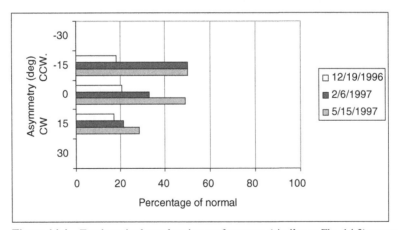

Figure 14.4 Trunk sagittal acceleration performance (similar to Fig. 14.3) compared at multiple times during the progression of the rehabilitation.

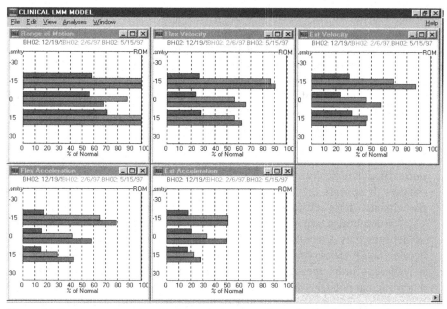

Figure 14.5 Range of motion, flexion velocity, extension velocity, flexion acceleration, and extension acceleration in the sagittal plane shown for patient over three different examination times. The horizontal axis shows the kinematic performance relative to asymptomatic individuals of the same age and gender.

extension velocity, flexion acceleration, and extension acceleration in the sagittal plane over three different examination times. This figure indicates that the type of information obtained by observing ROM is significantly different from that derived from motion measures. Note that the asymmetry in performance among the testing planes is only apparent when examining the higher order derivatives of motion (i.e., velocity and acceleration profiles). As with Fig. 14.4, these asymmetries in performance indicated nerve root compression on one side of the spine.

These results have confirmed that accurate, objective benchmarking of low back pain can be achieved by documenting motion (kinematic) characteristics. Trunk motion assessment data are rather simple to collect compared to the other systems that attempt to classify patients with low back pain. Five of the previous studies reporting sensitivity and specificity required EMG. This often requires disrobing and an application of strength (which may be limited by pain sensation in some participants). The other technique reporting sensitivity and specificity required testing of maximum torso strength (62). Although they reported respectable sensitivity and specificity, the safety associated with strength testing is often in question. For example, one study (73) found that they injured more participants using strength testing than the number of low back pain episodes they were able to prevent. Thus, the present method is easier to administer and has better accuracy than previous efforts.

Several features of this assessment suggest that the technique of quantifying low back pain using motion measures is a valid approach. First, a valid method should perform well over a large number of subjects. With a large data set, questionable subject performance would be diluted amongst the mass of the database. The study that was used to establish the validity of this impairment quantification method (21) represents the largest data set for evaluating the extent of a low back pain found in the literature to date. With over 700 participants and strong sensitivity and specificity findings, this study provides a stringent test of the methodology. Second, several validation and classification procedures were employed resulting in very similar error rates, sensitivities, and specificities. The convergence of the results indicates a very robust and consistent model. Third, compared to other available methods for identification of low back pain, this technique not only has a lower classification error but also has a much better balance between the strength of sensitivity and specificity. In fact, it is possible that this approach may outperform the "gold standards" used by the physicians for inclusion in this study.

Two limitations of this method should also be reported. First, the test can take up to a half hour to perform and requires the cooperation of the patient. Second, the test is intended for the nonacute phases of low back pain.

A sensitivity analysis of these study results (21) was performed to determine where misclassification errors occurred. These analyses indicated that patients misclassified as normal had statistically lower pain scores by an average of 43% than the correctly classified patients. It appears that the model did not misclassify randomly but specifically with participants whose self-reported pain was significantly less severe.

It should also be noted that the measure of low back pain discussed in this six-variable model uses only a small portion of the available variables. The individual velocity and acceleration profiles observed in specific asymmetries during the flexion–extension tasks may serve as further measures of specific structural problems (e.g., sensitivity of a nerve root at a particular point). A documented motion deficit in one of the specific asymmetries may indicate a specific disability and may be tracked as an indication of recovery. The value of motion measures may go well beyond the general assessment reported here.

This method provides a simple, easy-to-use, and sensitive measure that quantifies the extent of low back pain given the patient's age and gender. The analyses performed here evaluate the value of the motion measures in isolation from any other information. Under realistic usage conditions, one would expect the motion measures to be used in conjunction with other indicators of disease. For example, factors such as a medical history or straight leg raise ability may be used in conjunction with trunk motion measures to get a more complete picture of patient status.

This impairment measurement study demonstrated that, using this method, the distinction between muscle and structural source of low back pain is possible. Our studies have indicated that motion measure models have very different profiles when the origin of a low back pain is structural versus. muscular (21).

Finally, the results suggest that this quantification technique can be used as a tool to track patient progress during treatments. One would expect a sensitive measure to track changes in low back pain status over time. As a test of this expectation, 31 subjects were tested longitudinally on two different occasions separated by several weeks. The patients fell into two distinct patterns over this period. Fifteen patients improved, while 16 remained the same or became worse in terms of reported pain. As self-reported pain improved over observation time, there were significant changes in the velocity and acceleration measures (but not in the ROM measure) contrary to those who did not report improvement. Changes in ROM were not indicative of changes in pain status, confirming earlier findings (20). Another paper (8) thoroughly reports how the motion measures described here are able to track medical improvement in the LBP over observation periods of 3–6 months.

This quantitative measure of LBP can also serve as a means to track factors affecting low back pain in future studies. Now that a means to assess the extent of a low back pain has been established, this "benchmark" can be used as a means to assess and compare the effectiveness of various treatment modalities. In addition, the measure can also be used to determine when one might be a candidate for extreme treatments, such as surgery, or when one is ready to return to the workplace without exacerbation of the problem. Finally, this LBP quantification can be used in conjunction with workplace quantification measures so that the matching of the workplace to the person's capabilities can be approached more scientifically.

Currently, efforts are underway to adopt this assessment technique to different measurement systems including vision–based measurement tools (VICON).

14.3.2 Effort Sincerity

We have seen that the more quantitative methods attempt to document the functional capacity of the torso by observing the torso dynamic motion profile. These methods, in one way or another, attempt to monitor or summarize the functioning of the trunk's musculoskeletal system status. The musculoskeletal system's status can be defined in terms of muscle recruitment patterns, muscle size and strength, joint stiffness, experience that can be affected by psychological and psychosocial factors (such as depression or fear of re-injury), and any other factors that may influence kinematic and kinetic performance. A clear understanding of the musculoskeletal system status is needed if functional capacity is to be evaluated objectively.

A potential issue with these measurement systems is that the results are only useful if the patient cooperates and performs the functional task without unnecessarily magnifying the impairment and performing at a level that reliably reflects the status of the trunk's musculoskeletal system. Patients may magnify impairment for several reasons including fear, mistaken beliefs, maladaptive coping strategies, and active attempts to seek treatment (25). If patients with low back pain do not perform the task to the best of their ability during the functional test session, then the quantitative measure may erroneously document the musculoskeletal status of the trunk. Thus, it is important to judge whether the patient is magnifying the low back impairment when assessing trunk status.

Assessing impairment magnification during a functional capacity test for the back has been a challenge. Assessments for other parts of the body often compare an individual's performance between limbs or different sites of the body. For example, a comparison of grip force generation of dominant and nondominant hands has been able to assess sincerity of effort in maximal grip strength with excellent sensitivity and specificity (74). However, this method is not feasible for trunk performance evaluation.

Many researchers have attempted to assess maximal versus submaximal exertions of the back by observing variations in back strength. One study observed variations in force curves produced by the muscles in the back during isokinetic exertions along with heart rate and reported that only heart rate was acceptably repeatable (75,76). Strength variance was found to vary greatly as a function of effort level and not necessarily sincerity. Others observing nonisokinetic dynamic strength found that those with and without back pain produced equally consistent levels of force (60). It has also been observed that consistency of isometric exertions was not a good indicator of submaximal exertions (77–79). Still others observed variability in isokinetic torque parameters during flexion and extension and have found that the ratio between flexion and extension strength may be indicative of low back pain (80). Further attempts to identify submaximal isokinetic strength generation observed the coefficient of variation of torque generation. Such efforts resulted in reasonable sensitivity or specificity in identifying sincere efforts, but not both (81).

Another study represents one of the few studies that attempted to identify sincerity using a large population of subjects (82). A sufficiently large subject population is important so that the data can be considered representative of a normal distribution of participant performance. They found that patients suspected of producing submaximal isokinetic exertions had lower trunk extension and flexion torque levels relative to their body weight.

Table 14.3 summarizes the ability of these measures to identify submaximal back exertions. In general, this table indicates that few studies have included large samples of subjects in their evaluations and few have reported reasonably high sensitivity and

TABLE 14.3 Literature Review Summarizing the Ability to Identify Submaximal Back Exertions (Adapted From Reference 22)

Technique	Reference	Number of Subjects	Objective of Study	Methods	Statistical Methods and Major Findings	Sensitivity and Specificity
Lifting Simulation	62	30 normal	Distinguish effort level using force/distance curves	Cybex Trunk Extension/Flexion and Liftask tests at two effort levels	Need to combine variability in force/distance curves with visual assessment for acceptable classification	Sensitivity 65–96.7%, specificity 51.7%–87.9%
	63	44 normal	Find indices to distinguish between effort groups	Isometric, isokinetic, and isoinertial tests with Cybex Liftask at two effort levels	Isometric tasks were not significantly different. Isokinetic and isoinertial indices provided moderate classification accuracy	Sensitivity 73–78%, specificity 66–69%
	1	15 controls, 16 LBP patients	Establish validity of determining effort level by visual observation of lifting test	Video analysis of lifting and lowering task. Lift lower task performed five times at each weight	Maximum performance was significantly different between controls and patients for both genders.	Sensitivity 53.4%, specificity 95.8%
	2	41 previous musculoskeletal pathology	Investigate reliability and validity of lift test as indicator of sincere effort	EPIC Lift Capacity Test	t-test showed that there was a significant difference in maximum weight lifted between sincere and insincere	Sensitivity 94%, specificity 80%
Trunk strength	69	32 Normal, 115 sincere LBD, 40 suspect LBD	Determine effect of effort level on trunk strength deficits	Cybex Trunk Extension/Flexion at maximal effort	Suspect LBD subjects had lower trunk extension–flexion torque/body weight ratio than sincere LBD subjects	Not reported
	64	20 normal	Evaluate variability for isometric lumbar extension between effort groups	Static lumbar extension at 100% and 50% effort levels	High test–retest correlations in peak torque for both effort conditions. Therapist classification was unreliable	Sensitivity 63%, specificity 53–58%
	65	20 normal	Determine effect of instructions on consistency of submaximal effort	Isometric lumbar extension at maximal effort and feigning effort levels	Sincere effort had greater variability than feigned. Test–retest peak torque cannot indicate sincerity of effort	Not reported

70	270 LBD	Evaluate usefulness of CVs as an indicator of effort	Static trunk strength measures	CV may not be a reliable predictor of effort. May combination of measures	Not reported
68	12 normal 10, mild LBD, 13 severe LBD	Distinguish effort level through variability of trunk strength	Lidoback dynamometer isokinetic flexion/extension for 100% and 50% efforts	Using a single cutoff of CV for both patients and normals will misclassify those with severe LBD as low effort	Sensitivity 37–83%, specificity 31–94%
4	35 controls	Test index for differentiating maximal from feigned effort	Kincom, low velocity 10° per second, fast velocity 40° per second	ANOVA. The index identifies feigned effort from maximal effort in normal subjects, slightly more so in men than women.	Not reported
3	44 LBD	Measure trunk extension strength in LBD and test eccentric concentric ratio	Kincom low velocity 10° per second, fast velocity 40° per second	In LBD patient eccentric strength was greater than concentric strength	Not reported
Trunk dynamics					
66	44 LBD	Evaluate a protocol for detecting LBD feigning	B-200 testing of peak torque, velocity, and range of motion	Ratios of testing variables can act as flags for feigned effort if three or more variables are out of acceptable ranges	Sensitivity 98%, specificity 82%
5	100 Controls, 100 LBD	To determine if trunk motion characteristics can identify impairment magnification	Trunk range of motion, velocity, acceleration, and jerk	Discriminant function analysis. Combinations of higher order velocity and acceleration motion components distinguish between sincere and insincere efforts	Sensitivity 75–92%, specificity 75–92%

specificity. Hence, we have few methods to ensure the accuracy of quantitative measures of low back pain.

The underlying assumption associated with the use of trunk motion quantification is that deficits in motion reflect the status of the trunk's musculoskeletal system. As discussed earlier, the musculoskeletal status is believed to represent the "mental model" or "central set" (also called motor set) or recruitment and firing pattern of the trunk musculature. The central set is developed throughout one's life and is expected to remain relatively consistent unless one develops low back pain. When low back pain occurs, this recruitment and discharge pattern is altered and a new central set is established as one discovers the limits of the disorder.

Even though the muscle recruitment pattern has been changed as a result of the low back disorder, the pattern is believed to be consistent in its functioning (relative to the status of the back impairment) and thus repeatable. Specifically, one would expect that higher order derivatives of position such as velocity and acceleration would require more information processing on the part of the person to establish recruitment patterns. It was hypothesized that higher order motion measures at certain points in the motion would be well established and repeatable since they represent this "mental model" of movement that a person is willing to accept. When one magnifies their impairment, they would not rely on this mental model and movements would be more variable. Hence, we contend that one should be able to assess the impairment magnification of an effort by observing a repeatable musculoskeletal recruitment pattern that should be reflected in trunk motion.

A study was performed to test this assumption, where a large group of patients with low back pain as well as asymptomatic individuals were asked to provide "genuine" efforts of trunk motion as well as feign or exacerbate back pain during different trials. The repeatability of the motion kinematics was observed as just discussed (22). The results of this study were consistent with the hypothesis that a central set or mental model of how recruiting components of the musculoskeletal system would produce repeatable higher order motion profiles. Higher order derivatives of motion, such as velocity and acceleration, appear to be the key to this assessment.

It has been shown that people have great difficulty judging higher order derivatives of a musculoskeletal exertion (88). Neurophysiological studies (76) have demonstrated that the musculoskeletal coordination pattern is fine-tuned through experience, and everyday motion provides abundant opportunities for gaining experience. The generation of motion requires the processing (and differentiation) of great amounts of proprioceptive information; and since the experimental task was to be performed quickly, we feel that the participant must rely on established lower level neural control programs that must form this central set. It has been hypothesized that this central set is well established for common tasks such as trunk bending. One relies on these established motor recruitment programs and the motion components would be repeatable if the plane of motion was similar on each repetition (as in the unmagnified conditions). However, if one attempts to override this established central set (as during a magnification of impairment), the participant would need to reestablish the central set. When the task is performed quickly, the motion patterns would reflect this reprogramming in the form of a lack of consistency. Practically, this means that one would expect that if one was relying on the established mental model to govern trunk motion patterns, then repetitions of the same motions would be nearly identical in timing in terms of higher order kinematics. Thus, as the torso passes through a given angle, one would expect identical instantaneous velocity and acceleration to occur on repeated motions if one was relying on the same mental model to produce the motion. On the contrary, if one were trying to "override" this mental model and magnify ones symptoms, one would expect that their instantaneous velocity and acceleration profiles would be far less consistent as one passed through a given torso angle since one would

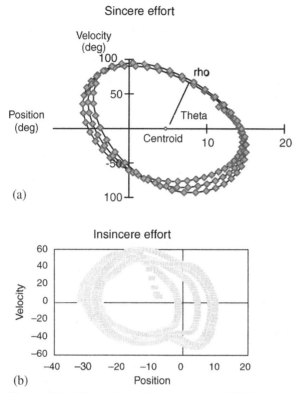

Figure 14.6   Phase plane of (**a**) a sincere and (**b**) insincere trunk motion efforts.

not be relying on an established "mental model" to control ones motions. Figure 14.6a and b shows an example of this variability through a phase plane of instantaneous trunk velocity in the sagittal plane versus. instantaneous trunk position for sincere (a) and insincere (b) efforts. The sincere efforts show much greater consistency on repeated flexion and extension.

Further analyses of the results verified that variability reduction in motions was primarily due to a reduction in variability at certain positions throughout movement. These analyses indicated that it is not just motion that is repeatable in the central set, but motion at particular points in space. For example, an acceleration profile may be highly repeatable for sincere conditions but only at the point where the subject changes direction. This finding is consistent with the idea that a mental model of recruitment pattern (central set) has been established.

It is also important to recognize that the characterization of motion pattern consistency is multivariate in nature. An individual motion parameter, in and of itself, would contain rich information about the central set. However, models consisting of multivariate parameters containing actions in all three cardinal planes of the body were capable of discrimination between the sincere versus insincere exertions when comparing performance in the various planes. Motion in the different cardinal planes requires different types of muscle recruitment patterns (concentric versus eccentric; agonist versus antagonist) and would be part of the central set that we are attempting to measure. Hence, differences in the interplay of motions (phase planes) would be elicited in a range of trunk exertions. This finding indicates that the central set is indirectly observable through motion profiles but is complex in its representation.

It is believed that the mental model or central set must be reestablished after injury but would be better established if the period in which the injury stabilizes is longer. Following this logic, we expect greater ability to identify magnified impairment efforts with asymptomatic participants (as demonstrated in this study) since asymptomatic subjects have established their motion patterns over a very long period. For the same reason, we also expect this technique to perform better with the patients with low back pain who are stabilized in their chronicity. This technique is not intended for the acute phases of low back pain.

These models indicate that it was indeed possible to distinguish between the groups of interest using motion generation information. These results also indicated that the error rate for identifying sincere and insincere efforts in persons without low back pain was much lower than that for patients with low back pain. This is probably due to a much better established central set for the asymptomatic subjects compared to the LBD subjects who needed to reestablish their central set to adapt to their injury. However, even for this low back pain group, the model was able to identify exacerbation of impairment 75% of the time. When the participant population was considered as a mixture of the two groups, the model performed better with an 18.5% error rate.

These results also produced an excellent balance between sensitivity and specificity. Although other models were found with better sensitivity *or* specificity, the emphasis of this study was to construct multivariate models that optimally identified both the sincere and insincere efforts. Ideally, one seeks a test that has 100% specificity and sensitivity, which indicates that the test agrees completely with the gold standard. In the case of sincerity, the gold standard is a function of how well the subjects complied with the experimental procedure. In addition, the subjects were not asked to vary their sincerity by any particular amount. Certain subjects may have chosen a level of insincerity that was close to their sincere level of effort and in this case it would be difficult to accurately interpret the meaning of the sensitivity and specificity measures. If participants were asked to choose a greater level of insincerity (e.g., pretend your back pain was severe), we would expect the distinction between the sincere and insincere conditions to be far better. Relative to other low back diagnostic measures, the sensitivity and specificity reported with torso motions compare very favorably. For example, commonly used neurological tests for lumbar disc herniation vary from single digits to 66% in terms of sensitivity and from 51% to 99% in terms of specificity (89).

These findings can be compared to previous studies that have tried to achieve these same goals. The summary of previous low back sincerity studies (Table 14.3) indicates that no previous study had employed a subject sample of sufficient size to adequately assess sensitivity or specificity.

14.4 SPINE LOADING OF THOSE EXPERIENCING LOW BACK PAIN

While multiple disorder pathways are potentially responsible for recurrent low back pain (6,90), a biomechanical source of low back disorders has historically been accepted as one potential pathway. Studies (91–93) have suggested that excessive mechanical loading on already compromised spinal structures can progressively affect disc degeneration, which may lead to chronic low back pain. Therefore, it is important to understand the mechanical loading of a LBP patient's spine during work tasks (such as lifting exertions) since this may represent a mechanism that further compromises the back's musculoskeletal system.

If one could understand, quantitatively, the characteristics of spine loading in patients with low back pain, then situations that might further exacerbate a low back disorder could be avoided. However, the mechanisms by which a history of low back pain increases risk have been poorly understood.

Several biomechanical studies have attempted to determine whether a history of low back pain results in greater spine loading and, potentially, an increase in low back pain risk. Many studies have identified differences in muscle recruitment patterns between individuals with low back pain and those not afflicted by low back pain (36,55,94,95). However, traditionally, it has been difficult to interpret these effects on spine loading (96). It has been suggested that, given the variability in muscle response in low back pain, the use of electromyography (EMG)-assisted models might be necessary to appreciate these differences (96). However, until recently, the use of EMG-assisted models with patients with low back pain has been problematic since there were no means to properly calibrate the EMG signal in such patients. This is true since patients with low back pain are reluctant to exert the maximum exertions necessary to calibrate the EMG signal.

Recently, an EMG normalization technique not requiring maximum exertions has been developed and validated that could be used with patients with low back pain (97,98). These advancements have permitted the first interpretation of spine loading for those suffering from low back pain (99). This study has demonstrated that after adjusting for differences in body mass (moment normalization), when patients with low back pain perform the exact same (kinematically controlled) lifting exertions as asymptomatic individuals, spine loading of patients with low back pain was 26% greater in compression and 70% greater in anterior–posterior (A/P) shear. Greater spine loading was due primarily to increases in muscle antagonistic coactivation presumably resulting from increased guarding and an increased need for stability. The study also found that when subjects were permitted to adapt their own lifting exertion style (as opposed to kinematically controlled exertions), patients with low back pain changed their kinematic patterns in an attempt to minimize the external moments (and spine loads) to which they were exposed. These findings suggest that subjects with low back pain have developed proprioceptive tolerance limits above which they are unwilling to load the body and, thus, adapt alternative lifting strategies. However, the realistic lifting environment often yields situations that make it difficult to employ alternative lifting strategies. In addition, since individuals with low back pain are typically heavier than asymptomatic individuals, they experience additional spine loading due to their greater body mass. This information suggests that lifting exertions performed by those with low back pain represent a substantially different situation compared to asymptomatic individuals.

An early investigation (99) of spine loading associated with patients with low back pain investigated controlled velocity sagittally symmetric lifts, exclusively, and compared LBP patients with asymptomatic individuals performing the same exertions. This investigation showed that even when the spine loadings were adjusted for the greater body mass of the LBP group (via moment normalization), significant increases in compression (26.3%) and lateral shear (75.5%) were present for the low back pain group, as shown in Fig. 14.7. In addition, the low back pain group exhibited statistically significant increases in muscle activities for all 10 muscles averaging 123% of the asymptomatic group values (Fig. 14.8). The coactivity index (a measure of the agonist muscle activities compared to antagonist muscle activities) for the low back pain group was also significantly larger compared to the asymptomatic group's index, suggesting that the low back pain group has nearly 50% more antagonistic muscle coactivation compared to the asymptomatic group. Hence, it appears that increased coactivation of the trunk muscles, also referred to as stability, has the effect of significantly increasing the compression and shear forces acting on the spine. These analyses indicate that when low back pain and asymptomatic subjects perform the same exact exertion, both the absolute and relative biomechanical costs to the patients with low back pain are much greater than for an asymptomatic individual. When this increase in spine loadings is coupled with the increased levels of proinflammatory cytokines (lower threshold for pain), we would expect that patients with low back pain are at a much greater risk of

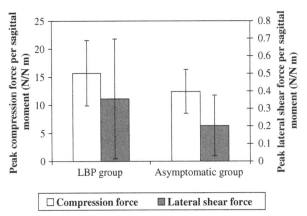

Figure 14.7   *Normalized lateral shear* and *Compression force* for individuals with low back pain and asymptomatic individuals for the controlled static exertions. (From reference 99).

recurrent low back pain. This situations has implications for the return to work for those suffering from low back pain.

Recent studies (100,101) have also suggested that spine tolerances to internal loads can also be compromised in those suffering from LBP. Excessive mechanical loading on already compromised spinal structures can progressively affect disc degeneration and may result in chronic low back pain. Therefore, it is important to understand, quantitatively, the mechanisms by which spine loading occurs in patients with low back pain so that we can compare spine loading due to patient activities with spine tolerance levels. This comparison would allow us to identify situations that might lead to further spine damage. Such an understanding would be useful for several purposes. First, it is important to understand spine loading in patients with low back pain so that they are not offered treatment modalities that might exacerbate the low

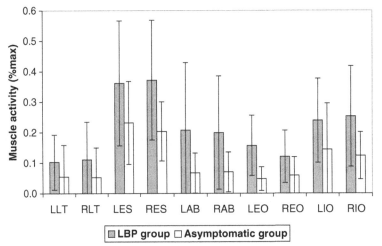

Figure 14.8   *Muscle activities* for the 10 trunk muscles (LLT—left latissimus dorsi, RLT—right latissimus dorsi, LES—left erector spinae, RES—right erector spinae, LRA—left rectus abdominus, RRA—right rectus abdominus, LEO—left external oblique, REO—right external oblique, LIO—left internal oblique, RIO—right internal oblique) for individuals with IBP and asymptomatic individuals for the controlled static exertions. (From reference 99).

back pain and result in pain chronicity. Second, this information would be important in matching the work performed by patients with low back pain to their spinal tolerance limits. Third, since we know that everyday activity is important for low back pain recovery, we can better understand the limits of these activities before further damage would be expected.

A recent study explored how three-dimensional spine loading compared in subjects experiencing low back pain compared to asymptomatic individuals among the variety of *unrestrained* lifting conditions and situations that would be expected of patients with low back pain as they returned to the workplace (102). The idea here was that the patient might compensate for their pain by changing their trunk kinematics and therefore compensate for the increased spine loads observed during the previous trunk velocity-controlled study. This study explored differences in vertical/horizontal lift origins as well as asymmetric lift origins between a relatively large group of patients and asymptomatic individuals (123 individuals).

Spine loads were significantly greater in the low back pain group compared to the asymptomatic group. Over all conditions, compression was about 11% greater and A/P shear about 18% greater in the patients with low back pain. Statistically significant increases in spine loading were noted as a function of lift origin region, lift asymmetry position, and the magnitude of the weight lifted for the low back pain group compared to the asymptomatic group among most of the dimensions of spine loading. Compression and A/P shear values were of greater magnitude and greater relative difference than the lateral shear values.

Figures 14.9 and 14.10 show the difference in compression and A/P shear, respectively, between the asymptomatic and low back pain groups as a function of lift origin region. Under all lift origin conditions, subjects with low back pain exhibited greater compression and A/P shear. However, the relative difference varied as a function of the region. Under the most biomechanically taxing lift origin region conditions, both compression and A/P shear differences between the subject groups were the smallest observed (10–13% difference in compression for the far-knee, far-waist, and knee regions, and 11–19% differences in A/P shear for the same lift origin regions), whereas the largest relative differences between the subject groups occurred at the least taxing lift origin regions (25–30% difference in compression for shoulder and waist regions and 24–35% difference in A/P shear for the same regions).

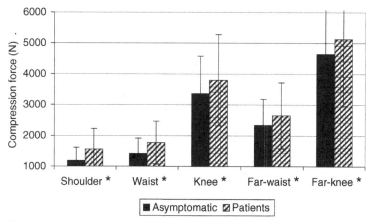

Figure 14.9 Compressive force as a function of lift origin and subject group (* indicates significant differences between groups, P < 0.05). (From reference 102).

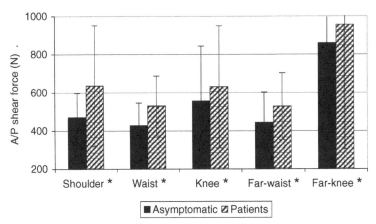

Figure 14.10 A/P shear force as a function of lift origin and subject group (* indicates significant differences between groups, $P < 0.05$). (From reference 102).

Similarly, patients with low back pain always exhibited greater compression and A/P shear loading under all symmetric/asymmetric conditions compared to the asymptomatic subjects. Figures 14.11 and 14.12 indicate that compression and A/P shear differences were greater between subject groups when lifting clockwise (CW) compared to lifting from counterclockwise (CCW) asymmetries (over twice as much compression difference between low back pain and asymptomatic groups when lifting in CW positions compared to CCW positions). The same trend held for A/P shear, but the differences were not as great, with greater differences between subject groups seen in CW lifts compared to CCW lifts (about 3% difference in increase between directions).

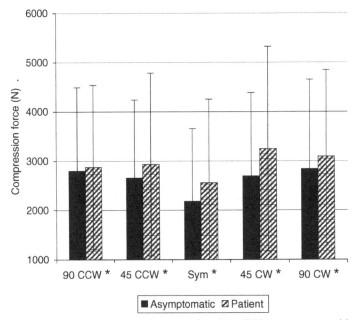

Figure 14.11 Compression force as a function of lift asymmetry position and subject group (* indicates significant difference between groups, $P < 0.05$). (From reference 102).

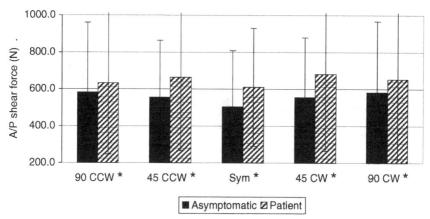

Figure 14.12   A/P shear force as a function of lift asymmetry position and subject group (* indicates significant difference between group, $P < 0.05$). (From reference 102).

A significant difference between low back pain and asymptomatic individuals also was present for the unique combinations (interaction) of lift origin region and asymmetry. Consistent with the previous patterns, patients with low back pain exhibited greater A/P shear loads under many of the condition combinations. As shown in Figs. 14.13 and 14.14, many of the lift origin/asymmetry combinations were significantly greater (20–30%) in A/P load for the low back pain group. Of particular interest were the differences in loads between subject groups at the far-knee origin region in combination with the CW and CCW asymmetries. Little difference existed in the symmetric A/P loads between subject groups. However, far greater A/P loads (15–30%) occurred at the asymmetric lifting positions under the far-knee lift origin regions. This condition was of particular concern since the loads approached or exceeded 1000 N in shear, which is often considered the tolerance limit for A/P shear (16).

Significant differences in compression and lateral shear occurred as a function of the weight handled between the low back pain and the asymptomatic group. In all cases, the low back pain group exhibited more loading compared to the asymptomatic group. However, the

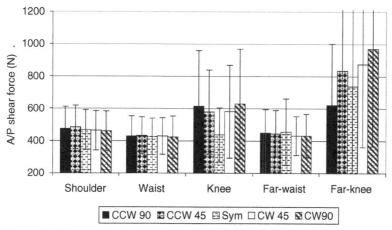

Figure 14.13   A/P shear lift origin by asymmetry position interaction for the asymptomatic group. (From reference 102).

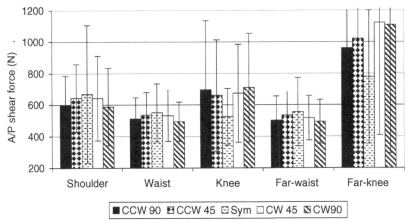

Figure 14.14 A/P shear lift origin by asymmetry position interaction for the patient group. (From reference 102).

differences in loading between subject groups were greatest at the lower weights of lift. Compression differences were approximately 3% different and lateral shear differences were about 5.3% different under the 4.5 kg lifting condition. As the weight increased, this difference in spine loading decreased to the point where at 11.4 kg the loading differences between subject groups were minimal due to weight lifted.

Significant muscle usage differences were observed between subjects groups. As with the earlier controlled trunk motion study, statistically greater activity was observed in the low back pain group for all muscle groups except for the erector spinae muscle group. Average increases in muscle activities in the low back pain group compared to the asymptomatic group were on the order of 32%.

This effort represents a step toward quantitatively matching a patient's specific abilities to an acceptable level of spine loading experienced during a lifting exertion. The load magnitudes selected for this study were purposely designed to represent the load magnitudes commonly recommended in return-to-work programs. The results demonstrate that in those suffering from low back pain, spine loading is increased relative to asymptomatic counterparts over a series of lifting exertions representative of those expected in a work environment.

Some of the most surprising findings of this study involved the nature of the relationship between the spine loadings of patients with low back pain and specific workplace conditions. The general pattern of spine loadings in asymptomatic individuals behaved as expected (103,104) varying as a function of lift origin region, lift asymmetry position, and weight lifted. However, the nature of the *differences* in spine loading patterns between patients with low back pain and asymptomatic subjects among the experimental conditions were not expected. These findings provide several significant insights into the functioning of the trunk's musculoskeletal system in response to the experience of low back pain. Several unique findings are worthy of discussion.

First, when the percent change in spine loading was considered as a function of lift origin region, larger differences between low back pain and asymptomatic groups were observed in lift origin regions that would be expected to be least stressful, biomechanically. In the cases of both compression and A/P shear, Figs. 14.9 and 14.10 indicated that the largest *difference* in loading between LBP patients and asymptomatic individuals occurred in the shoulder lift origin region followed by the waist lift origin region. In absolute terms, these lift origin regions are the least taxing on the biomechanical system. However, the relative increase in loading among subjects with low back pain compared to the asymptomatic group is large (25–35%) in these two regions. Thus, patients with low back pain pay a greater relative biomechanical cost for lifting in these regions. Most notably, the increased A/P shear observed in the shoulder lift origin region in the low back pain group resulted in a mean shear value that exceeded that in the knee lift origin region for both the low back pain and asymptomatic subjects, whereas A/P shear in the shoulder region was lower than that in the knee region for the asymptomatic subjects.

Examination of the kinematic profiles recorded during lifting exertions revealed that mean sagittal plane angular hip velocities and accelerations of patients with low back pain were equal to or even greater than those of the asymptomatic group under these presumably less taxing conditions. Hence, there appears to be a musculoskeletal trade-off where subjects with low back pain employ greater hip movement in lieu of torso motion. Examination of the EMG data recorded during the lifting exertions revealed significantly increased activities (up to 60%) for subjects with low back pain compared to the asymptomatic group in all muscles except the erector spinae group in the shoulder and waist lift origin regions. These findings indicate that the musculoskeletal system increases antagonistic coactivation as a means to control or stabilize or "guard" against this increased kinematic task demand. It is interesting that lesser erector spinae activity is displayed compared to the asymptomatic group. This indicates a very different coactivation strategy in the LBP group compared to the asymptomatic group. It is this "different" coactivation pattern that results in increases in spine loading in the LBP group.

Second, perhaps the most unexpected pattern involving *differences* in loading between the low back pain group and the asymptomatic group involved the asymmetric lift position variable. The differences in compression between the low back pain group and the asymptomatic groups were more than twice as large in the CW asymmetries compared to that in the CCW asymmetries. Such differences had not been reported earlier and indicate that we are either preprogrammed to prefer motions in the CCW direction, possibly as a function of hand preference, or we are conditioned to prefer CCW lift origins due to the physical layout of our environment.

Our results indicate little difference between CW and CCW compression values within the asymptomatic group, but show increases in compression in CW compared to CCW movements within the patients with low back pain. Further analyses revealed that spine lateral kinematics as well as pelvic rotation kinematics changed significantly between subject groups as a function of asymmetry position. Thus, indicating the adoption of alternative lifting strategies in the low back pain group. However, these adaptations occurred only as a function of CCW asymmetry. Kinematic measures were essentially the same during lifting in the CW direction for both groups of subjects. However, as was the case for differences observed as a function of lift origin region, the musculoskeletal system was taxed to a greater degree in the CW direction compared to the CCW direction. It is unclear why the low back pain group did not choose to adopt alternative lifting strategies in the CW direction as they did in the CCW direction.

Interesting differences in antagonistic coactivation also occurred as a function of the asymmetric lifting positions. Under most conditions, the low back pain group coactivated the trunk muscles to a much greater extent than did the asymptomatic group. Examination of the CW–CCW differences in EMG patterns indicated that patients with low back pain coactivated 8 of the 10 trunk muscles to a greater degree in the CW direction compared to the CCW direction. This greater muscle activation in the CW direction was responsible for the greater loading. It was also interesting that when the subject pain diagrams were reviewed, twice as many subjects reported right-side pain compared to left-side pain. Thus, the majority of subjects might have increased guarding when rotating CW. Certainly the increased tension in the trunk muscles resulting from this coactivation would place patients with low back pain at a greater risk of activating both the structural disruption and muscle function disruption pain pathways discussed in Chapter 5.

Third, to a lesser extent than expected, load weight magnitude also played a role in spine loading differences between low back pain and asymptomatic subjects. In general, larger differences between the low back pain and asymptomatic subjects groups were observed at the lower weight levels, but these differences were rather minor compared to the asymmetry and lift origin differences. As with the other significant spine loading differences, differences in loading could also be explained by differences in muscle coactivations. These findings again suggest that the *largest differences in spine loading between asymptomatic subjects and patients with low back pain are found in the least taxing conditions*.

One might question why the relative differences in loading were greater in the least taxing biomechanical conditions. It would appear that these less biomechanically taxing positions provide the opportunity for patients with low back pain to increase spine coactivity in an attempt to increase spine stability (105–107). There is no need for an intact (asymptomatic) individual to cocontract to the same degree as LBP patients in these postures. However, under the more taxing external loading conditions, both groups of subjects sense the need to control trunk motion and stability to a greater degree and, therefore, coactivate the trunk muscles. In addition, under greater external loading condition, system stability is inherent with greater magnitude loads. Thus, the difference between the groups is diminished. Hence, compared to asymptomatic workers, it appears that the least taxing activities would contribute relatively more to a cumulative trauma index compared to the more taxing tasks (108–110).

As a general example of this relationship, Fig. 14.15 shows our typical load–tolerance relationship for a range of low, medium, and high external loading magnitudes for a LBP patient and asymptomatic person. The figure shows the expected tolerance limits that would most likely be related to proinflammatory cytokine upregulation tolerance limits (at least for the LBP patient). By examining the relationship between load and tolerance for both LBP patients and asymptomatic workers, we see that the loading for the LBP patient is much greater than that for the asymptomatic worker under the low force conditions but approach the same levels of magnitude as those for the asymptomatic worker exposed to greater

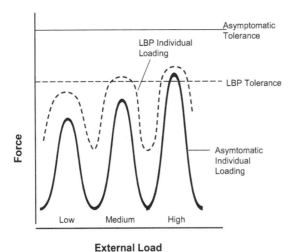

Figure 14.15 Load–tolerance relationship for different levels of external load applied to LBP and asymptomatic workers.

external loads. However, comparing the relationship of the load to the tolerances, we see that the load approaches or exceeds the tolerance for the LBP patient, although this occurs only at the high loads for the asymptomatic worker.

Thus, exertion conditions that would be considered relatively low stress, and would be considered good candidates for return to work tasks, may be more costly from a biomechanical perspective than expected. These findings are consistent with previous epidemiologic observations (99) that found that "pain associated with carrying out simple daily movements" was the best indicator of low back pain relapse. Hence, their findings may indicate that the patients were experiencing greater spine loading in these simple tasks than would be expected.

14.5   CAN KINEMATIC IMPAIRMENT ASSESSMENTS PREDICT CHANGES IN SPINE LOADING?

Given the increased spine loading expected of LBP patients during lifting exertions, it would be desirable to predict the degree to which patients with low back pain would increase their spine loading given their low back pain status, so that activity limitations could be quantitatively prescribed. Traditionally, strength-based functional capacity assessments have been employed in an effort to match the abilities of the patient with low back pain with task demands to determine when an individual may return to physically demanding activities. A multitude of capacity measures, such as strength and range of motion, have been employed to characterize the abilities of the patient with low back pain in an attempt to determine when a patient's abilities have returned to normal or determine when the patient's abilities meet job demands (57,111–115). However, these measures do not reflect the underlying changes in spine loading that occur in the individual with low back pain that might potentially result in exacerbation of low back pain. Thus, a void exists in that we have no means to estimate how the extent of low back pain impairment relates to the increases in spine loading associated with an exertion.

We have just seen that trunk kinematics has been shown to be related to occupational LBP risk (9–11) as well as spine loading (12–18) in asymptomatic subjects. Efforts have also been able to demonstrate that torso *kinematic compromise* is a sensitive indicator of the degree of low back pain impairment. The torso kinematic profile is believed to reflect the torso's motor recruitment patterns adopted by the patient (21,22,117). In addition, we have just seen that patients with low back pain experience significantly greater spine loads compared to asymptomatic individuals. Hence, it is reasonable to expect that spine kinematics deficits might relate to changes in spine load in the patient with low back pain, and this relationship might provide insight into the spine loads expected in the patient returning to the workplace.

To assess the relationship between an individual's kinematic status and spine loading, a study was performed where a kinematic pretest evaluated patients with low back pain and asymptomatic individuals for their degree of torso kinematic compromise using the validated kinematic testing methodology discussed earlier in this chapter (117). A laboratory study employing the same population of subjects evaluated spine loadings for both groups of subjects as they lifted a variety of loads from a spectrum of lift origin locations. Kinematic performance measures and lifting condition information were used to develop a model that predicted spine loads for all subjects. One hundred and twenty-three subjects participated in this study.

The relationship between the kinematic performance measures (describing low back impairment) and the spine loading measures obtained during the lifting exertions were evaluated for evidence of significant relationships. Variables were selected and used to develop a statistical model that described the relationship between $p(n)$, the physical characteristics of the

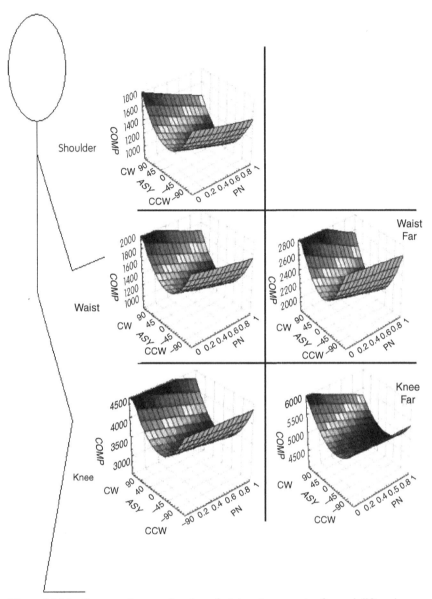

Figure 14.16   Compression as a function of $p(n)$ and asymmetry for each lift region ($pN = 1 = $ normal asymptomatic worker). (From reference 117).

experimental condition (lift origin, asymmetry, and weight) in predicting spine loading over the range of $p(n)$ for each loading dimension. Statistics indicating the degree of variability in spine loading explained by the kinematic compromise (pseudo-R^2 values) estimate that the degree of kinematic compromise (measure as $p[n]$) can explain 87%, 61%, and 65% of the variability in spine compression, A/P shear, and lateral shear, respectively.

As an example of this relationship, Figs. 14.16 and 14.17 describe the compression and A/P shear behavior, respectively, for this model as a function of lift asymmetry and the $p(n)$ measure for all lift origin regions. These figures indicate how spine loading is expected to vary as $p(n)$ goes from 0 (fully impaired) to 1.0 (average of the asymptomatic individual) for

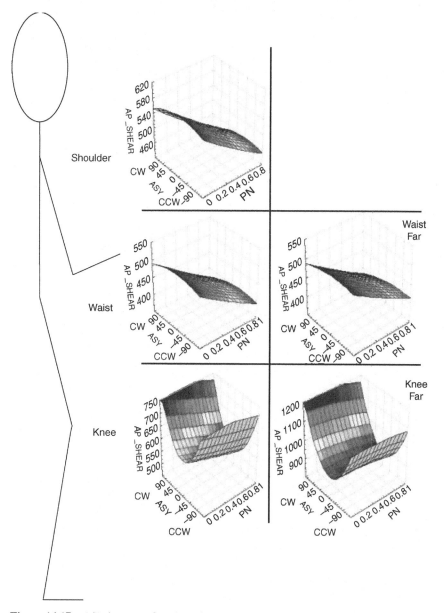

Figure 14.17   A/P shear as a function of $p(n)$ and asymmetry for each lift region (pN = 1 = normal asymptomatic worker). (From reference 117).

the combinations of different origins and asymmetries. Much greater differences between asymptomatic and low back pain spine compressions were observed when lifting from CW lift origins compared to CCW lift origins.

As seen in Fig. 14.18, compression could vary by more than 1000 N as kinematic capacity varies. Increases in spine loading in kinematically impaired subjects were as large as 79% over the range of $p(n)$ under some conditions. Figure 14.18 indicates how the $p(n)$ variable interacts with the load weight lifted to yield differences in spine compression. In general, compression increased by 2% for every 1 kg increase in weight lifted. Similar relationships were developed for A/P and lateral shear forces. A/P shear increased by 2% for

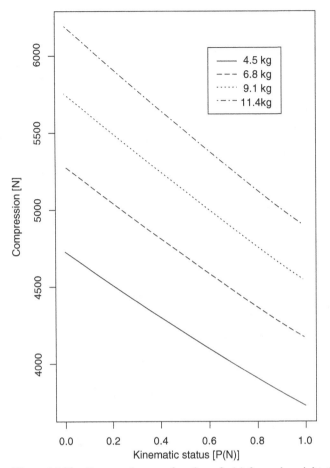

Figure 14.18   Compression as a function of $p(n)$ for each weight. (pN = 1 = normal asymptomatic worker). (From reference 117).

each kilogram increase in weight, whereas lateral shear force increased by nearly 3% for every kilogram increase in weight lifted.

This evaluation has been able to estimate the degree of increased spine loading expected as a function of kinematic compromise and the physical characteristics of the lifting situation of the patient with low back pain. Since the study contained a relatively large subject population (over 100 subjects) for a detailed biomechanical study, the statistical power permitted us to assess, in detail, the response of the musculoskeletal system.

Examination of the results indicated that when loading was increased in patients with low back pain compared to asymptomatic individuals there was a "mismatch" between kinematic task demands and the kinematic abilities of the patient with low back pain. The patient with low back pain responded with increased torso muscle coactivation resulting in significantly greater loading compared to an asymptomatic individual.

For example, under many lifting exertion conditions where the largest differences in loading between subject groups were noted (Fig. 14.14), the average peak sagittal velocity during lifting for both groups was about the same. However, the kinematic capacity (impairment assessment measures) of the two subject groups observed was significantly different with larger relative kinematic deficits seen with subjects with low back pain (relative to the asymptomatic subjects). Thus, a kinematic mismatch between task demands versus. subject kinematic status appears to reflect the differences in spine loading between the low back pain and asymptomatic group via a muscle coactivation mechanism.

Perhaps the most remarkable finding of this study was the ability to characterize these underlying mismatches and their subsequent effect on spine loading through a relatively simple model. The model reflects spine compression best (explaining 87% of the variability) and spine A/P shear moderately well (explaining 61% of the variability). Thus, this model can predict changes in spine loads (compared to an asymptomatic individual) given the lifting situation and the degree of a LBP patient's kinematic compromise.

These findings have significant implications for the return to work of individuals with low back pain in that given kinematic capabilities of a patient with low back pain, it would be possible to quantitatively determine which specific work activities might compromise the rehabilitation of the patient. Thus, patients with low back pain could return to work sooner if one could determine which specific tasks should be avoided. In addition, periodic remonitoring of the patient's kinematic status would reveal when the patient with low back pain would be able to return to more demanding tasks without risk of excessive mechanical spine loading. Hence, these findings suggest that it is possible to minimize exposure to activities that might be responsible for a recurring back problem exacerbated by mechanical loading.

Collectively, this study indicated that valuable information is contained within kinematic information relative to the recruitment pattern and functioning of the musculo-skeletal system. Based on these results, it is highly likely that trunk kinematic deficits are reflective of increase in trunk muscle coactivation that probably arise from a desire of the patient with low back pain to increase guarding and stability but also result in greater loading. These findings also suggest that those jobs that would be expected to impose the least amount of risk may involve far more spine loading than expected. It appears that patients with low back pain experience greater levels of coactivity (compared to asymptomatic subjects) under conditions where externally imposed loads are minimal. It is assumed that the increase in coactivity is intended to increase stability in situations where stability is marginal.

14.6   LIFTING EXPOSURE LIMITS FOR WORKERS WITH LBP

These previous investigations have demonstrated that spine loading is a function of back health status (impairment) as well as where (in space) a worker is lifting a load. The previously mentioned studies have shown that we can reasonably estimate spine loads if we simply know the origin of the lift as defined by different lifting "zones." Furthermore, if we understand the low back impairment status of the worker, we can also show how loading differs for an asymptomatic worker compared to a worker with LBP.

Recently, a study was performed for the Ohio Bureau of Workers' Compensation to identify safe lifting limits for workers who were returning to work after suffering a low back pain event (118). A large group of workers with muscle-based LBP as well as a large group of age- and gender-matched asymptomatic individuals were asked to lift from various lifting zones. Using the low back impairment tool described earlier (lumbar motion monitor based kinematic assessment), the LBP group was found to have an average impairment rating $p[n]$ of 0.13. The lifting zones varied in height off the floor (four zones) and distance from the spine (two zones) as well as asymmetric locations (five zones). A biologically assisted biomechanical model was used to analyze spine loads for compression, A/P shear, and lateral shear as the asymptomatic and LBP workers lifted from these different zones. Spine loads were compared with traditional spine tissue tolerance limits to identify acceptable lifting limits for the LBP workers compared to the asymptomatic workers.

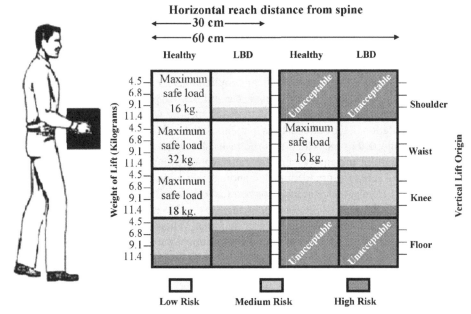

Guidelines for lifts involving
trunk-twisting angle* +/- 30 degrees

*Angle in which the person doing the lifting will twist (left and/or right)

Figure 14.19   Acceptable lifting limits for asymptomatic versus LBP workers when lifting in zones within ±30° of symmetric. (From reference 118).

The results of these investigations are reported in Figs. 14.19–14.21 for three asymmetric lift origins. The figures indicate the horizontal reach distance zones of 30 or 60 cm and vertical lift origins defined as floor, knee, waist, or shoulder levels. Each zone shows acceptable lifting load limits for both asymptomatic and workers with low back pain. These values vary from 4.5 to 11.4 kg for LBP workers and can range to 32 kg for asymptomatic workers. The values are pattern coded to indicate low risk, medium risk, or unacceptable zones and weight combinations. Note that acceptable lifting limits can vary up to a factor of 3 between LBP and asymptomatic workers. This demonstrates the strong influence of the muscle recruitment system (internal loads) to determine spine loading in asymptomatic workers compared to LBP workers. Thus, it is important to accommodate LBP workers and adjust their lifting exposure when they return to work.

14.7   RECURRENCE OF LBP AND WORK

One of the significant problems with interpreting recurrence rates concerns the lack of a standardized definition for recurrence. Some have proposed lost work time as a standard for

Guidelines for lifts involving
trunk-twisting angle*
between 30 and 60 degrees

*Angle in which the person doing the lifting will twist (left and/or right).

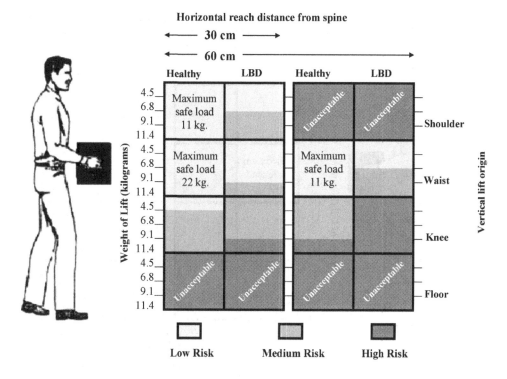

•Choose a column indicating whether the person has a lower-back disorder (LBD) or not (Healthy).

•Determine the region (zone) of the maximum horizontal reach distance (measured from spine to hands) and the vertical lift origin from the floor for each lift.

•The color-coded zones indicate degree of risk for LBD (green = low; yellow= medium; red = high).

•To minimize the risk of recurrent injury, change the lifting conditions so that the lifting weight is in the green areas.

Figure 14.20   Acceptable lifting limits for asymptomatic versus. LBP workers when lifting in zones between 30° and 60° of asymmetry (twisting). (From reference 118).

recurrence (119–121). Others have defined recurrence as report of an additional claim within a given period (5). Still others report recurrence as a function of pain symptom reports (121). One would expect different rates of recurrence depending on the nature of the definition adopted. Hence, the definition of low back pain recurrence should play a pivotal role in assessing predictors of recurrent low back pain.

As we have seen, the causal mechanisms behind low back pain are multidimensional, complex, and most likely, interactive. The source of low back pain can vary significantly and few low back pain reports can be associated with a specific anatomical problem. Causality sources range from muscular problems, to structural problems within the spine, to upregulation of cytokines at a specific site, and quite often are unknown. Each of these mechanisms may or may not initiate pain and each may have a very different potential for recurrence. One

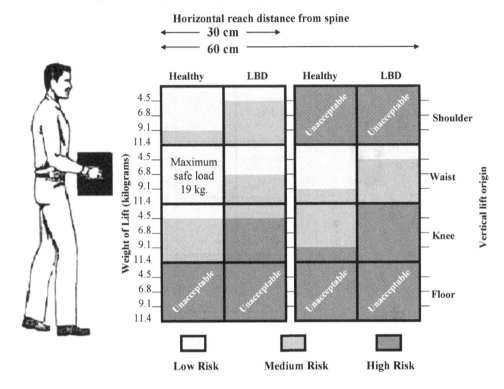

Guidelines for lifts involving
trunk-twisting angle*
between 30 and 60 degrees

*Angle in which the person doing the lifting will twist (left and/or right).

•Choose a column indicating whether the person has a lower-back disorder (LBD) or not (Healthy).

•Determine the region (zone) of the maximum horizontal reach distance (measured from spine to hands) and the vertical lift origin from the floor for each lift.

•The color-coded zones indicate degree of risk for LBD (green = low; yellow= medium; red = high).

•To minimize the risk of recurrent injury, change the lifting conditions so that the lifting weight is in the green areas.

Figure 14.21 Acceptable lifting limits for asymptomatic versus. LBP workers when lifting in zones between 60° and 90° of asymmetry (twisting). (From reference 118).

would expect that the mechanisms underlying recurrence might also be complex, multidimensional, and possibly different from the mechanisms involved in the initial onset of low back pain. Due to the complexity and many potential sources or initiators of pain, it is difficult to assess predictors of recurrence.

A recent study could help shed some light on the issue of recurrence (122). This study prospectively monitored workers who had reported a low back pain episode (due to work) as they returned to full duty work and identified, quantitatively, which factors and how much exposure to the contributing factors play a role in predicting low back pain recurrence as a function of four definitions of low back pain (symptoms, medical visits, lost time, and confirmed lost time) over the course of a 1-year period.

The study was designed to monitor industrial workers over the course of a 1-year period after returning to their full duty jobs following a low back pain report. When workers returned to full duty, five types of assessments were performed including (1) a low back kinematic functional assessments (discussed earlier in this chapter), (2) evaluation of the job physical demands, (3) psychosocial assessment of the job environment, (4) self-reported impairment including perception of symptoms and psychological measures, and (5) personal factors including anthropometry and low back pain history. Workers were monitored to assess recurrence according to the four different definitions of low back pain recurrence.

In this investigation, 206 patients were followed as they returned to their jobs in 41 different industrial work environments. Recurrence rates varied depending on the definition of recurrence. A monotonic decrease in recurrence reporting occurred as the definition of recurrence became more restrictive. For example, when recurrence was defined simply as the presence of pain, 58% of the population reported a recurrence. However, when recurrence was defined as lost workdays, which had to be confirmed with the employer, recurrence rates fell to 10%.

This investigation yielded several general observations worthy of mention. First, none of the psychosocial workplace measures yielded statistically significant differences for any of the LBP recurrence definitions.

Second, none of the physical workplace measures, by themselves, demonstrated a statistically significant difference among nonrecurrent and recurrent low back pain cases when the most restrictive definition of recurrence was used. However, as the definition of low back pain recurrence became more liberal, more of the physical workplace factors were able to distinguish between LBP recurrence groups, indicating that more subjective reports of low back pain were associated with a job's physical requirements.

Third, a large difference in the number of statistically significant kinematic functional assessment measures were noted between the recurrent and nonrecurrent low back pain groups as a function of the recurrence definition. The most liberal measure of recurrence (pain) yielded half the number of significant differences in kinematic functional abilities as compared to the three more restrictive definitions of low back pain recurrence.

Fourth, subjective symptom measures tended to be significantly different between recurrent and nonrecurrent groups regardless of the definition of recurrence. Specifically, the Million visual analog scale (VAS), which measures subjective impairment of activities of daily living, the McGill Pain Questionnaire Present Pain Intensity Score as well as several other subscores, the NASS symptom questionnaire, and several SF-36 Health Survey scores were equally responsive to all low back pain recurrence outcomes.

Fifth, of the personal/anthropometric measures, only marital status and education distinguished between recurrence groups for the most restrictive definition of low back pain recurrence (confirmed lost time), whereas hours worked, overtime, restricted days, and lost days (prior to return to work) indicated a statistically different profile between recurrence groups for the less restrictive definitions of recurrence (pain reporting and medical visits).

A multiple logistic regression model of recurrence based on the various recurrence definitions is shown in Table 14.4. This table shows the combination of variables that best distinguish between those patients who experience a low back pain recurrence based on the four definitions of recurrence. This table indicates that recurrence can be estimated with surprisingly good sensitivity and specificity. In addition, the multivariate models indicate that different variables are important in predicting different recurrence definitions. It is interesting to note that the most subjective definition of recurrence (pain) can be predicted using two self-reported perception of impairment variables, one variable from the kinematic functional assessment, physical workplace measures, and psychosocial measures. It is also interesting to note that some of the variables employed in the multivariate model contribute to prediction in combination with

TABLE 14.4   Model Parameters Derived from the Five Types of Assessments that Best Predict Recurrence (as Distinguished by the Different Definitions of Recurrence) (From Reference 122)

Model parameter	Pain	Medical visits	Lost time	Confirmed lost time
Million visual analog score	72.0*	45.0*	86.0*	86*
SF-36 physical function	26.5*			
Sagittal flexion velocity at 15 left		11.2*		
Sagittal extension acceleration at 15 left			63.1*	59.8*
Sagittal range of motion at zero			33.4*	
Clinical lateral velocity (deg/sec)	48.9*			
Lateral acceleration demand to capacity				1.44
Mean load (kg)		88		
Mean moment (N m)	36			
Hours worked		48*		
Supervisor support	3.38			
Workload variance		2.84		
Role conflict				2.82
Sensitivity	79%	78%	79%	80%
Specificity	73%	74%	78%	80%

*The sensitivity and specificity indicate the ability of the multiple logistic regression model to identify LBP recurrence. Indicates significance P > 0.05 for univariate analysis.

other variables but are not significant predictors by themselves. The next most liberal definition of recurrence also employs at least one variable from each category of measures to predict recurrence. However, when the more restrictive measures of recurrence are evaluated, the models rely heavily on a combination of worker's perception of impairment response and two quantitative descriptions of the kinematic capacity of the worker. It was also notable that the most restrictive definitions of recurrence produced the best balance between sensitivity and specificity with confirmed lost time being predicted with sensitivity and specificity of 80%.

The predictive ability of the individual variables entering into the multiple logistic regression models are reported in Table 14.5. It is notable that, in general, the more objective predictors resulted in stronger odds ratios as the recurrence definition became more restrictive.

This study indicates that the variables that predict recurrence are a complex mix of perceptual impairment, psychophysical, kinematic ability, and physical demand variables. These findings emphasize the highly multidimensional nature of low back pain recurrence. However, the combination of variables that best predict recurrence is also highly dependent on how one defines low back pain recurrence. It is notable that the significant predictor variables shifted from a broad mix of all combinations of variable categories (i.e., perceptual, workplace, functional status, etc.) to a combination of only subjective impairment and physical ability categorical variables as the definition of recurrence becomes more restrictive. Thus, low back pain recurrence prediction is highly dependent on how it is defined.

These analyses provide insight into the causality issues associated with recurrent low back pain. Several points are worth noting in this respect. First, perhaps the most useful point associated with recurrence prediction is the ability to define categories of variables that contribute to the prediction of recurrence. In these analyses, all categories of variables that might predict recurrent low back pain based on the literature were included. As discussed earlier, different combinations of variables predict different definitions of recurrence. This confirms some of the previous contentions stated in the literature (119–121). These findings

TABLE 14.5 Odds Ratios (95% Confidence Intervals) for Variables that Entered the Final Models (From Reference 122)

Model parameter	Pain	Medical visits	Lost time	Confirmed lost time
Million visual analog score	7.70 (2.88–20.62)	4.13 (2.17–7.86)	6.19 (2.47–15.52)	10.00 (3.62–27.62)
SF-36 physical function	6.29 (3.14–12.59)			
Sagittal flexion velocity at 15 left		4.18 (2.22–7.86)		
Sagittal extension acceleration at 15 left			9.81 (3.26–29.47)	15.37 (3.46–68.37)
Sagittal range of motion at zero			2.84 (1.10–7.34)	
Clinical lateral velocity (deg/sec)	3.85 (2.08–7.16)			
Lateral acceleration demand to capacity				6.53 (1.47–29.00)
Mean load (kg)		1.53 (0.84–2.78)		
Mean moment (N m)	1.01 (0.58–1.79)			
Hours worked		2.79 (1.50–5.17)		
Supervisor support	3.39 (1.23–9.31)			
Workload variance		2.32 (1.28–4.26)		
Role conflict				2.91 (0.65–13.04)

suggest difficulty in interpreting much of the previous literature regarding recurrence unless the definition of recurrence is clearly defined.

Second, we identified the specific categorical variables that produced the best models of recurrence. Our goal in model building was to produce models that had the least number of variables but that distinguished best between recurrence and nonrecurrence. With this understanding in mind, we observe that in the less restrictive definitions of recurrence, all classes of categorical variables play a role. It is interesting to note that some of these variables by themselves (e.g., psychosocial factors) do not play a role in identifying recurrence. However, when combined with other workplace, kinematic functional abilities, and perception of pain variables, they can identify pain reporting or visits to medical facilities well. Hence, pain reporting and experiencing symptoms severe enough to seek medical attention are driven by a number of psychometric impairment and physical factors, supporting a biopsychophysical model of pain recurrence. However, kinematic functional assessments played a major role along with perception in identifying lost time and confirmed lost time definitions of recurrence. It is interesting to note that the difference between these models is simply an addition of a (univariate) psychosocial role conflict variable and demand–capacity variable that in combination with perceptual and kinematic functional assessment variables produced the highest levels of sensitivity and specificity (80% each).

Third, the increasing importance of the kinematic functional assessments as a function of more restrictive definitions of recurrence suggests a greater biomechanical role in the more restrictive definitions of recurrence. While workplace analyses indicated that most jobs to which workers returned would be classified as moderate risk via quantitative work assessment tools (9,10), laboratory assessments of deficits in kinematic abilities have reported much greater spine loading of patients who suffered kinematic impairments compared to patients who possessed greater kinematic capacities (117). Hence, collectively, these findings suggest that patients returning to the workplace with less kinematic capacity were experiencing greater spine loadings as they performed their regular jobs. This suggests caution in early return to work unless the patient's kinematic functional abilities are near normal when they return to even moderately demanding jobs.

It should also be noted that the difference between lost time and confirmed lost time may be driven by the severity of the pain or reporting policy. Postreporting interviews with the patients described some unexpected reporting issues. Some patients felt their jobs would be in jeopardy if they reported a low back pain problem so they took a personal day off or a vacation day. In other instances, company policy was such that lost days were not associated with a report unless a minimum of two lost days occurred. Thus, some of the data in this category may reflect a more restrictive definition of recurrence than originally thought.

The differences among the trends associated with different definitions of low back pain recurrence are remarkable. It is interesting to observe how the individual variables, by themselves, related to recurrence. Surprisingly, psychosocial factors and many of the workplace physical factors played little role in predicting recurrence, especially when the more restrictive definitions of recurrence are considered. This may emphasize that low back pain recurrence is very different in nature from the initial low back pain event and is influenced by very different factors. Perceptions of pain and low back impairment, as well as objective measures of physical abilities (kinematic functional assessments), appear to play much greater role in predicting recurrence. These pain perceptions may be a result of the upregulation of cytokines and the resultant increase in sensitivity that is often observed once one develops low back pain.

14.8 A RETURN-TO-WORK STRATEGY

Considering these findings collectively provides some insight into a proper return-to-work strategy. First, since spine loading of workers returning to the workplace is heavily influenced by kinematic mismatch between the job-defined kinematics and the worker's kinematic ability, it is important to make sure the worker is returned to a job that is designed in such a way that risk to the low back is minimum from a kinematic standpoint. Chapter 11 discusses methods to assess the contribution of kinematics to overall risk. Next, it is important to assess the kinematic capacity of the worker. As shown in Fig. 14.17, kinematic compromise can seriously impact spine loading. Thus, the risk of recurrence is related to the kinematic capacity of the job compared to the abilities of the worker. Ideally, the worker's $p(n)$ should be above 0.5 (the value at which a person is classified as normal) before return to work. Finally, attitudes about the workers pain should be considered via the MVAS. Activities of daily living should not be a challenge to the worker when returning to work. As with most primary low back pain, this strategy represents a systematic approach to managing the various components and risk factors for low back pain.

14.9 CONCLUSIONS

This chapter has shown that secondary or recurrent low back pain represents a major challenge to those responsible for the design of work expected to accommodate someone recovering from low back pain. There appears to be a significant biomechanical cost to returning to the workplace with low back pain symptoms. Laboratory studies have indicated that spine loading is up to 70% greater (especially in shear) for the individual with low back pain compared to an asymptomatic individual performing the exact same task. This increased loading is due to increased coactivation of the torso muscles in the individual with low back pain, presumably in an attempt to stabilize and "guard" the back. However, this response requires a high biomechanical cost.

This assessment has also shown that it is possible to predict increases in spine loading by monitoring the patients kinematic capacity. Using these quantitative tools to assess the individual's capacity for natural kinematic motion and comparing this to the requirements of the work, it is possible to match the work requirements to the worker.

It is possible to predict low back pain recurrence, but it depends heavily on the definition of recurrence. The most accurate predictions can be made for the least subjective measures of recurrence and involve a multidimensional combination of patient kinematic capacity, task demands, subjective well-being, and psychosocial response. This information confirms that there are many factors that could activate low back pain pathways discussed earlier, and that these pathways are similar to that for the initial exposure to low back pain. However, a major difference with recurrent low back pain is that the load tolerance is greatly reduced before the activation of pain pathway. Thus, interventions that are beneficial for the recurrence of low back pain can also minimize the initial onset of low back pain.

Finally, these efforts simply begin to help us understand the mechanisms of recurrent low back pain and work. Future studies need to delineate the role of the interactions among risk factors in triggering the low back pain pathway. In addition, future studies need to define more precisely how much tissue loading is necessary to exceed the pain initiation thresholds (i.e., upregulation of cytokines, tissue damage, etc.).

KEY POINTS

- Spine loading is generally much greater in those suffering from low back pain due to cocontraction of the trunk muscles. This cocontraction is presumed to be a result of guarding and an attempt to increase stability.

- Kinematic deficits have also been noted in those suffering from low back pain, and this deficit can be quantified.

- The degree of kinematic deficits is linearly related to the increases in spine loading compared to an asymptomatic individual.

- Recurrence depends heavily on the definition of recurrence. More restrictive and objective definitions are a function of (1) perceptions about the ability to perform daily activities, (2) kinematic compromise of the back, (3) the kinematic demands of the job to which the worker is returning, and (4) the role conflict environment of the work.

- Return-to-work strategies should include (1) assessment of the kinematic and job requirements of the job to which the worker is returning, (2) an assessment of kinematic compromise, (3) evaluation of worker perceptions about their health, and (4) evaluation of psychosocial status (role conflict).

REFERENCES

1. SMEDLEY J, et al. Prospective cohort study of predictors of incident low back pain in nurses. Br Med J 1997;314 (7089):1225–1228.

2. van POPPEL MN, et al. Risk factors for back pain incidence in industry: a prospective study. Pain 1998; 77(1):81–86.

3. FERGUSON SA, MARRAS WS. A literature review of low back disorder surveillance measures and risk factors. Clin Biomech 1997;12:211–226.

4. PAPAGEORGIOU AC, et al. Influence of previous pain experience on the episode incidence of low back pain: results from the South Manchester Back Pain Study. Pain 1996;66(2–3):181–185.

5. MACDONALD MJ, et al. A descriptive study of recurrent low back pain claims. J Occup Environ Med 1997;39 (1):35–43.

6. NRC. Musculoskeletal disorders and the workplace: low back and upper extremity. Panel on Musculoskeletal Disorders at the Workplace. Washington (DC): National Academy of Sciences, National Research Council, National Academy Press; 2001 p.492.

7. HAMRICK C. CTDs Ergonomics in Ohio. International Ergonomics Association (IEA) 2000/Human Factors and Ergonomics Society (HFES) 2000 Congress; San Diego (CA): Human Factors and Ergonomics Society; 2000.

8. FERGUSON SA, MARRAS WS, GUPTA P. Longitudinal quantitative measures of the natural course of low back pain recovery. Spine 2000;25(15):1950–1956.

9. MARRAS WS, et al. Biomechanical risk factors for occupationally related low back disorders. Ergonomics 1995;38(2):377–410.

10. MARRAS WS. et al. The role of dynamic three-dimensional trunk motion in occupationally-related low back disorders. The effects of workplace factors, trunk position, and trunk motion characteristics on risk of injury. Spine 1993;18(5):617–628.

11. MARRAS WS. et al. Prospective validation of a low-back disorder risk model and assessment of ergonomic interventions associated with manual materials handling tasks. [in process citation]. Ergonomics 2000;43 (11):1866–1886.

12. FATHALLAH FA, MARRAS WS, PARNIANPOUR M. An assessment of complex spinal loads during dynamic lifting tasks. Spine 1998;23(6):706–716.

13. GRANATA KP, MARRAS WS. The influence of trunk muscle coactivity on dynamic spinal loads. Spine 1995;20(8):913–919.

14. GRANATA KP, MARRAS WS. Relation between spinal load factors and the high-risk probability of occupational low-back disorder. Ergonomics 1999;42(9):1187–1199.

15. MARRAS WS, DAVIS KG, SPLITTSTOESSER RE. Spine loading during whole body free dynamic lifting. Columbus (OH): The Ohio State University; 2001. p.84.

16. MARRAS WS, GRANATA KP. Spine loading during trunk lateral bending motions. J Biomech 1997;30(7):697–703.

17. MARRAS WS, GRANATA KP. Changes in trunk dynamics and spine loading during repeated trunk exertions. Spine 1997;22(21):2564–2570.

18. MARRAS WS, GRANATA KP. A biomechanical assessment and model of axial twisting in the thoracolumbar spine. Spine 1995;20(13):1440–1451.

19. MARRAS WS, WONGSAM PE, FLEXIBILITY velocity of the normal and impaired lumbar spine. Arch Phys Med Rehabil 1986;67(4):213–217.

20. MARRAS WS, et al. The classification of anatomic- and symptom-based low back disorders using motion measure models. Spine 1995;20(23):2531–2546.

21. MARRAS WS, et al. The quantification of low back disorder using motion measures. Methodology and validation. Spine 1999;24(20):2091–2100.

22. MARRAS WS, et al. Impairment magnification during dynamic trunk motions. Spine 2000;25(5):587–595.

23. WADDELL G, ALLAN D, NEWTON M. Clinical evaluation of disability in low back pain, In The Adult Spine: Principles and Practice. FRYMOYER JW, editor. Philadelphia: Lippincott-Raven; 1997.171–183.

24. TEASELL RW, HARTH M. Functional restoration. Returning patients with chronic low back pain to work—revolution or fad? Spine 1996;21(7):844–847.

25. DILLANE J, FRY J, KALTON G. Acute back syndrome: a study from general practice. Br Med J ,1966;2:82–84.

26. SPIELER EA, et al. Recommendations to guide revision of the guides to the evaluation of permanent impairment. J Am Med Assoc 2000;283(4):519–523.

27. Insurance. U.S. Board of Disability, Disability Evaluation Under Social Security; A Handbook for Physicians. U.S. Government Printing Office; 1970 .

28. FRYMOYER JW, A practical guide to current United States impairment rating: a critical analysis. In FRYMOYER JW, editor. The Adult Spine: Principles and Practice. New York: Raven Press; 1991.

29. SPRATT KF, et al. A new approach to the low-back physical examination. Behavioral assessment of mechanical signs. Spine 1990;15(2):96–102.

30. BRADLEY LA, et al. Comment on "personality organization as an aspect of back pain in a medical setting". J Person Assess 1978;42(6):573–578.

31. GRABINER MD, KOH TJ, EL GHAZAWI A. Decoupling of bilateral paraspinal excitation in subjects with low back pain. Spine 1992;17(10):1219–1223.

32. AHERN DK, et al. Comparison of lumbar paravertebral EMG patterns in chronic low back pain patients and non-patient controls. Pain 1988;34(2):153–160.

33. TRIANO JJ, SCHULTZ AB. Correlation of objective measure of trunk motion and muscle function with low-back disability ratings. Spine 1987;12(6):561–565.

34. PAQUET N, MALOUIN F, RICHARDS CL. Hip–spine movement interaction and muscle activation patterns during sagittal trunk movements in low back pain patients. Spine 1994;19(5):596–603.

35. WATSON PJ, et al. Surface electromyography in the identification of chronic low back pain patients: the development of the flexion relaxation ratio. Clin Biomech (Bristol, Avon) 1997;12(3):165–171.

36. HUBLEY-KOZEY CL, VEZINA MJ. Differentiating temporal electromyographic waveforms between those with chronic low back pain and healthy controls. Clin Biomech (Bristol, Avon) 2002;17(9–10):621–629.

37. NEWCOMER KL, et al. Muscle activation patterns in subjects with and without low back pain. Arch Phys Med Rehabil 2002;83(6):816–821.

38. LEINONEN V, et al. Back and hip extensor activities during trunk flexion/extension: effects of low back pain and rehabilitation. Arch Phys Med Rehabil 2000; 81(1):32–37.

39. NOUWEN A, VAN AKKERVEEKEN PF, VERSLOOT JM. Patterns of muscular activity during movement in patients with chronic low-back pain. Spine 1987;12 (8):777–782.

40. HODGES PW. Changes in motor planning of feedforward postural responses of the trunk muscles in low back pain. Exp Brain Res 2001;141(2):261–266.

41. PEACH JP, MCGILL SM. Classification of low back pain with the use of spectral electromyogram parameters. Spine 1998;23(10):1117–1123.

42. ROY SH, et al. Spectral electromyographic assessment of back muscles in patients with low back pain undergoing rehabilitation. Spine 1995;20(1):38–48.

43. KLEIN AB, et al. Comparison of spinal mobility and isometric trunk extensor forces with electromyographic spectral analysis in identifying low back pain. Phys Ther 1991;71(6):445–454.

44. MAYER TG, et al. Lumbar myoelectric spectral analysis for endurance assessment. A comparison of normals with deconditioned patients. Spine 1989;14(9):986–991.

45. BIEDERMANN HJ, et al. Power spectrum analyses of electromyographic activity. Discriminators in the differential assessment of patients with chronic low-back pain. Spine 1991;16(10):1179–1184.

46. LARIVIERE C, et al. Evaluation of measurement strategies to increase the reliability of EMG indices to assess back muscle fatigue and recovery. J Electromyogr Kinesiol 2002;12(2):91–102.

47. ODDSSON LI, De LUCA CJ. Activation imbalances in lumbar spine muscles in the presence of chronic low back pain. J Appl Physiol 2003;94(4):1410–1420.

48. KANKAANPAA M, et al. Back and hip extensor fatigability in chronic low back pain patients and controls. Arch Phys Med Rehabil 1998;79(4):412–417.

49. SHERMAN RA, Relationships between strength of low back muscle contraction and reported intensity of chronic low back pain. Am J Phys Med 1985;64 (4):190–200.

50. COOPER RG, et al. Increased central drive during fatiguing contractions of the paraspinal muscles in patients with chronic low back pain. Spine 1993;18 (5):610–616.

51. ALEXIEV AR. Some differences of the electromyographic erector spinae activity between normal subjects and low back pain patients during the generation of isometric trunk torque. Electromyogr Clin Neurophysiol 1994;34(8):495–499.

52. ROBINSON ME, et al. Lumbar iEMG during isotonic exercise: chronic low back pain patients versus controls. J Spinal Disord 1992;5(1):8–15.

53. LAMOTH CJ, et al. Effects of chronic low back pain on trunk coordination and back muscle activity during walking: changes in motor control. Eur Spine J 2006; 15(1):23–40.

54. PIROUZI S, et al. Low back pain patients demonstrate increased hip extensor muscle activity during standardized submaximal rotation efforts. Spine 2006;31(26): E999–E1005.

55. DANNEELS LA, et al. Differences in electromyographic activity in the multifidus muscle and the iliocostalis lumborum between healthy subjects and patients with sub-acute and chronic low back pain. Eur Spine J 2002;11(1):13–19.

56. MANDELL PJ, et al. Isokinetic trunk strength and lifting strength measures, Differences and similarities between low-back-injured and noninjured workers. Spine 1993; 18(16):2491–2501.

57. KISHINO ND, et al. Quantification of lumbar function. Part 4, Isometric and isokinetic lifting simulation in normal subjects and low-back dysfunction patients. Spine 1985;10(10):921–927.

58. KUMAR S, DUFRESNE RM, Van SCHOOR T. Human trunk strength profile in flexion and extension. Spine 1995;20 (2):160–168.

59. MAYER TG, et al. Use of noninvasive techniques for quantification of spinal range-of-motion in normal subjects and chronic low-back dysfunction patients. Spine 1984;9(6):588–595.

60. MCINTYRE DR, et al. A comparison of the characteristics of preferred low-back motion of normal subjects and low-back-pain patients. J Spinal Disord 1991;4(1): 90–95.

61. HULTMAN G, et al. Body composition, endurance, strength, cross-sectional area, and density of MM erector spinae in men with and without low back pain. J Spinal Disord 1993;6(2):114–123.

62. NEWTON M, et al. Trunk strength testing with isomachines. Part 2. Experimental evaluation of the Cybex II Back Testing System in normal subjects and patients with chronic low back pain. Spine 1993;18(7):812–824

63. LEE JH, OOI Y, NAKAMURA K. Measurement of muscle strength of the trunk and the lower extremities in subjects with history of low back pain. Spine 1995;20 (18):1994–1996.

64. ITO T, et al. Lumbar trunk muscle endurance testing: an inexpensive alternative to a machine for evaluation. Arch Phys Med Rehabil 1996;77(1):75–79.

65. BRADY S, MAYER T, GATCHEL RJ. Physical progress and residual impairment quantification after functional restoration: Part II. Isokinetic trunk strength. Spine 1994;19 (4):395–400.

66. RUDY TE, et al. Body motion during repetitive isodynamic lifting: a comparative study of normal subjects and low-back pain patients. Pain 2003;105(1–2):319–326.

67. DESCARREAUX M, BLOUIN JS, TEASDALE N. Force production parameters in patients with low back pain and healthy control study participants. Spine 2004;29 (3):311–317.

68. MELLIN G, et al. A controlled study on the outcome of inpatient and outpatient treatment of low back pain. Part II. Effects on physical measurements three months after treatment. Scand J Rehabil Med 1989;21(2):91–95.

69. JAYARAMAN G, et al. A computerized technique for analyzing lateral bending behavior of subjects with normal and impaired lumbar spine. A pilot study. Spine 1994;19(7):824–832.

70. McCLURE PW, et al. Kinematic analysis of lumbar and hip motion while rising from a forward, flexed position in patients with and without a history of low back pain. Spine 1997;22(5):552–558.

71. MARRAS WS, et al. A normal database of dynamic trunk motion characteristics during repetitive trunk flexion and extension as a function of task asymmetry, age and gender. IEEE Trans 1994;2(3):137–146.

72. HORAK F, DIENER H. Cerebellar control of postural scaling and central set in stance. J Neurophysiol 1994;72: 479–493.

73. BATTIE MC, et al. Isometric lifting strength as a predictor of industrial back pain reports. Spine 1989;14(8):851–856.

74. CHENGALUR SN, et al. Assessing sincerity of effort in maximal grip strength tests. A J Phys Med Rehabil 1990;69(3):148–153.

75. HAZARD RG, REEVES V, FENWICK JW. Lifting capacity. Indices of subject effort. Spine 1992;17(9):1065–1070.

76. HAZARD RG, et al. Isokinetic trunk and lifting strength measurements: variability as an indicator of effort. Spine 1988;13(1):54–57.

77. ROBINSON ME, et al. Reproducibility of maximal versus submaximal efforts in an isometric lumbar extension task. J Spinal Disord 1991;4(4):444–448.

78. ROBINSON ME, et al. Effect of instructions to simulate a back injury on torque reproducibility in an isometric lumbar extension task. J Occup Rehabil 1992;2:191–199.

79. SMITH G, et al. Validation of a protocol for determining submaximal efforts in back strength assessment. Int Soc Biomech 1991;397–399.

80. HUPLI M, et al. Isokinetic performance capacity of trunk muscles: Part I: The effect of repetition on measurement of isokinetic performance capacity of trunk muscles among healthy controls and two different groups of low-back pain patients. Scand J Rehabil Med 1996;28(4):201–206.

81. LUOTO S, et al. Isokinetic performance capacity of trunk muscles: Part II. Coefficient of variation in isokinetic measurement in maximal effort and in submaximal effort. Scand J Rehabil Med 1996;28(4):207–210.

82. REID S, HAZARD RG, FENWICK JW. Isokinetic trunk-strength deficits in people with and without low-back pain: a comparative study with consideration of effort. J Spinal Disord 1991;4(1):68–72.

83. RENEMAN MF, et al. Testing lifting capacity: validity of determining effort level by means of observation. Spine 2005;30(2):E40–E46.

84. JAY MA, et al. Sensitivity and specificity of the indicators of sincere effort of the EPIC lift capacity test on a previously injured population. Spine 2000;25(11):1405–1412.

85. SIMONSEN JC. Coefficient of variation as a measure of subject effort. Arch Phys Med Rehabil 1995;76(6):516–520.

86. DVIR Z, KEATING J. Identifying feigned isokinetic trunk extension effort in normal subjects: an efficiency study of the DEC. Spine 2001;26(9):1046–1051.

87. DVIR Z, KEATING JL. Trunk extension effort in patients with chronic low back dysfunction. Spine 2003;28(7):685–692.

88. KROEMER KH, MARRAS WS. Towards an objective assessment of the "maximal voluntary contraction" component in routine muscle strength measurements. Eur J Appl Physiol 1980;45(1):1–9.

89. DEYO RA, DIEHL AK. Lumbar spine films in primary care: current use and effects of selective ordering criteria. J Gen Intern Med 1986;1(1):20–25.

90. NRC. Work-related musculoskeletal disorders: report, workshop summary, and workshop papers. Steering Committee for the Workshop on Work-Related Musculoskeletal Injuries: The Research Base. National Academy of Sciences, National Research Council. Washington (DC): National Academy Press; 1999. p.229.

91. ADAMS MA, et al. Mechanical initiation of intervertebral disc degeneration. Spine 2000;25(13):1625–1636.

92. ADAMS MA, McNALLY DS, DOLAN P. 'Stress' distributions inside intervertebral discs. The effects of age and degeneration. J Bone Joint Surg Br 1996;78(6):965–972.

93. ADAMS MA, et al. Sustained loading generates stress concentrations in lumbar intervertebral discs. Spine 1996;21(4):434–438.

94. LU WW, et al. Back muscle contraction patterns of patients with low back pain before and after rehabilitation treatment: an electromyographic evaluation. J Spinal Disord 2001;14(4):277–282.

95. NG JK, et al. EMG activity of trunk muscles and torque output during isometric axial rotation exertion: a comparison between back pain patients and matched controls. J Orthop Res 2002;20(1):112–121.

96. LARIVIE'RE C, GAGNON D, LOISEL P. A biomechanical comparison of lifting techniques between subjects with and without chronic low back pain during freestyle lifting and lowering tasks. Clin Biomech (Bristol, Avon) 2002;17(2):89–98.

97. MARRAS WS, DAVIS KG. A non-MVC EMG normalization technique for the trunk musculature: Part 1. Method development. J Electromyogr Kinesiol 2001;11(1):1–9.

98. MARRAS WS, DAVIS KG, MARONITIS AB. A non-MVC EMG normalization technique for the trunk musculature: Part 2. Validation and use to predict spinal loads. J Electromyogr Kinesiol 2001;11(1):11–18.

99. MARRAS WS, et al. Spine loading characteristics of patients with low back pain compared with asymptomatic individuals. Spine 2001;26(23):2566–2574.

100. LOTZ JC. Animal models of intervertebral disc degeneration: lessons learned. Spine 2004;29(23):2742–2750.

101. LOTZ JC, CHIN JR. Intervertebral disc cell death is dependent on the magnitude and duration of spinal loading. Spine 2000;25(12):1477–1483.

102. MARRAS WS, et al. Spine loading in patients with low back pain during asymmetric lifting exertions. Spine J 2004;4(1):64–75.

103. MARRAS WS, et al. Effects of box features on spine loading during warehouse order selecting. Ergonomics 1999;42(7):980–996.

104. MARRAS WS, DAVIS KG. Spine loading during asymmetric lifting using one versus two hands. Ergonomics 1998;41(6):817–834.

105. CHOLEWICKI J, McGILL S. Mechanical stability of the in vivo lumbar spine: implications for injury and chronic low back pain. Clin Biomech (Bristol, Avon) 1996;11 (1):1–15.

106. CHOLEWICKI J, VANVLIET IJ. Relative contribution of trunk muscles to the stability of the lumbar spine during isometric exertions. Clin Biomech (Bristol, Avon) 2002;17(2):99–105.

107. PANJABI MM. The stabilizing system of the spine. Part I. Function, dysfunction, adaptation, and enhancement. J Spinal Disord 1992;5(4):383–389. discussion 397.

108. CALLAGHAN JP, SALEWYTSCH AJ, ANDREWS DM. An evaluation of predictive methods for estimating cumulative spinal loading. Ergonomics 2001;44(9): 825–837.

109. KUMAR S. Cumulative load as a risk factor for back pain. Spine 1990;15(12):1311–1316.

110. SEIDLER A, et al. The role of cumulative physical work load in lumbar spine disease: risk factors for lumbar osteochondrosis and spondylosis associated with chronic complaints. Occup Environ Med 2001;58 (11):735–746.

111. LINDSTROM I, et al. Mobility, strength, and fitness after a graded activity program for patients with subacute low back pain. A randomized prospective clinical study with a behavioral therapy approach. Spine 1992;17(6):641–652.

112. LINDSTROM I, OHLUND C, NACHEMSON A. Validity of patient reporting and predictive value of industrial physical work demands. Spine 1994;19(8): 888–893.

113. MELLIN G, et al. Outcome of a multimodal treatment including intensive physical training of patients with chronic low back pain. Spine 1993;18(7): 825–829.

114. HAZARD RG, et al. Functional restoration with behavioral support. A one-year prospective study of patients with chronic low-back pain. Spine 1989;14(2):157–161.

115. MAYER TG, et al. A prospective two-year study of functional restoration in industrial low back injury. An objective assessment procedure. J Am Med Assoc 1987;258(13):1763–1767.

116. McGILL S. Low Back Disorders: Evidence-Based Prevention and Rehabilitation. Vol. XV. Champaign (IL): Human Kinetics; 2002. p.295.

117. MARRAS WS, et al. Functional impairment as a predictor of spine loading. Spine 2005;30(7):729–737.

118. FERGUSON SA, MARRAS WS, BURR D. Workplace design guidelines for asymptomatic vs. low-back-injured workers. Appl Ergon 2005;36(1):85–95.

119. de VET HC, et al. Episodes of low back pain: a proposal for uniform definitions to be used in research. Spine 2002;27(21):2409–2416.

120. OLESKE DM, et al. Association between recovery outcomes for work-related low back disorders and personal, family, and work factors. Spine 2000;25 (10):1259–1265.

121. WASIAK R, PRANSKY GS, WEBSTER BS. Methodological challenges in studying recurrence of low back pain. J Occup Rehabil 2003;13(1):21–31.

122. MARRAS W, et al. Low back pain recurrence in occupational environments. Spine 2007; 32(21):2387–2397.

CHAPTER 15

CONCLUSIONS

The previous chapters have laid the foundation for a systematic understanding of how the various risk factors associated with low back pain can be integrated via a logical sequence of events and provide a potential explanation for how low back pain can occur due to exposures in the workplace. As noted at the beginning of this book, one must view these potential causal pathways as pieces of a puzzle that must be viewed in context for a comprehensive picture to emerge. The puzzle pieces begin with an understanding of which factors must be integrated into a working hypothesis. The literature is filled with epidemiologic evidence suggesting that physical work factor exposure, psychosocial/organizational work factor exposure, and individual risk factors interact to define the risk of low back disorders in the workplace. While it is difficult to act upon a person's individual risk factors within the work environment, it is imperative that we consider how they interact with work-related risk factors if we are to control the risk. The operative word in this statement is *interact*. While each one of these categories of risk factors are believed to independently influence risk, the key to understanding overall risk of low back pain is to appreciate how these various categories of risk factors might intermingle to exacerbate risk.

The next piece of the puzzle in understanding the working back is to appreciate the mechanisms by which these epidemiologically identified risk factors can interact. The line of reasoning in this effort suggests that biomechanical loading of the tissues can provide this common conduit. We have seen that, anatomically, there are many structures and tissues within the spine and general low back region that are capable of initiating a pain response. However, these tissues require stimulation, at least initially, to project a pain sensation to the brain. This is an important prerequisite for pain. It is highly unlikely that tissues become sensitized without any mechanical stimulation what so ever. While the pain may not be perceived immediately while the stimulus is present, the application of tissue load is the event that can initiate the sequence of events that result in pain perception. Though we have seen that numerous tissues are capable of transmitting a pain signal from the peripheral tissue, it is also clear that with enough stimulation, especially repeated stimulation, the tissue can become overly sensitized. Hence, the biomechanical stimulus need not be large in magnitude to perpetuate the pain. In addition, the pain literature has clearly shown that if the sensitization of the peripheral tissue continues, it is possible for the pain to become centralized, residing in the CNS and various locations in the brain. Thus, one must appreciate the temporal history of exposure and pain perception to understand how pain can be exacerbated at the workplace. The modern pain literature clearly shows that, given this progression of pain from peripheral to central, it is possible to experience pain even after the original tissue has recovered from an insult. This cascade of pain responses merely requires a restimulation of the tissue at a relatively low level to propagate the pain sequence.

Our knowledge of pain perception suggests that it is important to address the work factors that can result in pain early in the pain perception process. If one waits until low back pain is severe enough to result in lost work time before one addresses the work factors, then the chances that the pain has become centralized is greatly enhanced and it is far more difficult to control and problem. Thus, early intervention is the key to the control of work-related low back pain. However, given the interaction of physical, psychosocial/organizational, and individual factors in defining tissue load, interventions must be systematic in their approach. They must not only address physical workplace factors but must also address the organizational and psychological components of work.

Administrative interventions are often a necessary part of this systematic approach to address low back pain in the workplace. Administrative efforts operate at several levels (1). For one, administrative surveillance programs impact the attitude of the workers who are at risk. Shaping attitudes in terms of empowering workers to take control of their destiny and helping the workers to understand that they have control over their work environment and life are important factors in mediating the biomechanical and biochemical response of the individual to the workplace.

Next, administrative efforts are also necessary to quantitatively monitor potential risk "hot spots" in the work environment. Administrative surveillance can identify work situations in need of attention.

Another important role of administrative controls is to assist in rehabilitation at work. It is important for management to recognize the pain cascade for return to the workplace of workers who are recovering from a low back pain problem. We must be cognizant of the extraordinary sensitivity to pain that can be self-perpetuating once the pain becomes centralized. The returning worker must be understood psychologically as well as in the social and organizational context. Their sensitivity to load and perceived pain is real, and we know that they must deal with the issues of "pulling their own weight" and assimilating into the workplace amongst the potential ridicule of coworkers. We must understand that given the coactivity expected in the power-producing muscles of the torso when suffering from low back pain, the loading of the spine is greater when recovering workers perform the same work as asymptomatic workers. In addition, we know that a psychosocially stressful environment can impose additional loading due to coactivation of the torso muscles. Hence, we must better understand the biomechanical costs of work when workers recovering from low back pain return to the workforce. We must adjust the physical and psychosocial/organizational work environment accordingly. Quantitative techniques for addressing these issues have become available in recent years as outlined in Chapter 14.

The administrative controls should be coupled with engineering controls to optimally minimize risk. The common pain pathway between physical aspects of the work and mental aspects of the work involve the activation of the muscles that load the spinal tissue through biomechanical mechanisms. An understanding of biomechanical loading of the spine's tissues is essential to understanding how the pathways can lead to low back pain at work. Modeling approaches have evolved over the last several decades from single equivalent muscle static models to multiple muscle models, to biologically (EMG) assisted dynamic motion models to stability-driven models. While much of the current effort in biomechanical modeling within the field is focused on the influence of stability, stability-driven models appear to be more appropriate for large-magnitude loading. They have not yet proven useful in assessing the role of the majority of work (moderate external force manipulation) in loading the spine compared to person-specific biologically assisted models of the spine.

We are fortunate that over the past two decades, person-specific biologically assisted biomechanical models have been available to assess how individuals respond to the various physical and nonphysical risk factors to which workers are exposed. These person-specific models are essential to understand *how* risk factors can influence tissue loading. Coactivation of the trunk muscles appears to be the common link among the risk factors in exacerbating spine loading. Only multiple muscle biologically assisted models have been successful at evaluating the coactivation of muscles occurring with as a result of physical or psychosocial factors at work. Thus, currently, only these models are able to accurately interpret the impact of the host of risk factors (physical, psychosocial/organization, and individual) that load the pain-sensing tissue of the back. Biomechanical modeling continues to evolve with recent advances importing person-specific spine imaging into the model so that the roles of individual variations in bone, disc, and nerve status can be considered and their influence of spine loadings during work can be better understood.

These biologically assisted models have demonstrated how the physical and psychosocial/organizational risk factors can increase tissue load when the person is exposed to risk factors of sufficient magnitude. However, models of sufficient sensitivity are required to understand how these risk factors result in sufficient tissue loading due to work. Unfortunately, many of the biomechanical assessment techniques that have traditionally been used to assess risk in the workplace have not been sensitive enough to detect these changes in tissue loading with sufficient accuracy especially when considered over prolonged periods of exposure. Subsequently, some have concluded that there is little biomechanical relationship between low back pain and work. Had these studies used more sophisticated models as are used in modern laboratory assessments, it is likely that there would be a much stronger appreciation for the role of biomechanical loading in low back risk. In other words, it is *not* that biomechanical loading is incapable of initiating low back pain. Instead, the biomechanical assessments tools that have been used in the past have not been robust enough to pinpoint the loading profiles of the tissues with adequate accuracy. Therefore, to control risk a work, more sophisticated risk tools should be employed to assess risk due to the physical work environment.

This book has shown that there is indeed adequate evidence to support the contention that work can lead to low back disorders. The key to making this argument is to view the various dimensions of the evidence *in perspective*. Only through this systematic view of the pain-sensing process applied to the trunk's anatomy viewed in combination with a realistic view of how spine tissues are stimulated via the development of biomechanical forces acting within the trunk can we develop a realistic understanding of the back pain pathways. Once the pieces of this low back causal pathway puzzle are put in place, it is possible to see how the physical and organizational/psychosocial risk factors can potentially contribute to low back pain development and the exacerbation of back pain. An appreciation for the causal pathways, their ability to be influenced by workplace and personal risk factors, and the ability and limitations of current workplace assessment tools to assess risk should arm one with the knowledge necessary to make intelligent, well-educated assessments of how the workplace can contribute to risk. In addition, this understanding should enable one to take the necessary actions that are necessary to modify the risk. Most importantly, it is necessary to appreciate that when dealing with the working back, we are working with a system and to affect system change it must be addressed via a number of crucial points within the system. For the working back, these crucial points include understanding the individual's make up and knowing what and how to modify the physical and psychological aspects of the workplace.

15.1 SUMMARY

- Low back pain is a common problem in the workplace that is caused by:

  o factors inherent to the individual worker,

  o physical work factors,

  o psychosocial/organizational (psychological) work factors,

  o interaction of these risk factors.

- These factors manifest themselves through muscle recruitment patterns (muscle cocontraction), which influence force imposed on the tissues of the back and spine structures.

- Acute or repetitive forces imposed on the (peripheral) tissues act as a stimulus to sensitize the tissues. This sensitization results in pain.

- If stimulation is repeated or prolonged, the sensitization can become neropathic and even central (to the brain) and is capable of precipitating pain even after the peripheral insult to the tissue has ceased and the tissue has recovered.

- Sensitization of workers returning to the workplace after low back pain can result in increased loading of the tissues compared to asymptomatic workers.

- Administrative interventions including organizational and psychosocial changes in conjunction with changes in the physical work environment (engineering controls) can optimally minimize risk. However, only biomechanically and biologically sensitive assessment tools can provide useful information about risk.

- Back pain at work is a systems problem and the solutions to reduce risk and return workers to the workplace after low back injury must be approached at a systems level.

REFERENCES

1. IMADA A.Technology in organizations. In LUCZAK H, ZINK H.editors. Human Factors in Organizational Design and Management. Vol. VII. North Holland: Amsterdam; 2003. p.55–62.

INDEX

Abdominal fascia, 35
Action limit (AL), 214
Acute biomechanical measures, 126
Acute inflammation, 48, 49, 78
Acute pain phase, 253
Acute tissue loads, 92
Acute trauma pain pathways, 65, 66, 129
Adenosine diphosphate (ADP), 95
Adenosine triphosphate (ATP), 95
Alcohol, 20
  role of, 20
Alpha motor neuron, 78
American Society of Orthopaedic Surgeons, 11
Anatomical cross-sectional area (ACSA), 188
Anatomy, 9
Animal models, 51
Antagonistic muscle, 193, 238
  coactivation of, 193
  reductions in, 238
Anterior–posterior (A/P) shear, 96, 128, 135, 202,
    140, 161, 203, 273, 276
Anterior longitudinal ligament, 32
Anthropometry, 19, 187, 200
  differences in, 187
Articular facet joint, 40
Automation, 8
Autonomic nervous system, 77
Average absolute error (AAE), 104
Average peak sagittal velocity, 284

Back anatomy, 41
  brief description of, 41
Back pain, 12, 52, 120, 233
  patients, 52
  progressive nature of, 233
Back pain research community, 23
Biochemical tolerance, 7, 66, 112
Biomechanical assessment techniques, 300
Biomechanical factors, 175, 219
Biomechanical load–tolerance relationship, 7
Biomechanical modeling, 88

Blood delivery system, 54
  role of, 54
Blood vessels, 39
Bone tolerance, 67
Box-sorting operation, 179
Brain functioning, 52
  recent theories, 52
Brick-laying tasks, 151
Buttock pain, 54

Cardinal planes, 29
Carpal tunnel syndrome, 78
Case–control methodology, 126
Cellular dysfunction, 78
Central nervous system (CNS), 44, 47
Central pain sensitization, 44, 47, 52, 53
Central trigger point (CTrP), 75
Cervical curves, 32
Chronic inflammation, 49, 50
Cigarette smoking, 21
Ciliary neurotrophic factor receptor gene, 81
Cinderella fibers, 78
Committee members, 234
Compact bone, 30
Compensation costs, 233
Compression loading, 146
Conceptual model, 6
Constrained work postures, 164
Contact force tolerance, 67
Controllable workplace factors, 205
Cortical bone, 30
Counter clockwise (CCW), 29, 179
  asymmetries, 276
  lift origins, 283
Coupling multiplier (CM), 217
Cross-sectional data, 13
Cumulative biomechanical measures, 126
Cumulative exposure, 147
Cumulative loading, 5
Cumulative trauma, 5, 6
  core of, 6

Printed in the United States
By Bookmasters